Practical Fracture Treatment

Ronald McRae F.R.C.S.

Consultant Orthopaedic Surgeon, Southern General Hospital, Glasgow.
Honorary Clinical Lecturer in Orthopaedics, University of Glasgow.
Lecturer in Anatomy, Glasgow School of Chiropody.
Member of the Institute of Medical and Biological Illustration.

With original drawings and illustrations by the author

CHURCHILL LIVINGSTONE
EDINBURGH LONDON MELBOURNE AND NEW YORK 1981

CHURCHILL LIVINGSTONE
Medical Division of Longman Group UK Limited

Distributed in the United States of America by
Churchill Livingstone Inc., 1560 Broadway,
New York, N.Y. 10036, and by associated companies,
branches and representatives throughout the world.

First published 1981
  Reprinted 1983
  Reprinted 1984
  Reprinted 1986
  Reprinted 1987
  Reprinted 1988

ISBN 0 443 01694 1

British Library Cataloguing in Publication Data
McRae, Ronald
  Practical fracture treatment.
  1. Fractures
  1. Title
  617'.15   RD 101   80-41216

Produced by Longman Group (FE) Ltd
Printed in Hong Kong

Practical Fracture Treatment

Preface

This book has been written primarily for the medical student, and the introductory section assumes little prior knowledge of the subject. The second part, which deals with particular fractures, is set in places at a more advanced level; it is hoped that the book will thereby continue to prove of value to the student when he moves to his first casualty or registrar post.

In planning this volume, I have paid particular attention to two points. Firstly, the details of each fracture and a good deal of the introductory section have been arranged in a linear sequence. The material has been divided into small packets of text and illustration in order to facilitate comprehension and learning. These packets have been set out in a logical sequence which in most cases is based on the relative importance of the initial decisions which must be made in a case, and the order in which treatment procedures should be carried out. This format is in a few places restrictive, with an imbalance in the amount of information carried by either text or illustration. This must be accepted because of spatial and subject limitations. Generally, however, text and illustration will be found to complement one another. The text, although of necessity brief, is concise and, it is hoped, to the point.

Secondly, fracture treatment has been given in an uncommon amount of practical detail. As there is such a variety of accepted treatments for even the simplest of fractures, this has the danger of attracting the criticism of being controversial and didactic. This is far from my intention, and I have tried to avoid this in several ways. Firstly, as minor fractures and most children's fractures (together forming the bulk of all fractures) are most frequently treated conservatively, the conservative approach I have employed for these injuries should on the whole receive general approval. Secondly, in the more controversial long bone fractures in adults, and in fractures involving joints, I have on the whole pursued a middle course between the extremes of conservative and surgical management. The methods I have singled out for description are those which I consider safest and most reliable in the hands of the comparatively inexperienced. Where alternative methods appear to me to be equally valid I have generally included these. To conceal my own whims I have not always placed these in the order of personal preference. In consequence, I hope that any offence given by the methods described will be restricted to the most extreme quarters.

Conventions:

1. Where two sides are shown for comparison, the patient's *right* side is the one affected.

2. Where several conditions are described, and only one illustrated, the first mentioned is the one shown, unless followed by the abbreviation 'Ill'.

Abbreviations:

A = anterior
Ill = illustrated
L = lateral or left
M = medial
N = normal
P = posterior
R = right

Acknowledgements

I would like to thank Mrs Mary Kelly for her painstaking care in the preparation of the typescript, Mr T. H. Norton and Dr Wilson James for their kind help in tracing and allowing me to copy several of the radiographs accompanying the text, and Mr James Patrick and my Glasgow colleagues for a number of useful suggestions.

To Helen

Contents

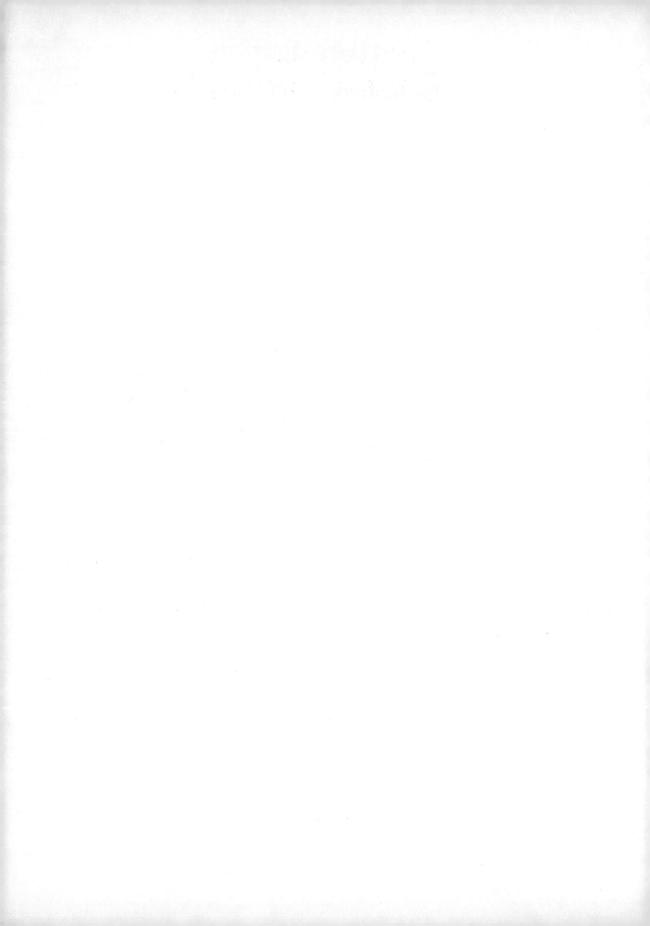

Section A:
General principles

1. Pathology and healing of fractures

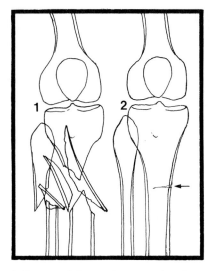

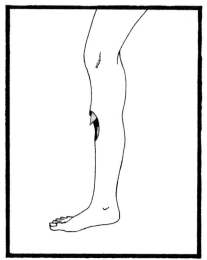

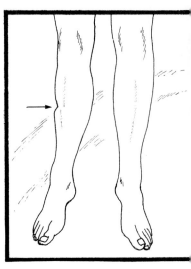

1. *Fracture:* A fracture is present when there is loss of continuity in the substance of a bone. The term covers all bony disruptions, ranging from (1) the highly comminuted fracture at one end of the scale to (2) hairline and even microscopic fractures at the other. The word is often erroneously associated with fragmentation.

2. *Compound fracture:* All fractures are either *simple or compound.* In a *compound (or open) fracture,* there is a wound in communication with the fracture, and the potential exists for organisms to enter the fracture site from outside. All compound fractures therefore carry the risk of becoming infected. In addition, blood loss from external haemorrhage may be significant.

3. *Simple fracture:* In a simple (or closed) fracture the skin is either intact, or if there are any wounds, these are superficial or unrelated to the fracture. So long as the skin remains intact, there is no risk of infection from outside. (Blood-borne infection of simple fractures is extremely rare.) Any haemorrhage is internal. The term 'simple' bears no relationship to the problems associated with the injury.

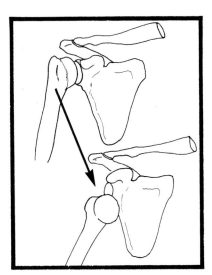

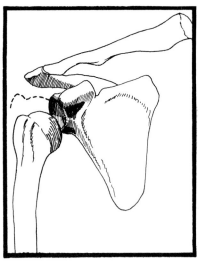

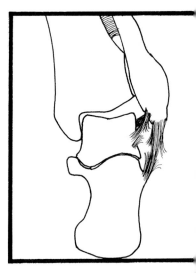

4. *Dislocation:* In a dislocation there is complete loss of congruity between the articulating surfaces of a joint. The bones taking part in the articulation are displaced relative to one another, e.g. in a dislocated shoulder the head of the humerus loses all contact with the glenoid. In the common anterior dislocation the head of the humerus is displaced anteriorly.

5. *Subluxation:* In a subluxation, the articulating surfaces of a joint are no longer congruous, but loss of contact is incomplete. The term is often used to describe the early stages in a condition which may proceed to complete dislocation (e.g. in a joint infection or in rheumatoid arthritis).

6. *Sprain:* A sprain is an incomplete tear of a ligament or complex of ligaments responsible for the stability of a joint, e.g. a sprain of the ankle is a partial tear of the external ligament, and is not associated with instability (as distinct from a complete tear). The term sprain is also applied to incomplete tears of muscles and tendons.

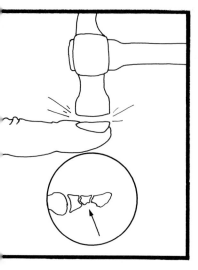

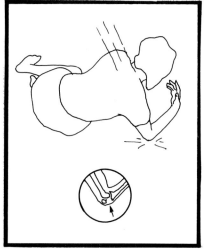

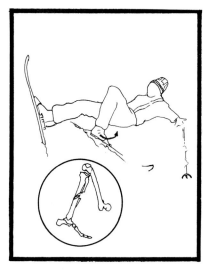

Direct violence (a) Fractures are caused by the application of stresses which exceed the limits of strength of a bone. Violence is the commonest cause. In the case of *direct violence*, a bone may be fractured by being struck by a moving or falling object—for example, a fracture of the terminal phalanx of a finger by a hammer blow.

8. *Direct violence* (b) A bone may also be fractured if it forcibly strikes a resistant object. For example, a fall on the point of the elbow may fracture the olecranon.

9. *Indirect violence:* Very frequently fractures result from indirect violence. A twisting or bending stress is applied to a bone, and this results in its fracture at some distance from the application of the causal force. For example, a rotational stress applied to the foot may cause a spiral fracture of the tibia. Indirect violence is also the commonest cause of dislocation.

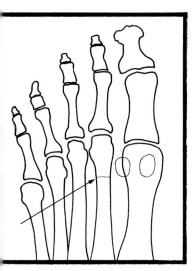

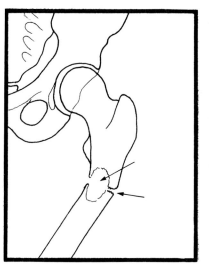

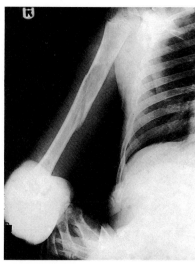

. *Fatigue fractures:* Stresses, repeated with excessive frequency to a bone, may result in fracture. This mechanism is often compared with fatigue in metals which break after repeated bending beyond their elastic limit. The commonest of these fractures involves the second metatarsal—the march fracture (so called because of its frequency in Army recruits).

11. *Pathological fractures* (a) A pathological fracture is one which occurs in an abnormal or diseased bone. If the osseous abnormality reduces the strength of the bone, then the force required to produce fracture is reduced, and may even become trivial. For example, a secondary tumour deposit may lead to a pathological fracture of the sub-trochanteric region of the femur—a common site.

12. *Pathological fractures* (b) Pathological fractures may also occur at the site of simple tumours—for example, a fracture of the humerus in a child with a simple bone cyst. The commonest causes of pathological fracture are osteoporosis and osteomalacia.

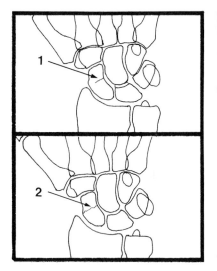

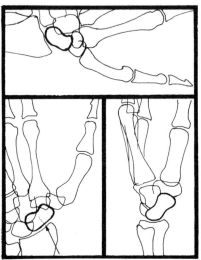

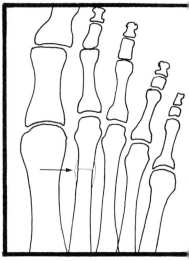

13. *Hair-line fractures* (a) Hair-line fractures result from minimal trauma: i.e. trauma which is just great enough to produce a fracture, but not severe enough to produce any significant displacement of the fragments. Such fractures may be (1) incomplete (2) complete.

14. *Hair-line fractures* (b) These fractures may be difficult to detect on the radiographs, and where there are reasonable clinical grounds for suspecting a fracture, the rules are quite clear. (1) Additional oblique radiographic projections of the area may be helpful. (2) Do not accept poor quality films. (3) Films repeated after 7–10 days may show the fracture quite clearly (due to decalcification at the fracture site).

15. *Hair-line fractures* (c) *Stress fractures* are generally hair-line in pattern, and are often not diagnosed with certainty until the is wisp of sub-periosteal callus formation, o increased density at the fracture site some 3–6 weeks after the onset of symptoms. Hair-line fractures generally heal rapidly requiring only symptomatic treatment: BU the scaphoid and femoral neck are notable exceptions.

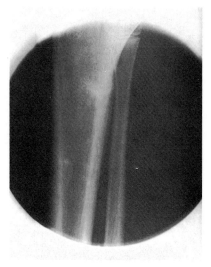

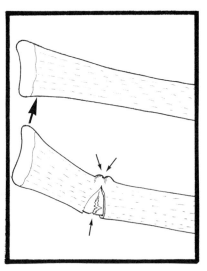

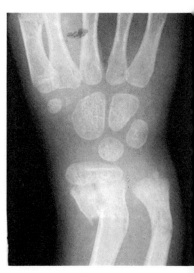

16. *Hair-line fractures* (d) Radiograph of upper tibia of an athletic adolescent with a 7-week history of persistent leg pain. Previous radiographs were reported as normal. Note the coned view to obtain optimal detail and the incomplete hair-line fracture revealed by bone sclerosis and sub-periosteal callus. A crepe bandage support only was prescribed, and the symptoms settled in a further 6 weeks.

17. *Greenstick fractures* (a) Greenstick fractures occur in children, but not all children's fractures are of this type. The less brittle bone of the child tends to buckle on the side opposite the causal force. Tearing of the periosteum and of the surrounding soft tissues is often minimal.

18. *Greenstick fractures* (b) This radiograp illustrates a more severe greenstick fractur of the distal radius and ulna. Note that although there is about 45° of angulation a the fracture site, that there is no loss of bor contact in either fracture. The clinical deformity is suggested by the clear soft-tissue shadow.

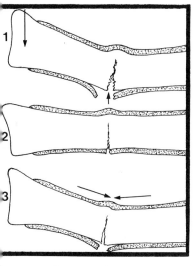

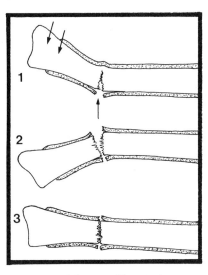

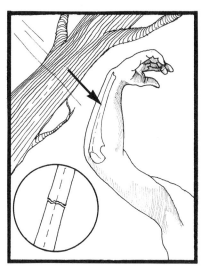

19. *Greenstick fractures* (c) Reduction of a greenstick fracture is facilitated by the absence of displacement and by the intact tissues on the concavity of the fracture. Angulation may be corrected by supporting the fracture and applying pressure over the distal fragment (1 and 2). The elastic spring of the periosteum may however lead to recurrence of angulation (3). Particular attention must therefore be taken over plaster fixation and after care.

20. *Greenstick fractures* (d) In the forearm in particular, where angulation inevitably leads to restriction of pronation and supination, some surgeons deliberately over-correct the initial deformity (1). This tears the periosteum on the other side of the fracture (2). This reduces the risks of secondary angulation (3). Healing in all greenstick fractures is rapid.

21. *Transverse fractures* (a) Transverse fractures run at right angles to the long axis of a bone. They are usually caused by direct violence: e.g. an isolated, transverse fracture of the ulna may be sustained in warding off a blow. Angulation may occur, but displacement is less common.

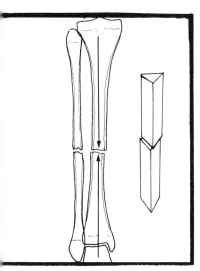

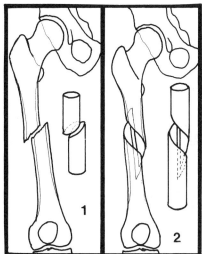

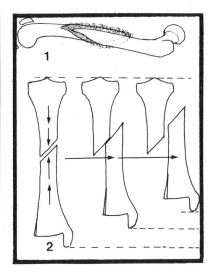

22. *Transverse fractures* (b) The inherent stability of this type of fracture (illustrated by the model on the right) reduces the risks of shortening and favours union. In the tibia, weight bearing may be permitted at a comparatively early stage. On the other hand, the area of bony contact is small, requiring very strong union before any external support can be discarded.

23. *Oblique fractures* (a) In an oblique fracture (1) the fracture line runs at an angle less than 90° to the long axis of the bone. *In spiral fractures* (2) the line of the fracture curves in a spiral fashion round the bone. Both these fractures may result from indirect violence. The spiral fracture in particular may be caused by torsional forces.

24. *Oblique and spiral fractures* (b) In spiral fractures, union can be rapid (1) as there is often a large area of bone in contact. In both oblique and spiral fractures, unopposed muscle contraction or premature weight bearing readily lead to shortening, displacement and sometimes loss of bony contact (2).

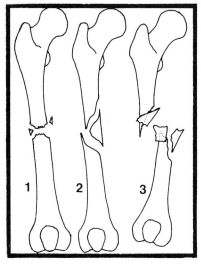

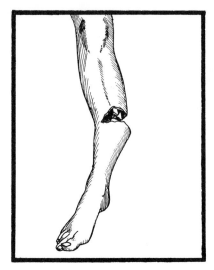

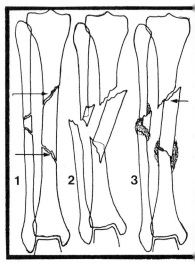

25. *Comminuted fractures* (a) A fracture is said to be comminuted when more than two fragments are present. Comminution ranges from (1) 'slight comminution at the fracture site' through (2) 'comminution at the fracture site with a large butterfly fragment' (so called from its shape) to (3) 'a highly comminuted fracture'.

26. *Comminuted fractures* (b) The presence of marked comminution indicates severe violence, and there is greater risk of damage to neighbouring muscle, vessels, nerves and skin. There may be accompanying injuries. Comminuted fractures are unstable. Delay in union and muscle damage may lead to joint stiffness and disability.

27. *Double fracture:* In a double fracture (1) the affected bone is fractured at two distinct levels. Double fracture must be distinguished from comminution. In the case illustrated, there is also a double fracture of the fibula. Instability (2) and difficulty in reduction and fixation are common. Internal fixation may further impair a dubious blood supply to the central segment, and non-union (3) is common at one level.

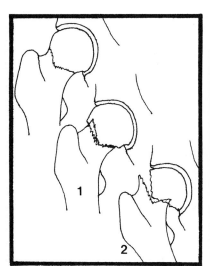

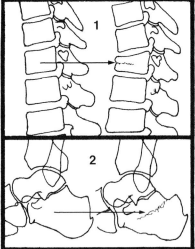

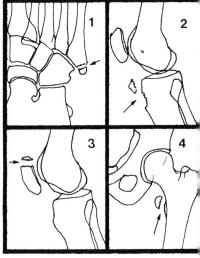

28. *Impacted fractures:* A fracture is impacted when one fragment is driven into the other (1). Cancellous bone is usually involved and union is often rapid. The *stability* of these fractures varies and is more implied than real. Displacement will occur if the fracture is subjected to deforming forces: e.g. without fixation, impacted femoral neck fractures frequently come adrift (3).

29. *Compression (or crush) fractures:* Crush fractures occur in cancellous bone which is compressed beyond the limits of tolerance. Common sites are (1) the vertebral bodies (as a result of flexion injuries) and (2) the heels (following falls from a height). If the deformity is accepted, union is invariably rapid. In the spine, if correction is attempted, recurrence is almost invariable.

30. *Avulsion fractures* (a) An avulsion fracture may be produced by a sudden muscle contraction—the muscle pulling off the portion of bone to which it is attached. Common examples include:
1. Base of fifth metatarsal (Peroneus Brevis).
2. Tibial tuberosity (quadriceps).
3. Upper pole of patella (quadriceps).
4. Lesser trochanter (ilio-psoas).

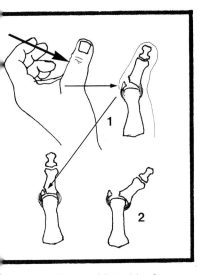

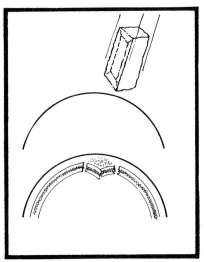

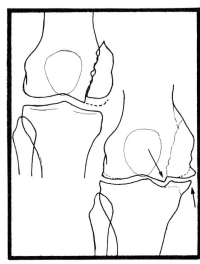

31. *Avulsion fractures* (b) Avulsion fractures may also result from traction on a ligamentous or capsular attachment: these are often witness of *momentary dislocation*: e.g. (1) an abduction force may avulse the ulnar collateral ligament attachment, with spontaneous reduction (2). *Late subluxation* (3) is common with this ('gamekeeper's thumb') and other injuries and is especially serious in the case of the spine.

32. *Depressed fracture:* Depressed fractures occur when a sharply localised blow depresses a segment of cortical bone below the level of the surrounding bone. Although common in skull fractures, this pattern is only rarely found in the limbs. There the tibia in the upper third is probably most frequently affected. Healing is rapid: complications are dependent on the site.

33. *Involving a joint:* When a fracture involves a joint, any residual articular irregularity may lead to secondary osteo-arthritis. *In all cases, there is risk of stiffness from intra-articular adhesions.* Sometimes complications may be minimised by accurate open reduction and internal fixation, but thereafter early mobilisation is essential if *increased* adhesions and stiffness are to be avoided. Prolonged physiotherapy is required as a rule in all these cases.

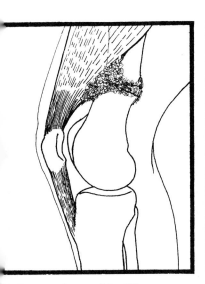

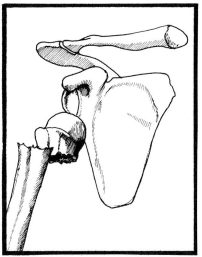

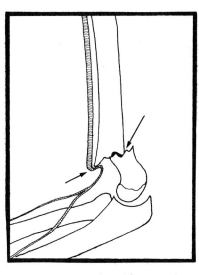

34. *Fracture close to a joint:* When a fracture lies close to a joint, stiffness may also be a problem due to tethering of neighbouring muscles and tendons by spread of callus from the healing fracture: e.g. in fractures of the femur close to the knee, the quadriceps may become bound-down by the callus, resulting in difficulty with knee flexion.

35. *Fracture-dislocation:* A fracture-dislocation is present when a joint has dislocated and there is in addition a fracture of one of the bony components of the joint. Illustrated is a fracture-dislocation of the shoulder, where there is an anterior dislocation with a fracture of the neck of the humerus. Injuries of this kind may be difficult to reduce and may be unstable. Stiffness and avascular necrosis are two common complications.

36. *Complex or complicated fractures:* A fracture is described as complicated if there is accompanying damage to major neighbouring structures. The diagram is of a complicated supracondylar fracture of the humerus. (Such an injury might also be described as a supracondylar fracture complicated by damage to the brachial artery.)

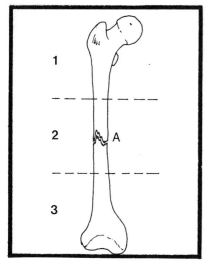

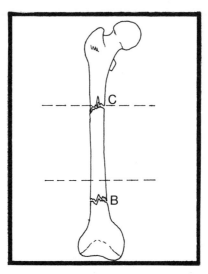

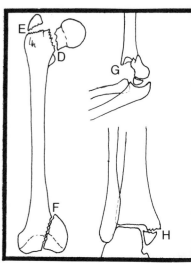

37. In the case of the long bones, the shaft is arbitrarily divided into thirds for descriptive purposes. A fracture at A would be described as a middle third fracture of the femur (or a mid-shaft fracture of the femur).

38. In the same way, a fracture as at B would be described as a fracture in the distal third and C would be described as a fracture at the junction of the proximal and middle thirds.

39. At the ends of the bones the nomenclature is either anatomical or refers to a personality whose name is associated with the fracture: D = fracture of the neck of the femur; E = fracture of the greater trochanter; F = intercondylar fracture; G = supracondylar fracture of the humerus; H = fracture of the medial malleolus, one type of Potts fracture of the ankle.

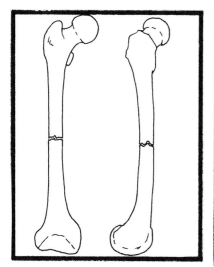

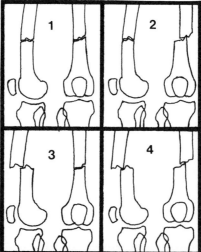

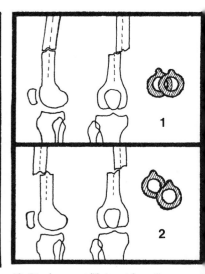

40. *Describing the deformity:* If there is no deformity—i.e. if the violence which has produced the fracture has been insufficient to cause any movement of the bone ends relative to one another—then the fracture is said to be in anatomical position. Similarly, if a perfect position has been achieved after manipulation of a fracture, it may be described as being in anatomical position.

41. *Displacement* (i) Displacement is present if the bone ends have shifted relative to one another. The direction of displacement is described in terms of movement of the distal fragment. For example, in these fractures of the femoral shaft at the junction of the middle and distal thirds there is (1) no displacement (2) lateral displacement (3) posterior displacement (4) both lateral and posterior displacement.

42. *Displacement* (ii) Apart from the direction of displacement, the degree must be considered. A rough estimate is usually made of the percentage of the fracture surfaces in contact. For example, (1) 50% bony apposition (2) 25% bony apposition. Good bony apposition encourages stability and union.

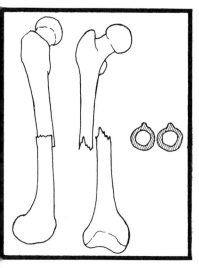

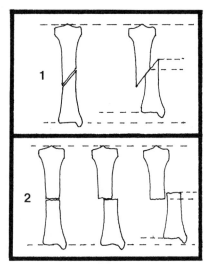

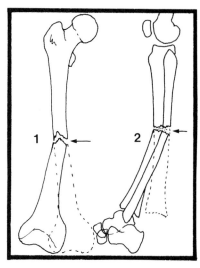

43. *Displacement* (iii) Where none of the fracture surfaces is in contact, the fracture is described as having 'no bony apposition' or being 'completely off-ended'. Off-ended fractures are (1) potentially unstable (2) liable to progressive shortening (3) liable to delay or difficulty in union (4) often hard to reduce, sometimes due to trapping of soft tissue between the bone ends.

44. *Displacement* (iv) (1) Displacement of a spiral or oblique fracture will result in shortening. Displacement of transverse fractures (2) will result in shortening only after loss of bony contact. The amount of shortening may be assessed from the radiographs (if an allowance is made for magnification). Speaking generally, displacement, whilst undesirable, is of much less significance than angulation.

45. *Angulation* (i) The accepted method of describing angulation is in terms of the position of the point of the angle. For example (1) fracture of the femur with medial angulation (2) fracture of the tibia and fibula with posterior angulation. (Both mid shaft fractures.) This method can on occasion give rise to confusion especially as deformity is described in terms of the distal fragment.

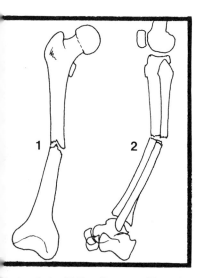

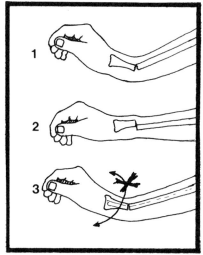

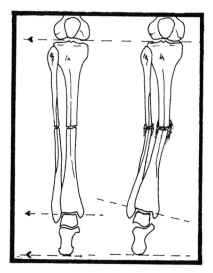

46. *Angulation* (ii) Equally acceptable, and perhaps less liable to error, would be to describe these fractures in the following way (1) a fracture of the middle third of the femur with the distal fragment tilted laterally (2) a fracture of the tibia and fibula in the middle thirds, with the distal fragment tilted anteriorly.

47. *Angulation* (iii) Significant angulation must always be corrected for several reasons. Deformity of the limb will be conspicuous (1) and regarded (often correctly) by the patient as a sign of poor treatment. Deformity from displacement (2) is seldom very obvious. In the upper limb, function may be seriously impaired, especially in forearm fractures where pronation/supination may be badly affected (3).

48. *Angulation* (iv) In the lower limb, alteration of the plane of movements of the hip, knee or ankle may lead to abnormal joint stresses, leading to the rapid onset of secondary osteo-arthritis.

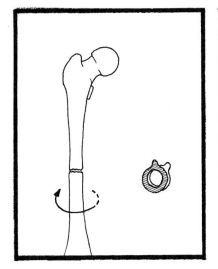

49. *Axial rotation* (i) A third type of deformity may be present: this is when one fragment rotates on its long axis, with or without accompanying displacement or angulation. This type of deformity may be overlooked unless precautions are taken and the possibility of its occurrence kept in mind.

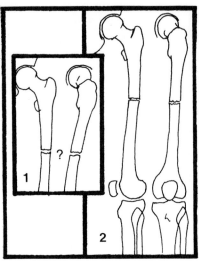

50. *Axial rotation* (ii) Radiographs which fail to show both ends of the bone frequently prevent any pronouncement on the presence of axial rotation (1). When both ends of the fractured bone are fully visualised on the one film rotation may be obvious (2). The moral is that in any fracture both the joint above and the one below should be included in the examination.

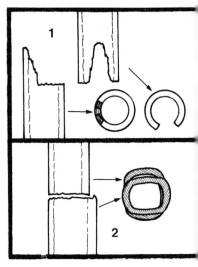

51. *Axial rotation* (iii) Axial rotation may also be detected in the radiographs by noting (1) the position of interlocking fragments (displaced fracture with 90° axial rotation illustrated). If a bone is not perfectly circular in cross section at the fracture site, differences in the relative diameters of the fragments may be suggestive of axial rotation (2). Axial rotation is of particular importance in forearm fractures.

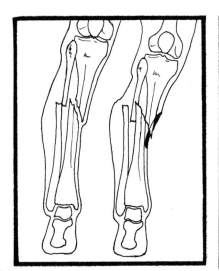

52. *Compound fractures* (i) Compound fractures are of two types: those which are compound from within out, and others which are compound from without in. In fractures which are *compound from within out* the skin is broached by the sharp edge of one of the bone ends. Compounding may occur at the time of injury, or later from unguarded handling of a simple fracture.

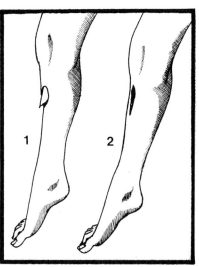

53. *Fractures compound from within out* (1) The case may be first seen with bone obviously still penetrating the skin which may be tightly stretched round it. (2) More commonly, the fracture having once broken the skin, promptly spontaneously reduces, so that what is seen is a wound at the level of the fracture.

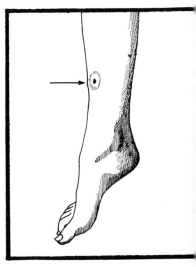

54. *Technically compound fracture:* Occasionally the skin damage is minimal, with a small area of early bruising in the centre of which is a tiny tell-tale bead of blood issuing from a puncture wound; this bead of blood re-appears as soon as it is swabbed. The risks of infection are much less in compound from within fractures. Within this group too the risks decrease in the order in which they have been described.

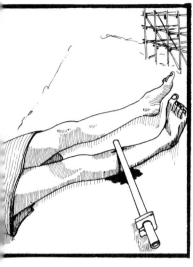

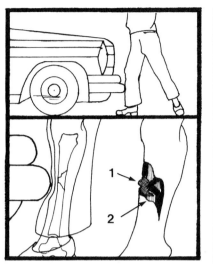

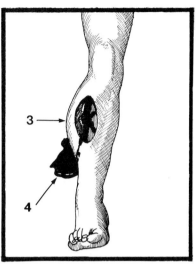

5. *Fractures compound from without in* (i) This type of injury is caused by direct violence: the causal force breaks the skin and fractures the underlying bone. Causes include injuries from falling objects (e.g. in the construction industry, mining, rock falls in mountaineering, etc.) and motor vehicle impacts.

56. *Compound from without in* (ii) The risks of infection are greater in this type of compound fracture as (1) dirt and fragments of clothing, etc. may be driven into the wound (2) the skin is often badly damaged; skin may even be lost. In either case, wound healing may be in jeopardy. Difficulty in closure must be anticipated.

57. *Compound from without in* (iii) In addition, there may be (3) damage to surrounding muscle, leading to oedema and further difficulty in wound closure (4) haemorrhage and shock may be greater than in corresponding within-out fractures. Note also that the fractures are often comminuted—with difficulty in reduction and fixation—and there may be vascular and neurological complications.

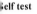**elf test**

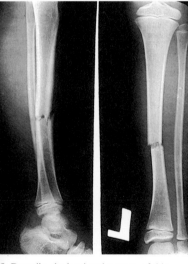

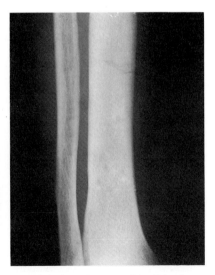

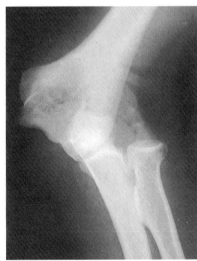

8. Describe the level and pattern of this child's fracture.

59. This is the radiograph of the tibia of a young man who was kicked whilst playing rugby. What is the pattern of fracture? What observations would you make regarding the detection of such a fracture?

60. Radiograph of the elbow of an adult injured in a fall. There is obvious clinical deformity. What is the injury?

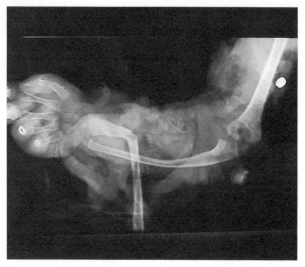

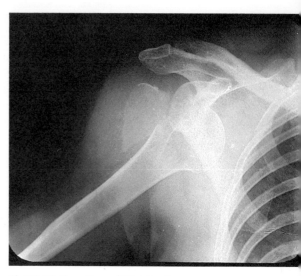

61. Radiograph of the arm of a child severely crushed in a run-over road traffic accident. Describe the injury.

62. What is the pattern of this injury?

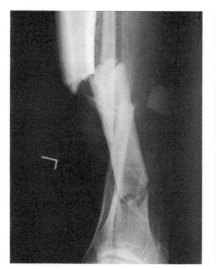

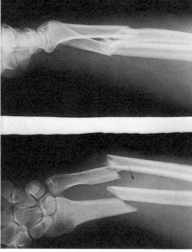

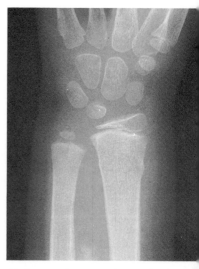

63. Describe this fracture. What problems might you anticipate with it?

64. Describe the level and any angulation or displacement that you see in this fracture.

65. Can you detect any abnormality in this A.P. radiograph of the wrist and forearm of a child?

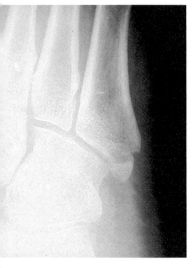

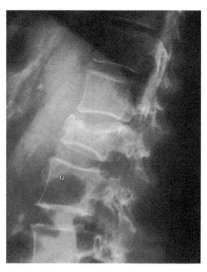

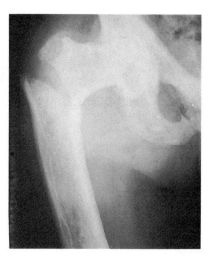

. These are the radiographs of a patient no complained of pain in the side of the ot following a sudden inversion injury. here is the fracture, and what is the attern of injury?

67. The history in this case is of pain in the back following a fall. What is the pattern of fracture?

68. This radiograph is of the hip of an elderly lady who complained of pain after a fall. What deformity is present? Have you any observations to make regarding any factors contributing to the fracture?

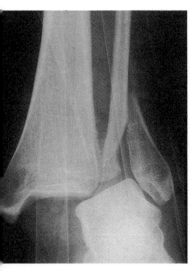

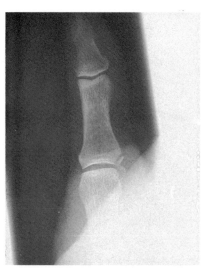

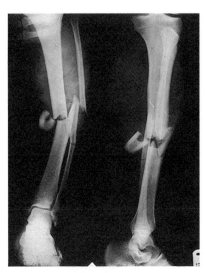

). What is this pattern of fracture? What is e importance of accurate reduction in this se?

70. What pattern of injury is illustrated in this thumb radiograph? What is its significance?

71. This injury was sustained in a road traffic accident. Describe the pattern of injury and the deformity.

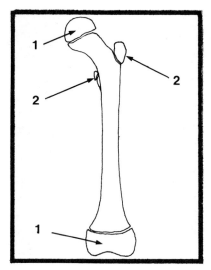

72. *Types of epiphyses.* There are two types of epiphyses: (1) *Pressure epiphyses*, which form part of the articulating surfaces of a joint, and (2) Traction epiphyses, which lie at muscle insertions, are non-articular, and do not contribute to the longitudinal growth of the bone.

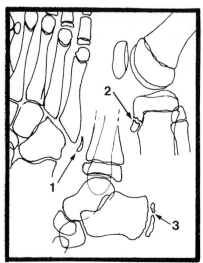

73. *Traction epiphyses ctd.:* Injuries to the traction epiphyses are nearly always avulsion injuries. The sites commonly affected include (1) the base of the fifth metatarsal (2) the tibial tuberosity (3) the calcaneal epiphysis. Traction injuries are probably the basic cause of Osgood Schlatter's and Sever's disease (2 and 3). Other sites include the lesser trochanter, ischium, and the anterior iliac spines.

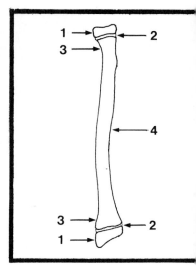

74. *Pressure epiphyses* (a) Pressure epiphyses are situated at the ends of the long bones and take part in the articulations. The corresponding epiphyseal plates are responsible for longitudinal growth of the bone. (Circumferential growth is controlled by the periosteum.)
Note: 1. epiphysis.
2. epiphyseal plate.
3. metaphysis.
4. diaphysis.

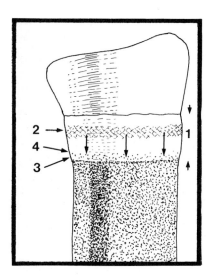

75. *Pressure epiphyses* (b) Within the epiphyseal plate (1) is a layer of active cartilage cells (2). The newly formed cells hypertrophy. Calcification and transformation to bone occur near the metaphysis (3). When there is an epiphyseal separation, it occurs at the weakest point, the layer of cell hypertrophy (4). The active region (2) remains with the epiphysis.

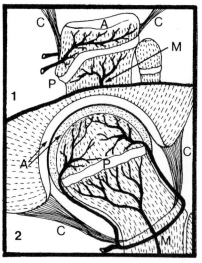

76. *Pressure epiphyses* (c) The metaphyseal side of the plate is nourished by vessels from the shaft (M). In the tibia (1) the epiphysis is supplied by extra-articular vessels. Vessels to the femoral head (2) lie close to the joint space and epiphyseal plate (P). Epiphyseal displacements may lead to avascular necrosis or growth arrest. The head of radius is similarly at risk. C = capsule
A = articular cartilage.

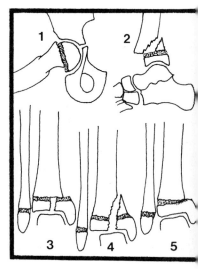

77. *Epiphyseal plate injuries* (Salter and Harris Classification)
Type 1. The whole epiphysis is separated from the shaft.
Type 2. The epiphysis is displaced, carrying with it a small, triangular metaphyseal fragment (the commonest injury).
Type 3. Separation of part of the epiphysis.
Type 4. Separation of part of the epiphysis, with a metaphyseal fragment.
Type 5. Crushing of part or all of the epiphysis.

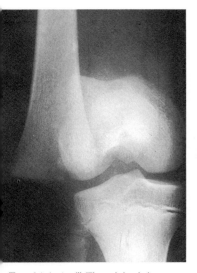

Type 1 injuries (i) The epiphysis is separated from the shaft without any accompanying fracture. This may follow trauma in childhood (illustrated is a traumatic displacement of the distal femoral epiphysis) or result from a birth injury. It may occur secondary to a joint infection, rickets or scurvy. Reduction by manipulation is usually easy in traumatic lesions, and the prognosis is good unless the epiphysis lies wholly within the joint.

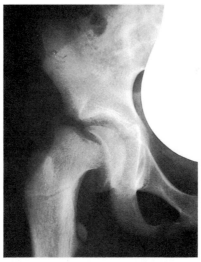

79. *Type 1 injuries* (ii) An endocrine disturbance is thought to be an important factor in the common forms of slipped upper femoral epiphysis. Avascular necrosis is not uncommon, especially if forcible reduction is attempted after a delay in diagnosis. Growth arrest is seldom a problem (as it occurs in adolescence towards the end of growth, and as most femoral growth is at the distal end).

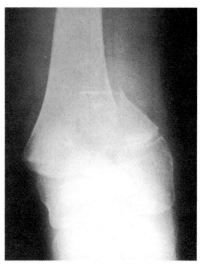

80. *Type 2 injuries:* The epiphysis displaces, carrying with it a small triangular fragment of the metaphysis (illustrated here in the distal femur). It is caused by trauma and is the commonest of epiphyseal injuries. Its highest incidence is in early adolescence. Growth disturbance is relatively uncommon. Reduction must be early—it becomes difficult after 48 hours by closed methods.

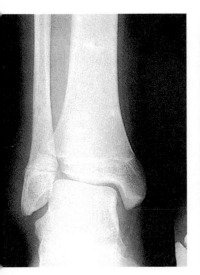

Type 3 injuries: Part of the epiphysis is separated. Accurate reduction is necessary in this type of injury to restore the smoothness and regularity of the articular surface. The prognosis is generally good unless the severity of the initial displacement has disrupted the blood supply to the fragment. The lower and upper tibial epiphyses are most commonly affected (note separated portion of tibial epiphysis behind lateral malleolus).

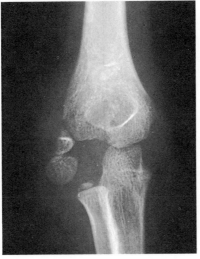

82. *Type 4 injuries:* Separation of part of the epiphysis with a metaphyseal fragment. The lateral condyle of the humerus is most commonly affected and must be accurately reduced—open reduction is usually necessary. Failure of reduction leads to bone formation in the gap and marked disturbance of growth.

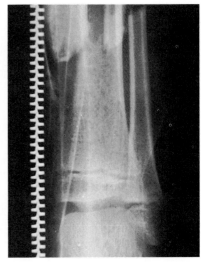

83. *Type 5 injuries:* Crushing or other damage to the epiphyseal plate. This radiograph of a child who was dragged along the road by a car shows the medial malleolus, part of the epiphyseal plate, and the adjacent tibia have been removed by abrasion. (The tibia is also fractured.) The epiphyseal plate may also be crushed in severe abduction and adduction injuries of the ankle.

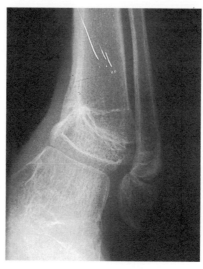

84. *Growth disturbances* (i) If growth is arrested over part of the epiphyseal plate only, there will be progressive angulatory deformity affecting the axis of movement of the related joint. There will be a little overall shortening. This radiograph shows the tilting of the plane of the ankle joint which occurred in the last case, with deformity of the foot and ankle. In the elbow, injuries of this type may lead to cubitus varus or valgus.

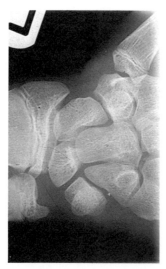
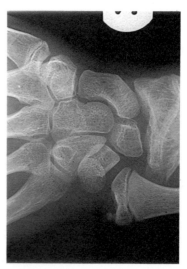

85. *Growth disturbances* (ii) If the whole epiphyseal plate is affected, growth will be arrested, leading to greater shortening of the bone. The final result will depend on the age at which epiphyseal arrest occurred, and the epiphysis involved: obviously the younger the child, the greater the growth loss. Arrest of one epiphysis in paired bones will lead to joint deformity. In the case illustrated, the radial epiphysis on the right has suffered complete growth arrest following a displaced lower radial epiphysis. The ulna has continued to grow at its usual rate: its distal end appears prominent on the dorsum of the wrist, and there is obvious deformity and impairment of function in the wrist. The normal left side is shown for comparison.

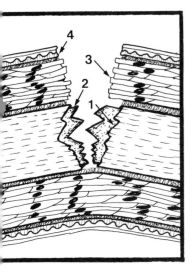

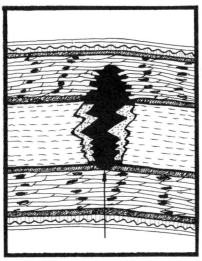

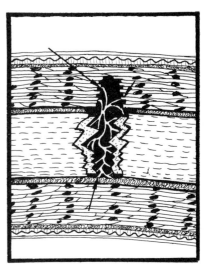

. As a result of the injury, (1) the
riosteum may be completely or partly
rn, (2) there is disruption of the Haversian
stems with death of adjacent bone cells,
there may be tearing of muscle,
pecially on the convex side of the fracture,
d damage to neighbouring nerves and
ood vessels, (4) the skin may be broached
compound injuries, with risk of ingress of
cteria.

87. *Fracture haematoma* (i) Bleeding occurs
from the bone ends, marrow vessels, and
damaged soft tissues, with the formation of a
fracture haematoma which clots. (Closed
fracture illustrated.)

88. *Fracture haematoma* (ii) The fracture
haematoma is rapidly vascularised by the
ingrowth of blood vessels from the
surrounding tissues, and for some weeks
there is rapid cellular activity. Fibrovascular
tissue replaces the clot, collagen fibres are
laid down, and mineral salts are deposited.

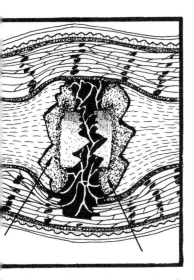

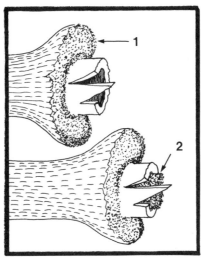

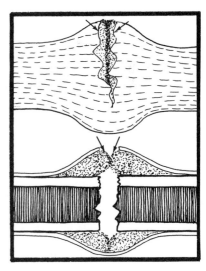

. *Sub-periosteal bone:* New woven bone is
rmed beneath the periosteum at the ends
the bone. The cells responsible are derived
om the periosteum, which becomes
retched over these collars of new bone. If
e blood supply is poor, or if it is disturbed
excessive mobility at the fracture site,
rtilage may be formed instead and remain
til a better blood supply is established.

90. *This primary callus response* (1) remains
active for *a few weeks only*. There is a much
less vigorous formation of callus from the
medullary cavity (2). Nevertheless, the
capacity of the medulla to form new bone
remains indefinitely throughout the healing
of the fracture.

91. *Bridging external callus* (i) If the
periosteum is incompletely torn, and there is
no significant loss of bony apposition, the
primary callus response may result in
establishing external continuity of the
fracture ('bridging external callus'). Cells
lying in the outer layer of the periosteum
itself proliferate to reconstitute the
periosteum.

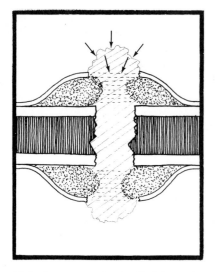

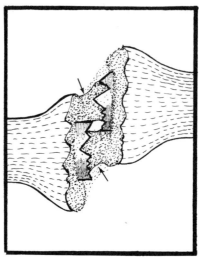

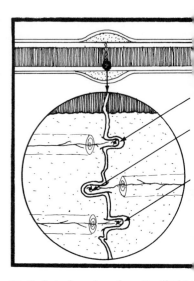

92. *Bridging external callus* (ii) If the gap is more substantial, fibrous tissue formed from the organisation of the fracture haematoma will lie between the advancing collars of sub-periosteal new bone. This fibrous tissue may be stimulated to form bone ('tissue induction'), again resulting in bridging callus. The mechanism may be due to a change of electrical potential at the fracture site or to a (hypothetical) wound hormone.

93. *Bridging external callus* (iii) If the bone ends are offset, the primary callus from the sub-periosteal region may unite with medullary callus. The net result of the three mechanisms just described is that the fracture becomes rigid, function in the limb returns and the situation is rendered favourable for endosteal bone formation and re-modelling.

94. *Endosteal new bone formation* (i) If there is no gap between the bone ends, osteoclasts can tunnel across the fracture line in advance of ingrowing blood vessels and osteoblasts which form new Haversian systems. Dead bone is re-vascularised and may provide an invaluable scaffolding and local mineral source. This process cannot occur if the fracture is mobile.

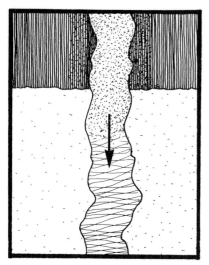

96. *Endosteal new bone formation* (iii) Where the bone ends are supported by rigid internal fixation, there is no functional requirement for external bridging callus: as a result external bridging callus may not be seen, or be minimal. Healing of the fracture occurs slowly through the formation of new cortical bone between the bone ends. It is therefore essential that internal fixation devices are retained until this process is complete.

Remodelling: After clinical union, new Haversian systems are laid down along the lines of stress. In areas free from stress, bone is removed by osteoclasts. Eventually little trace of external bridging callus will remain. The power to remodel bone in this way is great in children, but not so marked in the adult. In a child, most or all traces of fracture displacement (including even off-ending) will disappear. There is also some power to correct angulation, although this becomes progressively less as the child approaches adolescence. Any axial rotation, however, is likely to remain. In the adult, there is virtually no correction of axial rotation or angulation. It is, therefore, important that axial rotation deformity is always corrected, and that angulation, particularly in adults, should not be accepted.

95. *Endosteal new bone formation* (ii) The formation of new cortical bone, with re-establishment of continuity between the Haversian systems on either side cannot occur if fibrous tissue remains occupying the space between the bone ends. If this is present, it must be removed and replaced with woven bone. This is generally achieved by ingrowth of medullary callus which remains active through the healing phase.

8. Transverse fracture of the tibia in the middle third. There is no significant displacement or angulation, and the fibula is intact. The fracture is of adult pattern and is not a greenstick fracture.

9. Hair-line fracture of the tibia in the lower middle third. Coned-down views are often helpful; if the initial radiographs appear normal, they should be repeated after an interval if there is continued suspicion that a fracture is present.

0. Dislocation of the elbow. The radius and ulna are displaced laterally in relation to the humerus (and also posteriorly, although this is not shown on the single radiograph).

1. This injury cannot be anything but *compound* as the right-angled angulation of the greenstick fracture of the radius (at the junction of its middle and lower thirds) indicates. The mottling of the soft-tissue shadows due to air is confirmatory. In addition, there a greenstick fracture of the ulna in its middle third (note the posterior angulation) and dislocation of the elbow (the ulna appears lateral and the humerus A.P.).

2. Fracture dislocation of the shoulder. The head of the humerus is not congruous with the glenoid. Lateral to it is a large fragment of bone, the avulsed greater tuberosity of the humerus.

3. Double fracture of the tibia. The upper fracture is virtually transverse and in the middle third. The distal fracture is also transverse and situated in the distal third. The fibula is fractured, and the tibia is displaced medially. Bony apposition has probably been lost at the upper fracture. Problems with reduction, fixation and non-union at one level are to be anticipated.

4. Fracture of the radius and ulna in the distal third. In the lateral projection, there is some slight anterior angulation (posterior tilting) of the ulna. In the A.P. view, there is lateral (or radial) displacement of the distal fragments which are virtually off-ended. There is some medial (ulnar) angulation (or the distal fragments are tilted laterally). The radial fracture is oblique with a slight spiral element. The ulnar fracture is transverse.

65. There is a greenstick fracture of the radius. Note the ridging of the radius both medially and laterally just proximal to the epiphysis.

66. Fracture of the base of the fifth metatarsal. This is an avulsion fracture, produced by the peroneus brevus which is inserted into the fifth metatarsal base.

67. The radiograph shows deformity of the body of the first lumbar vertebra which has been reduced in height anteriorly. This is an anterior wedge or crush fracture.

68. There is an oblique fracture of the proximal femur, running between the lesser and greater trochanters, with a coxa vara deformity (the distal femur is tilted medially). The hip is arthritic, and the disturbance in bone texture in the pelvis and femur is typical of Paget's disease (i.e. this is a pathological fracture).

69. There is an oblique fracture of the fibula, which is displaced laterally, accompanied by the talus. The distal end of the fibula is tilted laterally (medial angulation). Unless accurately reduced, this fracture involving a joint is liable to lead to secondary osteo-arthritis.

70. The small fragment of bone detached from the base of the proximal phalanx has been avulsed by the ulnar collateral ligament of the M.P. joint. It indicates that the thumb has been dislocated, and that there is potential instability at this level.

71. There is a comminuted fracture of the tibia, with 4 main fragments. There is a double fracture of the fibula. Both fractures are in the mid third. Soft tissue shadows indicate, as might be anticipated, that this is a compound injury. There is lateral angulation (i.e. the distal fragment is tilted medially). During the taking of the A.P. and lateral radiographs there has been some alteration of position of the fracture: note that in the lateral projection there is considerable *axial rotation* (the foot is lateral, but the upper tibia is almost in the A.P. plane). Axial rotation is not a feature of the A.P. projection.

2. The diagnosis of fractures and principles of treatment

1. History

In taking the history of a patient who may have a fracture, the following points may prove to be helpful, especially when there has been a traumatic incident.

1. What activity was being pursued at the time of the incident? (e.g. taking part in a sport, driving a car, working at a height, etc.)

2. What was the nature of the incident? (e.g. a kick, a fall, a twisting injury, etc.)

3. What was the magnitude of the applied forces? (e.g. if a patient was injured in a fall, it is helpful to know how far he fell, if his fall was broken, the nature of the surface on which he landed, and how he landed; trivial violence may lead one to suspect a pathological fracture: severe violence makes the exclusion of multiple injuries particularly important.)

4. What was the point of impact and the direction of the applied forces? In reducing a fracture, one of the principle methods employed is to reduplicate the causal forces in a reverse direction. If a fracture occurs close to the point of impact, additional remotely situated fractures must be excluded.

5. Is there any significance to be attached to the incident itself? (For example, if there was a fall, was it precipitated by some underlying medical condition, such as a hypotensive attack, which requires separate investigation?)

6. Where is the site of any pain, and what is its severity?

7. Is there loss of functional activity? For example, walking is seldom possible after any fracture of the femur or tibia; inability to weight bear after an accident is of great significance.

Diagnosis: In some cases the diagnosis of fracture is unmistakable; for example, when there is gross deformity of the central portion of a long bone or when the fracture is visible as in certain compound injuries.

In the majority of other cases, a fracture is suspected from the history and clinical examination, and confirmed by radiography of the region.

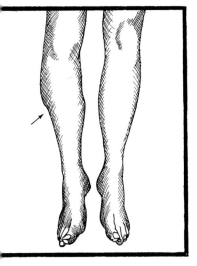

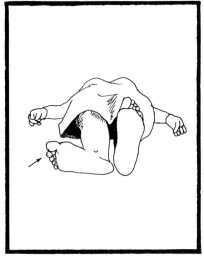

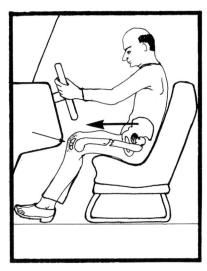

Inspection (i) Begins by inspecting the limb most carefully, comparing one side with the other. Look for any *asymmetry of contour*, suggesting an underlying fracture which has displaced or angled.

3. *Inspection* (ii) Look for any persisting *asymmetry of posture* of the limb: for example, persisting external rotation of the leg is a common feature in disimpacted fractures of the femoral neck.

4. *Inspection* (iii) Look for local bruising of the skin suggesting a *point of impact* which may direct your attention locally or to a more distant level. For example, bruising over the knee from dashboard impact should direct your attention to the underlying patella, and also to the femoral shaft and hip.

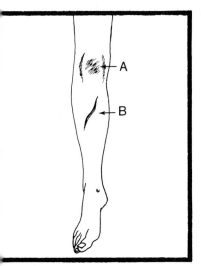

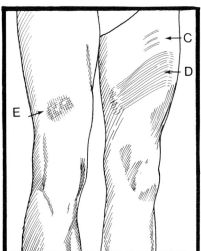

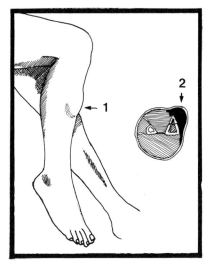

Inspection (iv) Look for other tell-tale skin damage: for example, (A) grazing, with or without ingraining of dirt in the wound, or friction burns, suggesting an impact followed by rubbing of the skin against a resistant surface. (B) Lacerations, suggesting impact against a hard edge, tearing by a bone end, or splitting by compression against a hard surface.

6. *Inspection* (v) Note the presence of: (C) skin stretch marks; (D) band patterning of the skin, suggestive of both stretching and compression of the skin in a run-over injury; (E) pattern bruising, caused by severe compression which leads the skin to be imprinted with the weave marks of overlying clothing. Any of these abnormalities should lead you to suspect the integrity of the underlying bone.

7. *Inspection* (vi) If the patient is seen shortly after the incident, note any localised swelling of the limb (1). Later, swelling tends to become more diffuse. Note the presence of any haematoma (2). A fracture may strip the skin from its local attachments; the skin comes to float on an underlying collection of blood which is continuous with the fracture haematoma.

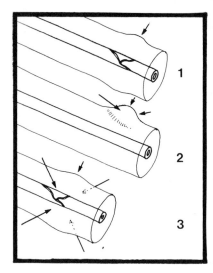

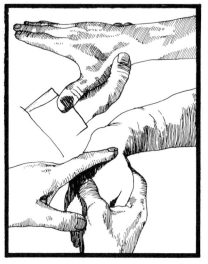

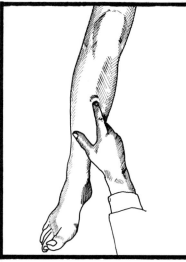

8. *Tenderness* (i) Look for tenderness over the bone suspected of being fractured. Tenderness is invariably elicited over a fracture (1), but tenderness will also be found over any traumatised area, even though there is no underlying fracture (2). The important distinguishing feature is that in the case of a fracture tenderness will be elicited when the bone is palpated on any aspect.

9. *Tenderness* (ii) In eliciting tenderness, once a tender area has been located, the part should be palpated at the same level from another direction. For example, in many sprained wrists, tenderness will be elicited in the anatomical snuff-box—but not over the dorsal and palmar aspects of the scaphoid which are tender if a fracture is present.

10. *Palpation:* The sharp edge of a fracture may be palpable. Note also the presence of localised oedema. This is a particularly useful sign over hairline and stress fractures. The development of oedema may however take some hours to reach detectable proportions.

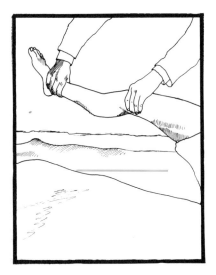

11. *Other signs:* If the fracture is mobile, moving the part may produce angulation or crepitus from the bone ends rubbing together. In addition, the patient will experience severe pain from such movement. These signs may be inadvertently observed during routine examination of the patient, but should not be sought unless the patient is unconscious and the diagnosis is in doubt.

12. *Radiographic examination:* In every case of suspected fracture, radiographic examination of the fracture is mandatory. Radiographs of the part will generally give a clear indication of the presence of a fracture and provide a sound basis for planning treatment. In the case where there is some clinical doubt, radiographs will reassure patient and surgeon and avert any later medico-legal criticism.

Radiographers in the United Kingdom receive thorough training in the techniques for the satisfactory visualisation of any suspect area, but it is essential that they in turn are given clear guidance as to the area under suspicion. The request form must be quite specific, otherwise mistakes may occur. At its simplest, the request must state *both the area to be visualised, and the bone suspected of being fractured.* It need hardly be stressed that a thorough clinical examination should precede the completion of the radiographic request if repetition and the taking of unnecessary films are to be avoided.

The following Table gives some of the commonest errors in requesting (diagnostic errors have been excluded):

13.

Area suspected of fracture	Typical request	Error	Correct request
Scaphoid	'X-ray wrist, ? fracture'	Fractures of the scaphoid are difficult to visualise: a minimum of 3 specialised views is required. A fracture may not show on the standard wrist projections	'X-ray scaphoid, ? fracture'
Calcaneus	'X-ray ankle, ? fracture' 'X-ray foot, ? fracture'	A tangential projection is necessary for satisfactory visualisation of the calcaneus. This is not performed routinely in radiographs of the foot and ankle	'X-ray calcaneus, ? fracture'
Neck of femur	'X-ray femur, ? fracture'	Poor centring of the radiographs may render the fracture invisible	'X-ray hip, ? fracture neck of femur' or 'X-ray to exclude fracture of femoral neck'
Tibial table or tibial spines	'X-ray tibia, ? fracture'	Poor centring may render the fracture invisible, or the area may not be included on the film	'X-ray upper third tibia to exclude fracture of tibial table'

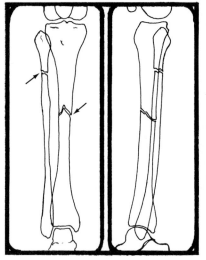

14. *The standard projections:* These are an *antero-posterior (A.P.) and lateral.* Ideally the beam should be centred over the area of suspected fracture, with visualisation of the proximal and distal joints. This is especially important in the paired long bones where, for example, a fracture of the tibia above the ankle may be accompanied by a fracture of the neck of the fibula.

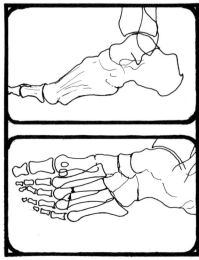

15. *Oblique projections:* In the case of the hand and foot, an oblique projection may be helpful when the lateral gives rise to confusion due to the superimposition of many structures. Such oblique projections may have to be specifically requested when they are not part of an X-ray department's routine.

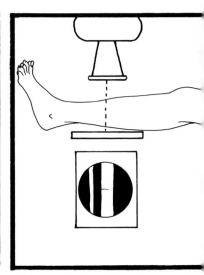

16. *Localised views:* Where there is marked local tenderness, but routine films are normal, coned-down localised views may give sufficient gain in detail to reveal for example a hair-line fracture: if such films are also negative, the radiographs should be repeated after an interval of 10–14 days if the symptoms are persisting (see also Hair-line fracture).

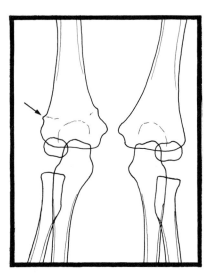

17. *Comparison films:* Where there is some difficulty in interpreting the radiographs (for example, in the elbow region in children where the epiphyseal structures are continually changing, or where there is some unexplained shadow, or a congenital abnormality) films of the other side should be taken for direct comparison.

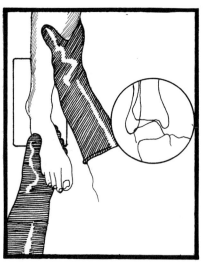

18. *Stress films* (i) Stress films can be of value in certain situations. (a) When a complete tear of a major ligament is suspected: for example, where the lateral ligament of the ankle is thought to be torn, radiographs of the joint taken with the foot in forced inversion may demonstrate instability of the talus in the ankle mortice. (Local or general anaesthesia may be required in fresh injuries.)

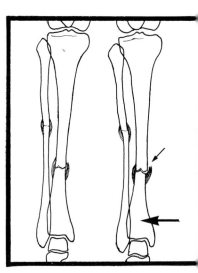

19. *Stress films* (ii) (b) For clarification of doubtful union or possible re-fracture of a uniting fracture.

There are many other radiological techniques. In particular, tomography and cineradiography are often of value in the investigation of spinal injuries. Special techniques are discussed under the appropriate regional sections.

Pitfalls

A number of fractures are missed with great regularity—sometimes with serious consequences. You should always be on the look-out for the following:

1. An elderly patient who is unable to weight bear after a fall must be examined most carefully. The commonest cause by far is a fracture of the femoral neck, and this must be eliminated in every case. If the femoral neck is intact, look for a fracture of the *pubic rami*. Note that on the rare occasion, a patient with an impacted fracture of the femoral neck may be able to weight bear, albeit with pain.

2. If a car occupant suffers a fracture of the patella or femur from a dashboard impact, always eliminate the presence of a dislocation of the hip which is sometimes silent.

3. If a patient fractures the calcaneus in a fall, examine the other side most carefully. Bilateral fractures are extremely common, and the less painful side may be missed.

4. If a patient complains of a 'sprained ankle' always examine the foot as well as the ankle. Fractures of the base of the fifth metatarsal frequently result from inversion injuries, and are often overlooked. The mistake of not performing a good clinical examination in these circumstances is compounded by requesting radiographs of the ankle (which do not show the fifth metatarsal bone).

5. In the unconscious patient, injuries of the cervical spine are frequently overlooked. *It pays* to have routine screening films of the neck, chest and pelvis in the unconscious patient.

6. Impacted fractures of the neck of the humerus are often missed, especially when one view only is taken. Conversely, in children, the epiphyseal line is often wrongly mistaken for fracture.

7. Posterior dislocation of the shoulder may not be diagnosed when it should be at the initial attendance. This is because the humeral head comes to lie directly behind the glenoid, and is not detected if only a single A.P. projection is taken. If there is a strong suspicion of injury, and especially if there is deformity of the shoulder, a second projection is *essential* if no abnormality is noted on the A.P. film.

8. Apparently isolated fractures of either the radius or ulna should be diagnosed with caution. The Monteggia and Galeazzi fracture-dislocations are still frequently missed. In the same way, it is unwise to diagnose an isolated fracture of the tibia until the whole of the fibula has been visualised: fracture of the tibia close to the ankle is, for example, often accompanied by fracture of the fibular neck.

9. At the wrist, greenstick fractures of the radius in children are often overlooked due to lack of care in studying the radiographs.

10. In adults, fractures of the radial styloid or Bennett's fracture may be missed or treated as suspected fractures of the scaphoid. Complete tears of ulnar collateral ligament of the M.P. joint of the thumb are frequently overlooked, sometimes with severe resultant functional disability.

The treatment of fractures

Primary aims: The primary aims of fracture treatment are:

1. The attainment of sound bony union without deformity.

2. The restoration of function, so that the patient is able to resume his former occupation and pursue any athletic or social activity he wishes.

To this might be added 'as quickly as possible' and 'without risk of any complications, whether early or late'. These aims cannot always be achieved, and in some situations are mutually exclusive. For example, internal fixation of some fractures may give rapid restoration of function, but at the expense of occasional infection. The great variations that exist in fracture treatment are largely due to differences in interpretation of these factors.

Priorities of treatment: If a fracture is a patient's sole injury, it is usually possible to proceed with its treatment without undue delay (although unfitness for anaesthesia may sometimes upset this ideal). If, however, a fracture is complicated by damage to other structures, or involvement of other systems, then treatment of the fracture usually takes second place. Immediate action must be taken to correct any life-endangering situation which may be present or anticipated. Therefore, when the patient is first seen, a rapid overall examination must be made to detect any condition which merits priority in treatment. The following situations may require consideration:

1. *Respiratory obstruction or impairment.* (i) Any blood, mucus or vomit must be removed from the mouth and upper respiratory passages by suction or swabbing. Dentures should be looked for and extracted. It may be necessary to pass an endotracheal tube to obtain a satisfactory airway while at the same time facilitating toilet of the upper respiratory passages and protecting them from aspiration. If there is evidence of the inhalation of vomitus, bronchoscopy may be required.

Support of the jaw, a simple airway, and turning the patient on his side may be effective in the more minor situation.

(ii) An open chest wound must be immediately covered to reduce the risk of tension pneumothorax; a simple adhesive dressing is usually quite adequate in the emergency situation.

(iii) If there is evidence of tension pneumothorax, pneumothorax or haemothorax, the appropriate chest cavities should be drained by intercostal catheters connected to water-seal drains.

(iv) If there is evidence of paradoxical respiration due to flail rib segment blood gas levels should be estimated; slight impairment of respiratory function may be managed by giving oxygen by inhalation and analgesics with caution. When the blood gas levels are seriously disturbed, and especially in the presence of a concurrent head injury, some form of assisted respiration is usually the best method of management.

2. *Haemorrhage and shock.* (i) External haemorrhage may be severe and if so must be brought under rapid control. Local padding or packing with firm bandaging is usually adequate, but in the uncommon situations where this fails, a tourniquet may be required. This must be adequately applied; too little pressure will increase the blood loss by preventing venous return,

and too great a pressure will endanger underlying nerves. A pneumatic tourniquet should always be applied in preference to any other type.

(ii) Internal haemorrhage: There may be significant internal haemorrhage from the extravasation of blood into the soft tissues in the area of a fracture. This is especially the case in fractures of the pelvis and femur and where there are multiple fractures. Serious blood loss may also occur in chest injuries where there may be rapid bleeding into the chest cavities and the formation of a haemothorax. In the abdomen, there may also be serious loss from rupture of the spleen and liver, and from mesenteric tears. Where there is major intra-abdominal haemorrhage, urgent exploration may be required.

(iii) Oligaemic shock: In any significant injury the pulse and blood pressure should be charted at 15-minute intervals, a sample of blood taken for grouping and cross matching, and a good intravenous line set up. An attempt should be made to work out how much blood the patient is likely to have lost and the amount and rapidity of future losses. Great accuracy cannot be expected, but it is important to have a clear idea of the replacement likely to be required and to strive to remain in control of the situation. Oligaemic shock should not be allowed to occur; it should be anticipated and prevented; but if present, it must be properly and adequately treated. If the estimated total loss is a litre or less (in an adult) replacement should not be required, and plasma or a plasma expander held in reserve. If the estimated loss is 2 litres, $1-1\frac{1}{2}$ litres may be replaced in the form of plasma and/or a plasma expander; 1 litre of cross matched blood may be held in reserve. If the losses are much in excess of 2 litres, whole blood will be required, but a decision that has frequently to be made is whether the patient can wait until full cross matching can be carried out. In many cases, if blood loss is slow and controlled, and there has been a good response to initial infusions of plasma or a plasma expander, the patient's condition may be maintained by the administration of up to 2 litres of plasma—during the waiting period. In other cases, where for example the patient arrives exsanguinated, it may be essential to resuscitate using substantial quantities of unmatched group O Rh −ve blood.

The following figures have been suggested in estimating blood losses:

Closed fracture of the femoral shaft	$\frac{1}{2}-1$ litre
Open ring fractures of the pelvis	2−3 litres
Intra-abdominal haemorrhage	2−3 litres
Haemothorax	1−2 litres

To this must be added the volume of any external haemorrhage. The total loss from two or more injuries is less than the sum of the individual losses.

3. *Head injury:* (i) Where there is a head injury present which requires urgent investigative procedures or operative intervention (for example an extra-dural haemorrhage with deterioration in the level of consciousness) this will take priority over the local treatment of most fractures. A combined procedure may often be planned with advantage but certainly in all cases some estimate should be made as to when definitive treatment of the fracture is likely to be possible; depending on that interval is the choice of a variety of initial procedures which may include the application of sterile dressings or light packing of compound wounds; supporting an injured limb with sandbags or an inflatable splint in such a position that the distal circulation

is maintained; or the use of light temporary plaster splintage.

(ii) Where there is a head injury in which the immediate prognosis is hopeless any temporary splintage of the fracture should be retained but no fresh treatment planned.

(iii) Where no active neurosurgical treatment is contemplated and the prognosis regarded as very poor but not absolutely hopeless, it is usually possible to devise some simple measures to give reasonable support to the injured part but at the same time permitting more definitive treatment in the near future should unexpected improvement occur.

4. *Cardiac tamponade: intrathoracic rupture of the aorta.* Prompt drainage of an intra-pericardial haematoma may be a life-saving measure. Aortic rupture may not be immediately fatal and be detected by the characteristic squaring-off of the mediastinal shadow on radiographs of the chest. Arrangements should be made without delay for exploration; as by-pass facilities will be required, in some cases this will require transfer of the patient to a specialist unit.

5. *Visceral complications.* Injury to the solid abdominal organs (especially the liver, spleen and kidneys) may give rise to severe intra-abdominal haemorrhage. Haemorrhage may also follow mesenteric tears and ruptures of the stomach and intestine with which the problems of perforation are also associated. Abdominal exploration takes priority over fracture treatment (see also complications of fracture).

Treatment of the fracture itself

The initial stages are clear:

Undue movement at the fracture site should be prevented by the use of temporary splintage till radiographic and any other examination is complete. This will reduce pain and haemorrhage and minimise the chances of a simple fracture becoming compound.

In the case of the lower limb, support with pillows and sandbags may be adequate. In both the upper and lower limbs inflatable splints are invaluable

Compound fractures should be protected with sterile dressings.

The fracture should be fully assessed by clinical and radiological examination: the site, pattern, displacement and angulation should be noted Involvement of the skin, and damage to related structures such as important nerves or blood vessels should be assessed.

With this information the following key decisions must be made:

1. Does the fracture require reduction?
2. If reduction is required, how is it planned to carry this out?
3. What support is required till union occurs?
4. If the fracture is compound, how will this influence treatment?
5. Does the patient require admission to hospital?

Some observations about these decisions will be made in sequence.

1. **Does the fracture require reduction?** It is obvious that an undisplaced fracture does not require reduction: but unfortunately, one still sees fractures in anatomical position subjected to manipulation, although only rarely are they displaced as a result of this.

If a fracture is only slightly displaced, reduction may nevertheless be highly desirable, as for example in Potts fractures involving the ankle joint, where even slight persisting deformity may lead to the development of osteoarthritic changes in the joint. In other situations, some displacement may often be accepted, depending on (a) the site involved (b) where good remodelling may be anticipated (especially in children) (c) if the patient is very old, when the risks of anaesthesia, etc., may be considered to outweigh a problematical improvement.

If the fracture is appreciably angled or rotated, reduction is generally essential for cosmetic and functional reasons (but see under appropriate fractures).

2. **If the fracture requires reduction, how is it planned to carry this out?** (a) The commonest method is by the application of traction, followed by manipulation of the fracture, under general anaesthesia. General anaesthesia has most to offer in terms of muscle relaxation, duration and overall versatility, but for minor procedures regional anaesthesia and intravenous diazepam are popular and useful measures, with the advantage that waiting time may be reduced.

(b) Continuous traction is used to achieve a reduction in fractures of the femur and fracture dislocations of the cervical spine. It is used less commonly for a number of other fractures.

(c) Open reduction of the fracture is carried out (i) as an obvious part of the treatment of a compound fracture—i.e. debridement of the wound exposes the fracture which may be reduced under vision (ii) where conservative methods have failed to give a satisfactory reduction (iii) where it is considered that the best method of supporting the fracture involves internal fixation, and exposure of the fracture is a necessary part of that procedure.

3. **What support is required until union of the fracture occurs?** *(a) Non rigid methods of support:* Arm slings, bandages and adhesive strapping may be used, and serve some of the following purposes.

(i) Firm support, in the form for example of crepe bandaging or circular woven bandaging, may help to limit swelling and oedema, and restrict the spread of haematoma.

(ii) Slings are often employed for elevation purposes, especially to limit gravitational swelling of the hand and fingers in upper limb injuries.

(iii) Pain may be relieved by the restriction of movement.

(iv) By restriction of limb movement, forces acting on the bone ends may be reduced to a level at which relative movement is unlikely, or insufficient to interfere with healing. This applies particularly to impacted fractures.

(b) Continuous traction: Traction may be maintained for several weeks, while holding a fracture in reduction. Fractures of the femoral shaft are frequently treated by this method. Traction may be effected through the skin (skin traction) by, for example, adhesive strapping, or through bone (skeletal traction) by, for example, a Steinman pin.

(c) Plaster fixation: Plaster of Paris, generally in the form of plaster impregnated bandages, is the commonest method of supporting a fracture. The plaster is carefully moulded to fit the contours of the limb, and the quick setting properties of the plaster allow the limb to be held without undue strain in the correct position until setting has occurred. For a plaster to

achieve its purpose, care must be taken over its application and subsequent supervision. A disadvantage of plaster splints is that they soften if they are allowed to become wet. There are a number of plaster substitutes now available to overcome this problem, but none as yet combine the unique properties of plaster with moderate cost.

(d) Internal fixation: Internal fixation is indicated (i) Where a fracture cannot be reduced by closed methods (e.g. a fracture of the tibia with soft tissue between the bone ends or many fractures of the forearm bones)

(ii) Where a reduction can be achieved but it cannot be satisfactorily held by closed methods (e.g. fractures of the femoral neck)

(iii) Where a higher quality of reduction and fixation is required than can be obtained by closed methods (e.g. some fractures involving articular surfaces).

In addition, there is a controversial area where the risks of internal fixation in a particular set of circumstances are outweighed, in the experience and opinion of the surgeon in charge, by the advantages. Some of the factors involved may include:

(i) The possibility of achieving and maintaining a high quality reduction.

(ii) Earlier mobilisation of joints, with less risk of permanent stiffness, disuse osteoporosis, etc.

(iii) Earlier discharge from hospital, and earlier return to full function (including work, athletic activities, etc.).

Some of the disadvantages of internal fixation are:

(i) The possibility of introducing infection. The consequences may be serious (e.g. chronic bone infection with non-union, which may sometimes necessitate amputation).

(ii) Internal fixation techniques require a degree of mechanical aptitude and experience on the part of the surgeon if the occasional serious failure is to be avoided.

(iii) To cover a wide range of fracture situations, a fairly formidable number of instruments and fixation devices will be required.

(iv) As on the whole the time under anaesthesia is much longer than when conservative measures are employed, the patient's general condition and health is of greater concern: the services of an expert anaesthetist are more frequently required.

The methods of achieving internal fixation include the use of a wide range of devices (screws, nails, plates, etc.).

(e) External skeletal fixation: With this method the bone fragments are held in alignment by skeletal pins. The central portion of each pin lies in the bone, while the ends protrude from the skin. 1–3 pins are fixed in each bone fragment. The fracture is reduced with the pins in situ (at open operation, or by using an image intensifier). The pins are then held in proper relation to one another by a rigid external support. Plaster may be used for this purpose, or a rigid mechanical system of clamps and connecting rods.

Such systems are of particular value in the management of compound fractures where the state of the skin and other factors may make the use of internal fixation devices undesirable. They are sometimes followed, even in closed fractures, by pin track infections. The quality of the fixation is also dependent on the pins remaining tight in bone, and there is some risk of non-union.

(f) Cast-bracing: Cast-bracing techniques are sometimes employed some weeks after the initial conservative management of a fracture. The method is used particularly in the treatment of fractures of the femur and tibia. In the case of fractures of the femur, one method employs two supports—one for the thigh and one for the leg below the knee—linked together by hinges at the side of the knee. Sufficient fixation may be achieved thereby to allow early ambulation.

4. **If the fracture is compound, how will this influence treatment?** The following points will require separate consideration:

(a) As debridement of the wound will almost certainly be needed, general anaesthesia and theatre facilities are essential.

(b) In every case, potential difficulty in skin closure and skin cover of the fracture must be anticipated, and at least one possible line of treatment worked out prior to the patient being taken to theatre.

(c) If the wound is badly soiled, and the skin damage substantial, the use of large implants is discouraged. The wider stripping of the tissues required for the insertion of some internal fixation devices may disseminate any infecting organisms and cause further (albeit local) tissue damage. The presence of inert material in the tissues may act as a nidus for infection, so that it is difficult for any local infection to be overcome. The bulk of an internal fixation device may make wound closure more difficult, and subsequent swelling is more likely to lead to sloughing of devitalised skin over any prosthesis.

If wound contamination is judged to be slight, if sound closure of the wound can be obtained, and if good primary healing can be justifiably anticipated, internal fixation of the fracture is often carried out where it is felt to contribute to the chances of union and a successful outcome.

(d) Compound fractures are usually associated with greater damage to surrounding soft tissues than is found in closed fractures. Post-operative swelling is invariable, is often severe, and may lead to circulatory impairment in the limb. Special precautions must be taken over the type of splintage, and the limb must be elevated. Admission for observation of the patient and of the limb circulation is almost invariably required.

(e) As a rule, compound fractures are associated with greater violence, more initial deformity, and more direct soft tissue damage. Neurological and vascular damage is more common, and should be looked for; if found, then the appropriate additional treatment will be required.

(f) Where contamination of the wound is substantial, prophylactic antibiotics are usually administered routinely. Generally a broad spectrum antibiotic to which the penicillin-resistant staphylococcus is sensitive is advised; it should be given at the earliest opportunity, before the patient goes to theatre for wound debridement. Attention must also be paid to tetanus prophylaxis.

If wound contamination is judged to be slight, antibiotics may or may not be given, depending to some extent on the assessment of the particular circumstances of the case and of unit policy.

5. **Does the patient require admission to hospital?** In most cases the decision is an easy one being related to the seriousness of the injury, the nature of the treatment, and the need for continuous observation. The main

criteria for admission very frequently overlap, and include the following:

(a) Admission dictated by treatment: Admission may be dictated by problems associated with anaesthesia—undue delay before anaesthesia, a prolonged anaesthetic, or where the anaesthetic is administered very late at night and recovery would be occurring at an inconvenient time in the early morning.

Admission will also obviously be required if the patient is being treated by continuous traction, partly because of the continuous use of special equipment, and partly because of the expert supervision required.

Most commonly, admission will be required when as a result of his injury the patient must be confined to bed.

(b) Admission for observation: Where there is appreciable risk of complications developing, admission may be required for continuous observation. This is obvious in the case of associated head injury, abdominal injury, or the case of general multiple trauma.

Of particular relevance is admission for observation of the circulation in an injured limb. The majority of tibial fractures in adults, and ideally all supracondylar fractures in children should be admitted for elevation of the limb and observation of the circulation.

After compound injuries (with the possible exceptions of fingers and toes) admission is advisable so that any developing infection can be detected and dealt with as early as possible.

(c) Admission for general nursing care: Many fracture cases may or may not require special treatment, but are nevertheless completely dependent on good nursing care. This applies particularly to fractures of the pelvis and spine where the patient is confined to bed. It also applies to other less obvious situations, such as the patient with fractures of both arms, who may be rendered virtually helpless with two comparatively minor injuries.

(d) Admission for mobilisation: Admission may be required for a period until the patient adapts to the limitations of his fracture and his splintage: for example, until a patient becomes sufficiently adept in the use of his crutches that he can manage in his own home.

(e) Admission for social reasons: Many elderly and infirm people, living alone or with equally affected relatives, may just be able to cope with life prior to injury. Even a minor fracture may render them unable to return to their normal environment. Admission is a necessity if no other help is available, and of course treatment is aimed at getting them fit to return home. Opportunity may be taken of their admission to investigate and treat any concurrent physical problem. If recovery is poor, assistance from hospital and domiciliary occupational therapists, social workers, or geriatricians may be required.

3. Closed reduction and fixation of fractures

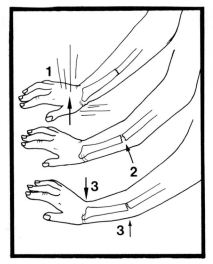

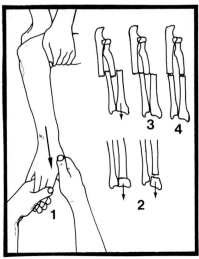

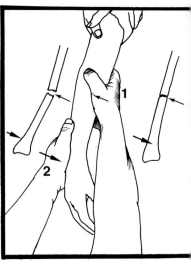

1. *Closed reduction of fractures: Basic techniques* (1) The direction and magnitude of the causal force (1) and the deformity (2) are related, and may be worked out from the history, the appearance of the limb, and the radiographs. Any force required to correct the displacement of a fracture is applied in the opposite direction (3).

2. *Basic techniques* (2) The first step in most closed reductions is to apply traction—generally in the line of the limb (1). Traction will lead to the disimpaction of most fractures (2) and this may occur almost immediately in the relaxed patient under general anaesthesia. Traction will also lead to reduction of shortening (3), and in most cases to reduction of the deformity (4).

3. *Basic techniques* (3) Any residual angulation following the application of traction may be corrected by using the heel of the hand under the fracture (1) and applying pressure distally with the other (2).

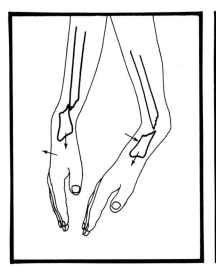

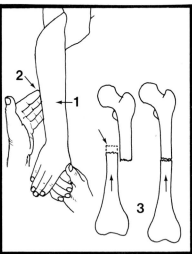

6. *Basic techniques* (6) After reduction of th fracture it must be prevented from re-displacing until it has united. The methods include the following:
Plaster fixation (7–36).
Skin and skeletal traction (for examples, see Femur 7–12).
Thomas splint (see Femur 13–36).
Cast bracing (see Femur 38–41 and Tibia 26–28).
Rigid external fixation (see Tibia 40–41).

4. *Basic techniques* (4) In some fractures there may be difficulty in reduction due to prominent bony spikes or soft tissue interposition. Reduction may sometimes be achieved by initially increasing the angulation prior to manipulation. This method of unlocking the fragments must be pursued with care to avoid damage to surrounding vessels and nerves.

5. *Basic techniques* (5) The effectiveness of reduction may be assessed by noting the appearance of the limb (1), by palpation, especially in long bone fractures (2), by absence of telescoping (i.e. axial compression along the line of the limb does not lead to further shortening) (3), and by check radiographs.

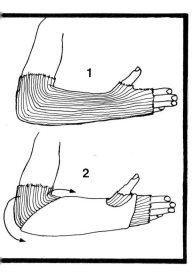

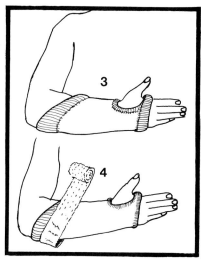

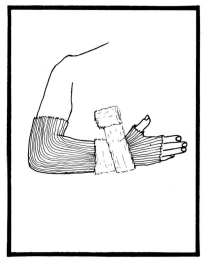

Protection of the skin: Stockingette: A ~yer of stockingette is usually applied next the skin (1). This has several functions: it lps prevent the limb hairs becoming ught in the plaster, it facilitates the nduction of perspiration from the limb, it moves any roughness caused by the ends the plaster and it may aid in the bsequent removal of the plaster. After the aster has been applied, the stockingette is ~ned back (2).

8. *Stockingette ctd.:* After the stockingette has been reflected, excess is removed, leaving 3–4 cm only at each end (3). The loose edge of stockingette is then secured with a turn or two of a plaster bandage (if a complete plaster is being applied) or with the encircling gauze bandage in the case of a slab.

9. *Wool roll:* A layer of wool should be used to protect bony prominences (e.g. the distal ulna). In complete plasters, where swelling is anticipated, several layers of wool may be applied over the length of the limb: the initial layer of stockingette may be omitted. Wool roll is also advisable where an electric saw is used for plaster removal.

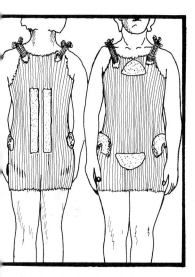

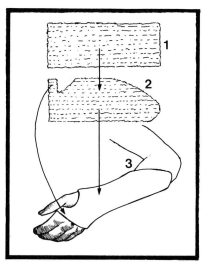

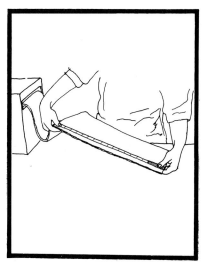

~. *Felt:* Where friction is likely to occur ~er bony prominences, protection may be ~en with felt strips or felt cut-outs, ~shioned to isolate the area to be relieved ~g. the vertebral and iliac spines, the pubis ~d manubrium in plaster jackets). Adhesive ~t should not be applied directly to the skin ~kin eruptions are to be avoided.

11. *Plaster slabs* (1) These consist of several layers of plaster bandage and may be used for the treatment of minor injuries or where potentially serious swelling may be anticipated in a fracture. In their application, slabs are cut to length (1) trimmed as required (2) to fit the limb before being applied (3). Slabs may also be used as foundations or reinforcements of complete plasters.

12. *Plaster slabs* (2) If a slab dispenser is available, measure the length of slab required and cut to length. A single slab of 6 layers of bandage will usually suffice for a child. In a large adult, two slab thicknesses may be necessary. In a small adult, one slab thickness may be adequate with local reinforcement.

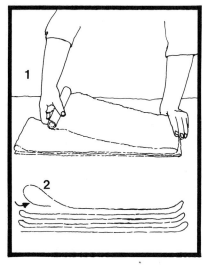

13. *Plaster slabs* (3) Alternatively, manufacture a slab by repeated folding of a plaster bandage, using say 8–10 thicknesses in an adult and 6 in a child as described (1). Turn in the end of the bandage (2) so that when the slab is dipped, the upper layer does not fall out of alignment.

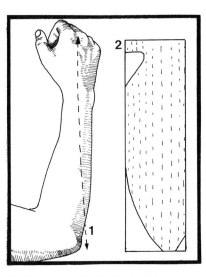

14. *Plaster slabs* (4) Ideally the slab should be trimmed with plaster scissors so that it will fit the limb without being folded over. For example, a slab for an undisplaced greenstick fracture of the distal radius should stretch from the metacarpal heads to the olecranon. It may be measured (1) and trimmed as shown, with a tongue (2) to lie between the thumb and index.

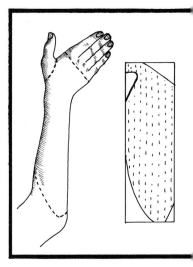

15. *Plaster slabs* (5) In a Colles fracture where the hand should be placed in a position of ulnar deviation, the slab should be trimmed to accommodate this position, stage that is often omitted in error. The preceding two plaster slabs are examples of dorsal slabs.

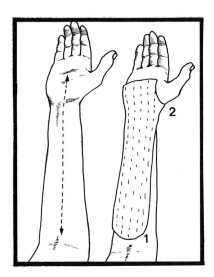

16. *Plaster slabs* (6) An anterior slab may be used as a foundation for a scaphoid plaster, or to treat an injury in which the wrist is held in dorsiflexion. (Measuring from a point just distal to the elbow crease with the elbow at 90°, to the proximal skin crease in the palm.) The proximal end is rounded (1) while the distal lateral corner is trimmed for the thenar mass (2).

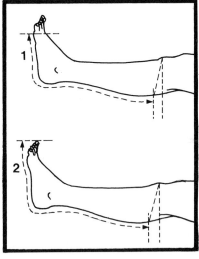

17. *Plaster slabs* (7) For the ankle (1) a plain untrimmed slab may be used, measuring from the metatarsal heads to the upper calf, 3–4 cm distal to a point behind the tibial tubercle.

For the foot (2) where the toes require support, choose the tips of the toes as the distal point.

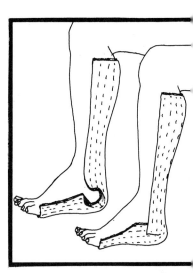

18. *Plaster slabs* (8) Due to the abrupt change in direction of the slab at the ankle the slab requires cutting on both sides so that it may be smoothed down with local overlapping.

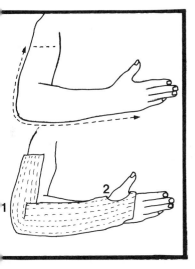

. *Plaster slabs* (9) The same technique of de cutting is required for long arm plaster abs (1). These are measured as indicated om the upper arm to the metacarpal heads, ith a cut-out at the thumb as in a Colles aster slab (2).

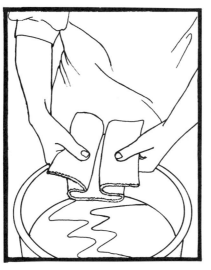

20. *Plaster slabs* (10) Wetting the slab: Hold the slab carefully at both ends, immerse completely in tepid water, lift out, and momentarily bunch up at an angle to expel excess water. Plaster setting time is decreased by both hot and soft water.

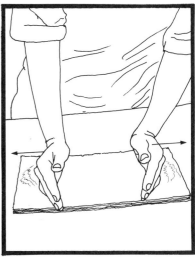

21. *Plaster slabs* (11) Now consolidate the layers of the slab. If a plaster table is available, quickly place the slab on the surface, and with one movement with the heels of the hands, press the layers firmly together. (Retained air reduces the ultimate strength of the plaster, and leads to cracking or separation of the layers.)

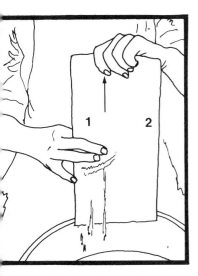

2. *Plaster slabs* (12) Alternatively, onsolidate the layers by holding the plaster t one end and pulling between two dducted fingers (1). Repeat the procedure om the other edge (2).

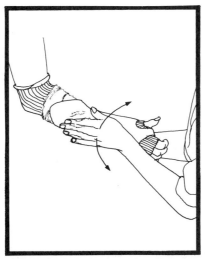

23. *Plaster slabs* (13) Carefully position the slab on the limb and smooth out with the hands so that the slab fits closely to the contours of the limb without rucking or the formation of sore-making ridges on its inferior surface.

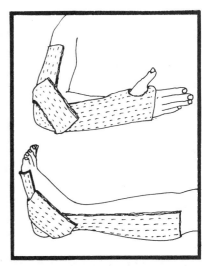

24. *Plaster slabs* (14) At this stage any weak spots should be reinforced. Where there is a right-angled bend in a plaster—for example at the elbow or the ankle—two small slabs made from 4″ (10 cm) plaster bandages, may be used as triangular reinforcements at either site. A similar small slab may be used to reinforce the back of the wrist.

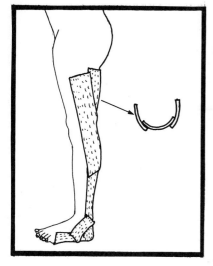

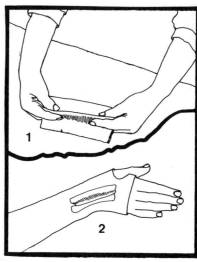

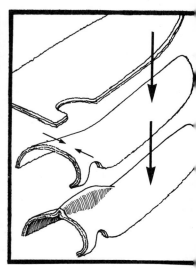

25. *Plaster slabs* (15) In the case of a long leg plaster slab, additional strengthening at the thigh and knee is always necessary, and this may be achieved by the use of two additional 6″ (15 cm) slabs.

26. *Plaster slabs* (16) Where even greater strength is required, the plaster may be girdered. For example, for the wrist, make a small slab of 6 thicknesses of 4″ (10 cm) bandage and pinch up in the centre (1). Dip the reinforcement, apply, and smooth down to form a T-girder over the dorsum (2).

27. *Plaster slabs* (17) Girdering may also be achieved without a separate onlay. The base plaster slab is pinched up locally after being applied to the limb. Care must be taken to avoid undue ridging of the inferior surface.

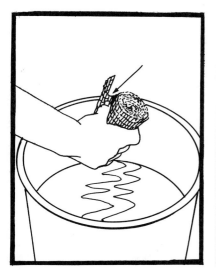

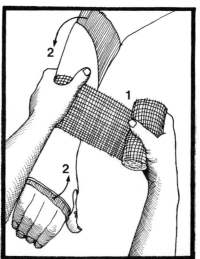

30. *Complete P.O.P. technique:* (1) The skin should be protected as previously described using where applicable stockingette, wool roll and felt. (2) The following sizes of plaster bandage are recommended for normal application:

Upper arm and forearm	6″ (15 cm)
Wrist	4″ (10 cm)
Thumb and fingers	3″ (7.5 cm)
Trunk and hip	8″ (20 cm)
Thigh and leg	8″ (20 cm)
Ankle and foot	6″ (15 cm)

28. *Bandaging* (1) Bandages used to secure plaster slabs should be of open weave (cotton or muslin) and be thoroughly wetted. This is to avoid tightening from shrinkage after coming in contact with the slab. Secure the end of the bandage between the thumb and fingers, and squeeze several times under water.

29. *Bandaging* (2) Apply to the limb firmly, but without too much pressure (1). Do not use reverse turns which tend to produce local constrictions. The ends of the underlying stockingette may be turned back and secured with the last few turns of the bandage (2). On completion, secure the bandage with a small piece of wetted plaster bandage.

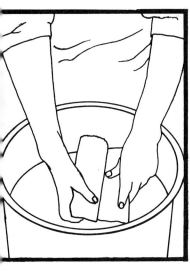

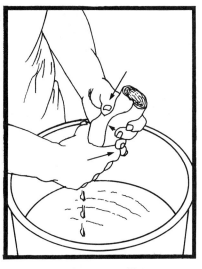

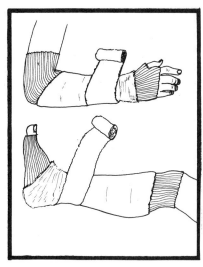

1. *Plaster bandage wetting* (1) Plaster bandages should be dipped in tepid water. Secure the end of the bandage with one hand to prevent the end becoming lost in the mass of wet bandage. Hold the bandage lightly with the other without compression. Immerse at an angle of 45°, and keep under water until the bubbles stop rising.

32. *Plaster bandage wetting* (2) Remove excess water by gently compressing in an axial direction and twisting slightly. Alternatively, pull the bandage through the encircled thumb and index while lightly gripping the bandage.

33. *Plaster bandage application* (1) Most moulding of the plaster will be required at the wrist in upper limb plasters, and at the ankle in lower limb plasters. It is often useful to apply the more proximal parts first, so that moulding can be more profitably carried out against a set or nearly set cuff of plaster on the forearm or calf (i.e. start a forearm plaster at the elbow, and a below knee plaster at the tibial tubercle).

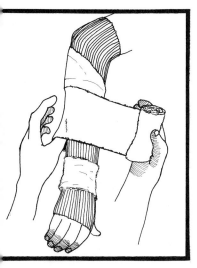

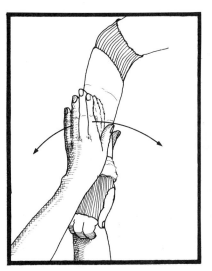

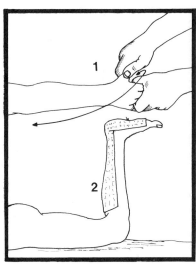

34. *Plaster bandage application* (2) Roll each bandage without stretching if there is no wool beneath: if there is a layer of wool, and no swelling is anticipated, a little even pressure may be applied to compress the wool to half thickness. Plain tucks may be used distally to ensure a smooth fit, but figure of eight or reverse turns should not be used if local constriction is to be avoided.

35. *Plaster bandage application* (3) After the application of each bandage smooth the layers down to exclude any trapped air and consolidate the plaster. A second and if necessary a third bandage may be applied to complete the proximal portion. Each bandage should extend 2–3 cm distal to the previous, and be well smoothed down. The distal part may then be completed, and the hand or foot portion moulded before setting is complete.

36. *Plaster bandage application* (4) Where possible the assistant should hold the limb in such a way that the surgeon has a clear run while applying the plaster (1). Where support must be given to a part included in the plaster, the flats of the hands should be used, and the hands eased proximally and distally to avoid local indentation. Where slabs are used, try to let gravity assist rather than hinder (2).

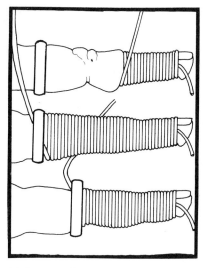

37. *Removal of rings* (1) Wherever possible rings should be removed in case finger swelling leads to distal gangrene. A tight ring can generally be coaxed from a finger if it is well coated with olive oil or a similar lubricant. If this fails, the finger may sometimes be sufficiently compressed by binding it with, for example, macrame twine to allow removal as shown.

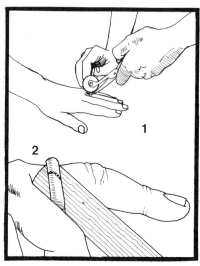

38. *Removal of rings* (2) Otherwise a ring may be cut with a ring cutter (1) or a saw cut may be made with a fine tooth hack-saw on to a spatula (2) to spring the ring. Ring removal is nevertheless sometimes obsessively pursued. If significant swelling is unlikely, the ring loose below the knuckle, the patient intelligent, and if the potential danger is indicated, it may be retained with acceptable safety.

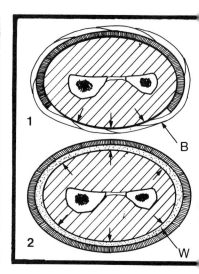

39. *Plaster precautions* (1) After an acute injury, if much swelling is anticipated (1) use a plaster slab in preference to a complete plaster. The retaining bandages have more 'give' than plaster, and are more readily cut in an emergency. (2) If a slab does not give sufficient support, then allow for swelling with a generous layer of wool beneath the plaster. (W = wool; B = bandage.)

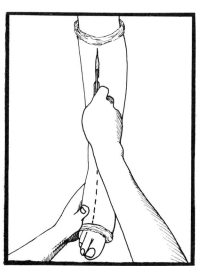

40. *Plaster precautions* (2) (3) Consider splitting any complete plaster. This should be done *routinely* after any operative procedure when swelling may be considerable (from tourniquet release, post-operative oedema, etc.). Use a sharp knife and cut down through the plaster to the underlying wool. (The wool protects the skin.) This should be done immediately after application of the plaster before it has had time to dry out.

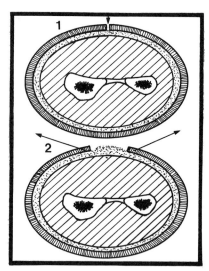

41. *Plaster precautions* (3) ctd. Be sure the plaster has been *completely* divided down to the wool along its whole length (1). (Any remaining strands will act dangerously as constricting bands.) You should be able to see the wool quite clearly. The plaster edges should spring apart by 5–10 mm or they may be eased apart by the handle of the knife thereby dynamically relieving any underlying pressure (2).

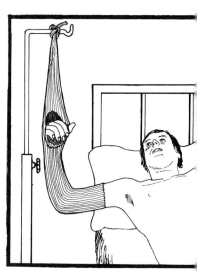

42. *Elevation* (1) Wherever possible, the injured limb should be elevated. In the case of the hand and forearm in a patient who has been admitted, the limb may be secured in stockingette (or in a roller towel using safety pins) attached to a drip stand at the side of the bed. Elevation should be maintained at least until swelling is beginning to resolve.

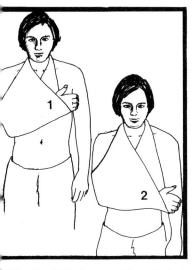

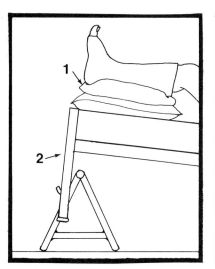

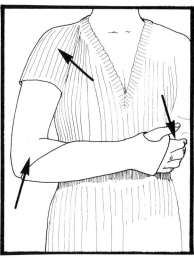

3. *Elevation* (2) In the case of the ambulant patient a sling may be used, provided the arm is kept high enough (1). If the sling is too slack the arm will hang down, encouraging oedema (2).

44. *Elevation* (3) In the case of the lower limb, the leg may be elevated on pillows (1). The end of the bed may be raised on an A-frame or on chairs (2). The ambulant patient should be advised to keep the foot as high as possible on a couch or chair whenever he is at rest.

45. *Exercise:* Those parts free of plaster should be exercised as frequently as possible: for example, the fingers in a Colles fracture (and later the elbow and shoulder). The patient should be shown how she should curl the fingers into full flexion and then fully extend them. She should be given clear instructions as to how frequently she should perform these exercises (e.g. for 5 minutes every waking hour).

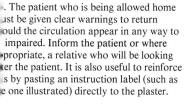

Instructions for Patients in Plaster of Paris Splints

A. (1) If fingers or toes become swollen blue, painful or stiff, raise limb.

(2) If no improvement in half an hour call in Doctor or return to hospital immediately.

B. (1) Exercise all joints not included in plaster—especially fingers and toes

(2) If you have been fitted with a walking plaster walk in it.

(3) If plaster becomes loose or cracked—report to hospital as soon as possible.

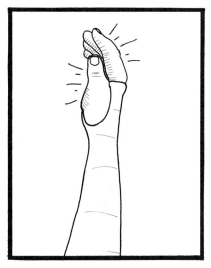

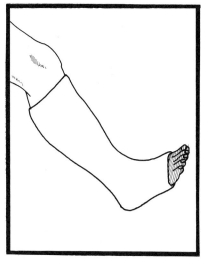

. The patient who is being allowed home must be given clear warnings to return should the circulation appear in any way to be impaired. Inform the patient or where appropriate, a relative who will be looking after the patient. It is also useful to reinforce these by pasting an instruction label (such as the one illustrated) directly to the plaster.

47. *After care of patients in plaster:* Note the following: (i) *Is there swelling?* Swelling of the fingers or toes is common in patients being treated in plaster, but the patient must be examined carefully for other signs which might suggest that circulatory impairment is the cause, rather than the local response to trauma. If there is no evidence of circulatory impairment, the limb should be elevated and movements encouraged.

48. (ii) *Is there discolouration of the toes or fingers?* Compare one side with the other; bluish discolouration, especially in conjunction with oedematous swelling distally, suggests that swelling of the limb within the plaster has reached such a level as to impair the venous return, and appropriate action must be taken.

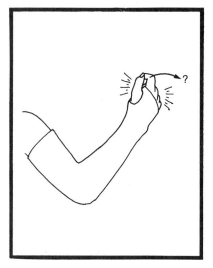

49. (iii) *Is there any evidence of arterial obstruction?* Note the 5 Ps: Intense PAIN, PARALYSIS of finger or toe flexors, PARAESTHESIAE in fingers or toes, PALLOR of the skin with disturbed capillary return, and 'PERISHING COLD' feel of the fingers and toes. Arterial obstruction requires *immediate*, positive action.

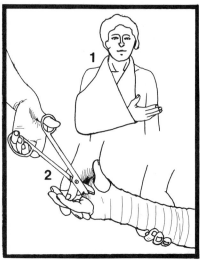

50. *Treatment of suspected circulatory impairment* (1) (a) Elevate the limb (1). (b) In the case of a plaster slab, cut through the encircling bandages and underlying wool (2) until the *skin is fully exposed*, and ease back the edges of the plaster shell until it is apparent that it is not constricting the limb in any way.

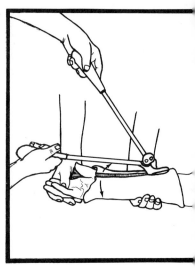

51. *Treatment* (2) Where the plaster is a complete one, split the plaster throughout it entire length. *Ease* back the edges of the ca to free the limb on each side of the mid-line *Divide* all the overlying wool and stockingette, and turn it back till skin is exposed. The same applies to any dressing swabs hardened with blood clot.

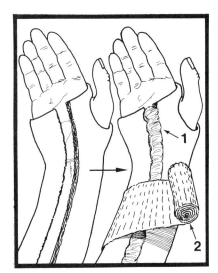

52. *Treatment* (3) If the circulation has been restored, gently pack wool between the cut edges of the plaster (1), and firmly apply an encircling crepe bandage (2). If this is not done, there is risk of extensive skin ('plaster') blistering locally. If the circulation is not restored, re-appraise the position of the fracture and suspect major vessel involvement. *On no account adopt an expectant and procrastinating policy.*

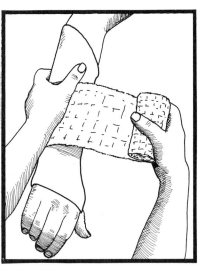

53. (iv) *Can the plaster be completed?* If the plaster consists of a back-slab or shell, completion depends on your assessment of the present swelling, and your prediction of any further swelling. Most plasters may be completed after 48 hours; but if swelling is very marked, completion should be delayed for a further 2 days, or until it is showing signs of subsiding.

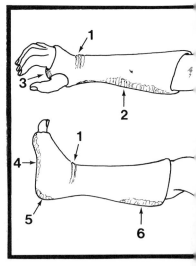

54. *Is the plaster intact?* Look for evidence of cracking, especially in the region of the joints (1). In arm plasters, look for anterior softening (2) and softening in the palm (3). In the leg, look for softening of the sole piece (4), the heel (5) and calf (6). Any weak areas should be reinforced by the application of more plaster locally.

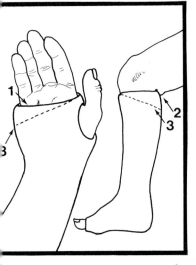

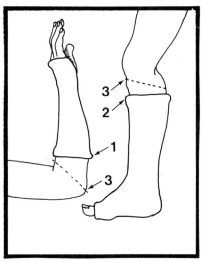

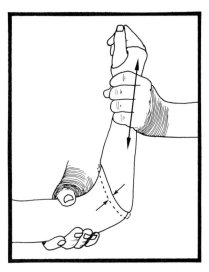

. (vi) *Is the plaster causing restriction of ovement?* Look especially for croachment of the palm piece on the ulnar de of the hand, restricting M.P. joint xion (1). In forearm plasters, look also for striction of elbow movements. In below nee plasters, note if the plaster is digging in hen the knee is flexed (2). Trim the plaster appropriate (3).

56. (vii) *Is the plaster too short?* Note especially the Colles-type plaster with inadequate grip of the forearm (1); note the below-knee plaster which does not reach the tibial tuberosity (2) and which apart from affording unsatisfactory support of an ankle fracture, will inevitably cause friction against the shin. Extend the defective plasters where appropriate (3).

57. (viii) *Has the plaster become too loose?* A plaster may become loose as a result of the subsidence of limb swelling and from muscle wasting. If a plaster is slack, then the support afforded to the underlying fracture may become inadequate. Assess looseness by attempting to move the plaster proximally and distally, while noting its excursion in each direction.

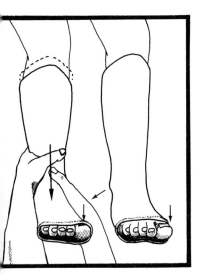

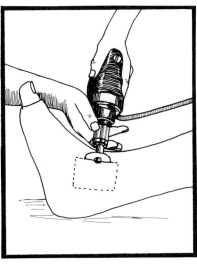

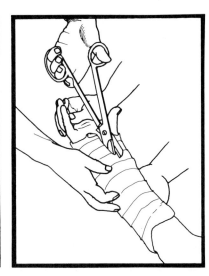

. *Has the plaster become too loose? ctd.:* the leg, grasp the plaster and pull it stally: note how far the toes disappear into e plaster. If a plaster is loose, it should be nanged unless (a) union is nearing mpletion, and risks of slipping are inimal, or (b) a good position is held, and e risks of slipping while the plaster is being nanged are thought to be greater than the sks of slipping in a loose plaster.

59. (ix) *Is the patient complaining of localised pain?* Localised pain, especially over a bony prominence, may indicate inadequate local padding, local pressure and pressure sore formation. In a child it may sometimes suggest a foreign body pushed in under the plaster. In all cases, the affected area should be inspected by cutting a window in the plaster and replacing it after examination.

60. *How to remove a plaster: Plaster slabs:* Plaster shells or slabs are easily removed by cutting the encircling open weave bandages which hold them in position. Care must be taken to avoid nicking the skin, and Bohler scissors are helpful in this respect.

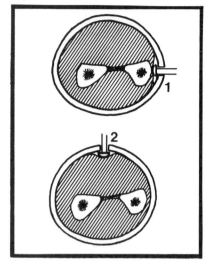

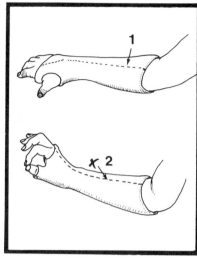

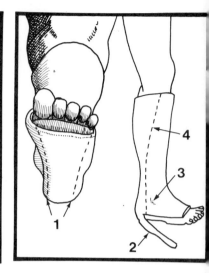

61. *Removing complete plasters: Using shears* (1) The heel of the shears must lie between the plaster and the limb. Subcutaneous bony prominences such as the shaft of the ulna (1) should be avoided to lessen the risks of skin damage and pain. Instead, the route of the shears should be planned to lie over compressible soft tissue masses (2).

62. *Using shears* (2) If possible, avoid cutting over a concavity. If the wrist is in moderate palmar flexion as in a Colles plaster, the plaster should be removed by a dorsal cut (1). In a scaphoid plaster, the dorsal route should be avoided (2) and the plaster removed anteriorly.

63. *Using shears* (3) Where there is the right angled bend of the ankle to negotiate, it is often helpful to make two vertical cuts down through the sole piece (1) and turn it down (2). This then gives access for the shears to make a vertical cut behind the lateral malleolus (3) and then skirt forwards over the peronei (4). The remaining plaster may then be sprung open.

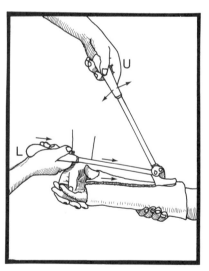

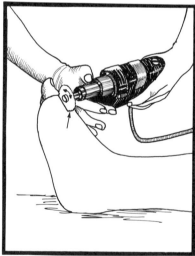

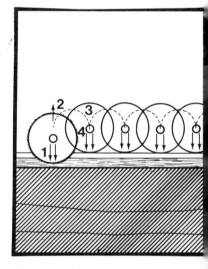

64. *Using shears* (4) Keep the lower handle (L) parallel to the plaster, or even a little depressed. Lift up the upper handle (U); push the shears forward with the lower handle so that the plaster fills the throat of the shears. Maintaining a slight pushing force, all the cutting action may be performed with the upper handle, moving it up and down like a beer pump.

65. *Using a plaster saw* (1) Plaster saws may be used for removing or cutting windows in plasters: but they should be used with caution and treated with respect. Do not use a plaster saw unless there is a layer of wool between the plaster and the skin. Do not use it over bony prominences: and do not use if the blade is bent, broken or blunt. Note: the blade does not rotate but oscillates.

66. *Using a plaster saw* (2) Electric saws are noisy, and the apprehensive patient should be reassured. Cut down through the plaster at one level (1): the note will change as soon as it is through; remove the saw (2) and shift it laterally about an inch (2.5 cm) (3) and repeat (4). *Do not* slide the saw laterally in shallow cuts; the cutting movement should be up and down.

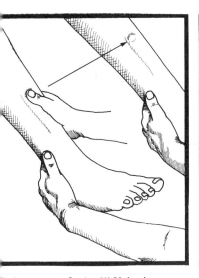

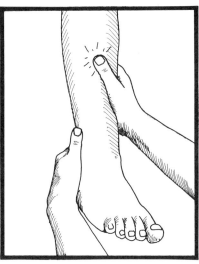

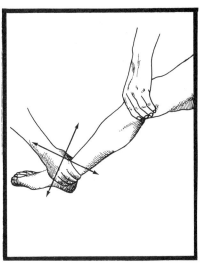

7. *Assessment of union* (1) Union in a
acture cannot be expected until a certain
mount of time has elapsed, and it is
ointless to start looking too soon. (See
dividual fractures for guidelines.) When it
reasonable to assess union, the limb
ould be examined out of plaster. Persistent
dema at the fracture site suggests union is
complete.

68. *Assessment of union* (2) Examine the
limb carefully for tenderness. Persistent
tenderness localised to the fracture site is
again suggestive of incomplete union.

69. *Assessment of union* (3) Persistent
mobility at the fracture site is certain
evidence of incomplete union. Support the
limb close to the fracture with one hand, and
with the other attempt to move the distal
part in both the anterior and lateral planes.
In a uniting fracture this is not a painful
procedure.

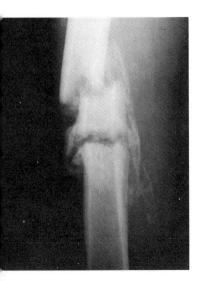

70. *Assessment of union* (4) Although clinical assessment is often adequate in many fractures
of cancellous bone, it is advisable in the case of the shafts of the femur, tibia, humerus, radius
and ulna to have up-to-date radiographs of the region. The illustration is of a double fracture
of the femur at 14 weeks. In the proximal fracture, the fracture line is blurred and there is
external bridging callus of good quality: union here is fairly far advanced. In the distal
fracture, the fracture line is still clearly visible, and bridging callus is patchy. Union is
incomplete, and certainly not sufficient to allow unprotected weight bearing.

In assessing radiographs for union, be suspicious of unevenly distributed bridging callus, of
a persistent gap, and of sclerosis or broadening of the bone ends. Note that where a
particularly rigid system of internal fixation has been employed, bridging callus may be
minimal or absent, and endosteal callus may be very slow to appear.

If in doubt regarding the adequacy of union, continue with fixation and re-examine in 4
weeks.

Note that in all cases you must assess whether the forces the limb is exposed to will result
in displacement or angulation of the fracture, or cause such mobility that union will be
prevented: you must balance the following equation:

external forces $<$ degree of union + support supplied by any internal fixation device and/or
external splintage.

4. Compound fractures: internal fixation

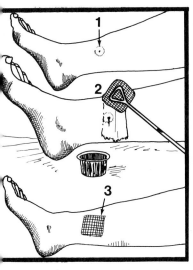

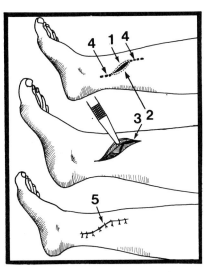

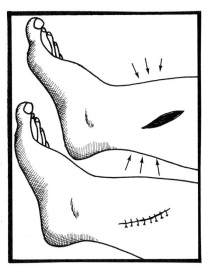

Compound fractures: The skin requires careful assessment in any compound injury. Various grades of damage may be recognised:
Grade 1: The fracture is technically compound only (1). The risks of infection are unlikely to be lessened by wide exposure—indeed there is greater risk of introducing infection. Thorough local cleaning (2) and the application of a sterile dressing (3) is all that is required unless the underlying fracture dictates otherwise.

2. *Grade 2:* The overlying wound has clean or minimally bruised, viable edges; and there is no gross swelling of the limb (1). The skin edges may be minimally excised (2). The deeper aspects of the wound should be inspected and cleaned (3); this usually involves extension of the wound (4). Primary closure may then be carried out (5).

3. *Grade 2 ctd.:* The overlying wound has clean or has minimally bruised edges, but there is marked swelling of the limb: if excision of the skin edges will lead to difficulty in closure, and they are macroscopically clean and viable, the wound should be sutured without carrying out preliminary excision.

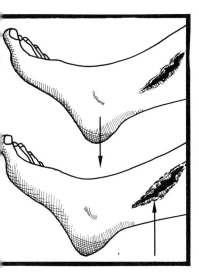

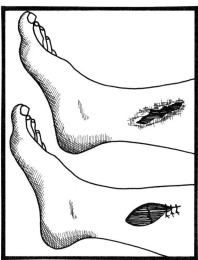

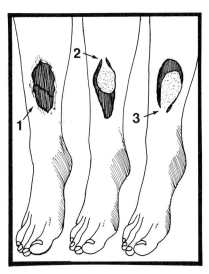

Grade 3: The skin edges are ingrained with dirt or very ragged and potentially necrotic. Swelling of the limb is not marked. The skin edges should be excised back to viable tissue, and closure by direct suture without undue tension aimed for. Do not excise widely or this will not be possible.

5. *Grade 4:* The skin edges are damaged over a wide area and a good deal of skin must be removed before viable tissue is reached—and/or there is marked swelling of the limb so that direct closure of the wound is not possible unaided.

6. *Grade 5:* There is a substantial area of skin damage, either by actual loss or crushing (1) or by the production of non-viable skin flaps, either with very narrow (2) or distally based (3) pedicles.

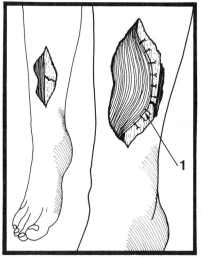

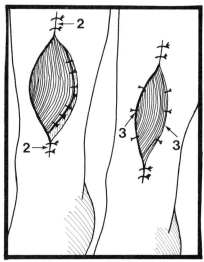

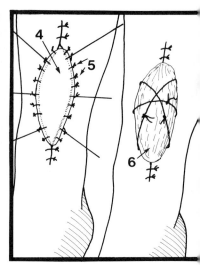

7. *Treatment* (a) In Grade 4 and 5 injuries, every effort should be made (other things being equal) to obtain bone cover, preferably in two layers. In many situations it is possible to draw related muscle across the fracture, and anchor it with deeply placed absorbable sutures to periosteum or other neighbouring tissue (1).

8. *Treatment* (b) Close as much of the skin as possible without undue tension (2). The remaining skin edges may be anchored with absorbable sutures to prevent their retraction (3). If there has been a fair amount of contamination the rest of the wound may be lightly packed with vaseline gauze: there is then free drainage for any infection while at the same time favourable conditions are established for granulation and secondary split skin-grafting.

9. *Treatment* (c) Alternatively, if contamination has been slight, a primary split skin graft may be applied to the defect (4) secured with sutures (5) and maintained in contact with its bed with ties placed over flavine emulsion soaked wool (6). A considerable number of alternative plastic procedures are available, but the possibilities may be restricted by the site and stability of the fracture.

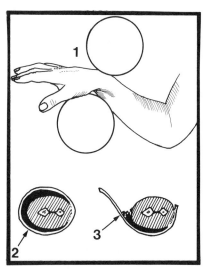

10. *Degloving injuries* (1) In a degloving injury, an extensive area of skin is torn from its underlying attachments and thereby deprived of its blood supply. In the hand or arm it is commonly caused by the limb being crushed between rollers (1); in the leg it may result from the shearing effect of a vehicle wheel passing over the limb in a run-over accident.

11. *Degloving injuries* (2) The skin may remain unbroken (2 in previous diagram), in which case the limb feels like a fluid-containing bag, due to the presence of an extensive haematoma between the skin and fascia. If the skin is torn (3), the effect is the creation of a large flap of full-thickness skin. In either case, massive sloughing is likely unless the injury is properly managed. A number of plastic surgical procedures are available. Probably the best method, if facilities are to hand, is the following: (a) The flap should be excised, first marking it (and the defect) so that it may be re-orientated later. (b) The flap is stored in a sterile container in a refrigerator (storage temperature is important). (c) The wound should be debrided, and the conditions optimised for the formation of a local bed of granulation tissue. (d) After 1–2 weeks the stored skin is replaced as a single sheet graft, after the deeper layers have been removed using special equipment.

In any compound injury, it is vital to keep in mind the risks of serious infection, particularly tetanus and gas gangrene. The appropriate protective measures should be taken; in addition, in many centres prophylactic broad spectrum antibiotics are used routinely, administration preferably commencing on admission of the patient and prior to surgery.

12. Principles of internal fixation and common fixation methods

When it is intended to implant materials for the treatment of fractures, the following criteria must be satisfied:

1. **Freedom from tissue reaction:** It is self-evident that if foreign material is being implanted in the tissues that it should be biologically inert, and not give rise to toxic reactions, local inflammatory changes, fibrosis, foreign-body giant cell reactions, etc., which in turn are likely to produce local pain, swelling, and impairment of function.

2. **Freedom from corrosion:** Implanted material should be free from corrosion. Where stainless steel is used it should have no impurities and be of such a type that corrosion does not spread if the surface skin is broken during handling or as a result of flexion after implantation. It is essential to avoid electrolytic degradation, and in practice this means that if more than one implant is used at the same site (e.g. a plate and screws) that identical materials are employed.

3. **Freedom from mechanical failure:** Implants must satisfy the purposes for which they are intended. To withstand the forces to which they will be subjected demands a satisfactory compromise between the materials used and the design of the implant. In the treatment of fractures, implants generally must have great mechanical strength in association with small physical bulk—which implies that they must be made of metal. Of the suitable metals, the most frequently employed are (1) certain stainless steels; (2) alloys of chromium, cobalt and molybdenum (e.g. Vitallium, Vinertia); (3) titanium. The chrome-cobalt alloys are biologically very inert, but are difficult to machine so that most inplants, including screws, are microcast, using the lost wax technique; this adds to their cost. The stainless steels are less inert, but are easier to machine and cheaper.

Fixation devices and systems: Fractures vary enormously in pattern: bones vary in their size, texture, and strength. To cope with even the most common situations and be a match for every subtle variation of circumstance requires an impressive range of devices and instruments for their insertion. The design of fixation devices has in the past been somewhat haphazard, and aimed at the treatment either of one fracture or the solution of a single fixation problem. There have been attempts to produce integrated systems of fracture fixation: sets of devices which can contend with any fracture situation. The most outstanding system, now firmly established, is that developed by the Association for the Study of Internal Fixation (ASIF or AO). Apart from the development of a series of screws, plates and other devices, and the corresponding instrumentation, the Association is responsible for some change in emphasis in the philosophy of fracture treatment. They feel that the common aim, a return to full function in the shortest time, can often best be achieved by the use of internal fixation devices, of such strength and design that external splintage can frequently be discarded permitting immediate joint freedom, early weight bearing, short-term hospitalisation, and early return to work and other activities. These ideals are often achieved, but some reluctance in universal acceptance of the AO system is due to fear of poor results from infection or a discrepancy between the complexities of the system and the technical abilities of the operator. It would be reasonable to accept that disappointments from fault technique will lessen with better training in the use of the equipment.

With any form of internal fixation great importance must always be placed on recognising which cases are best treated in this way. It is equally important to recognise which cases are not suited to treatment by internal fixation, and those which may be dealt with either surgically or conservatively.

It is in the last group that there is often some difficulty, and it is important to remember the hazards of infection; even although it may be uncommon, it must always be a feared complication which on occasion can turn a comparatively minor fracture into a disaster. As in many branches of surgery, the core problem is in deciding how many excellent results are required to balance the occasional serious failure, and the compromise to be made between the particulars of a case and the outlook and judgement of the surgeon.

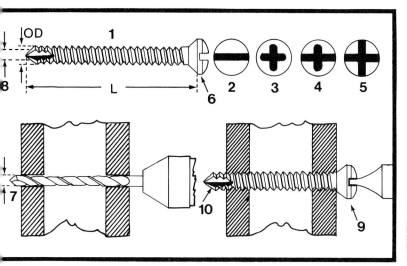

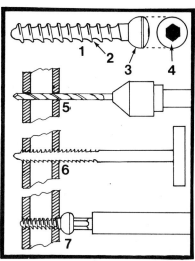

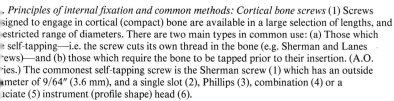

. *Principles of internal fixation and common methods: Cortical bone screws* (1) Screws
signed to engage in cortical (compact) bone are available in a large selection of lengths, and
estricted range of diameters. There are two main types in common use: (a) Those which
: self-tapping—i.e. the screw cuts its own thread in the bone (e.g. Sherman and Lanes
ews)—and (b) those which require the bone to be tapped prior to their insertion. (A.O.
ies.) The commonest self-tapping screw is the Sherman screw (1) which has an outside
meter of 9/64″ (3.6 mm), and a single slot (2), Phillips (3), combination (4) or a
iciate (5) instrument (profile shape) head (6).
sertion: A 7/64″ (2.8 mm) hole (7) (just marginally larger than the core diameter (8)) is
lled through the bone and is followed after depthing by the screw (9) whose fluted end (10)
ts its thread into the bone.

14. *Cortical bone screws* (2) The standard
A.O. cortical screw (1) has a buttress form
thread (2) of 1.75 mms pitch ($\bar{c}$ 15 T.P.I.)
and is 4.5 mms in diameter. The head has a
hemispherical underside (3) and a hex
socket (4) for its insertion. A 3.2 mm hole is
drilled in the bone to clear the core, and
this is then threaded with the corresponding
tap (6) before the screw is driven home (7).

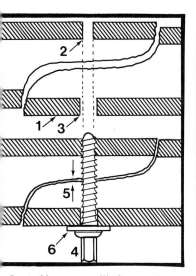

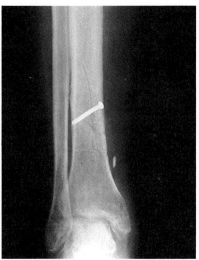

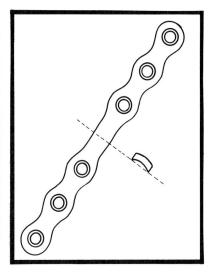

. *Cortical bone screws* (3) If a screw is
ng used to draw two bone fragments
ether, the threads should not have any
rchase on the near cortex (1). After the
ping hole (2) has been drilled (and tapped
ecessary), a clearance hole is made (3).
htening the screw (4) draws the
gments together (5). The screw head may
countersunk or fitted with a cup washer

16. *Cortical bone screws* (4) Screws used in
isolation can seldom serve as more than a
weak internal splint; some form of external
support is generally required to prevent the
screw breaking out: e.g. if an isolated screw
is used to stabilise a tibial fracture, plaster of
Paris will be required till union is well
advanced.

17. *Screws and plates* (1) Only occasionally
will the obliquity of a long bone fracture
permit stabilisation by screws alone;
generally a plate will be required to bridge
the fracture. The Sherman plate (ill.) is
lightweight and of slender construction. The
fixed position of the holes may in certain
circumstances prevent close apposition of
the bone ends (e.g. when there is bone
absorption at the fracture site).

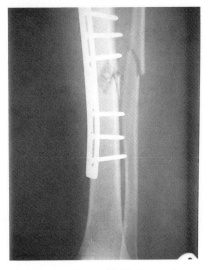

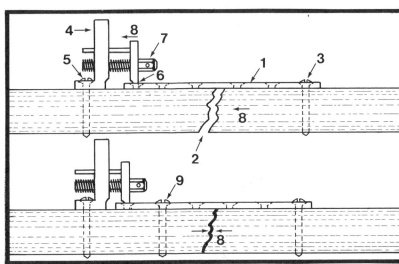

18. *Screws and plates* (2) The Eggar plate, which is slotted, is designed to overcome this problem: the screws are not fully tightened so that the bone ends have the opportunity to remain in close contact. Note how the plate has been bent to follow the contour of the bone, a necessity in treating most fractures. Both the Sherman and Eggar plates generally require additional (usually plaster) support.

19. *Screws and plates* (3) When rigid fixation is required (e.g. to let external splintage be discarded) the plate must be very strong and ideally the fracture surfaces should be compressed together so that even slight movement becomes impossible: e.g. (a) *Using a Mueller tensioning device:* The fracture is reduced and held in alignment. The plate (1) is applied across the fracture (2) and anchored to one fragment with a screw (3). The tensioning device (4) is temporarily fixed to the other fragment with a screw (5). A lug on the device engages the last hole of the plate (6). By turning the end of the screw (7) the two fragments are compressed (8). The position can then be maintained by inserting a screw on the clamp side (9). The other screws are inserted—the last after removal of the tensioner.

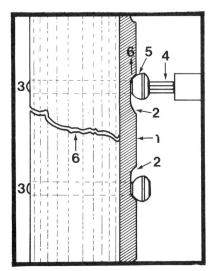

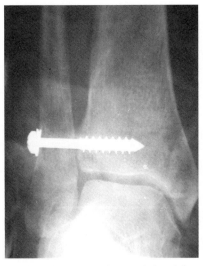

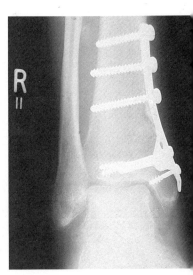

20. *Screws and plates* (4) (b) *Using a dynamic compression plate:* Compression may also be obtained by the use of an A.O. dynamic compression plate (1). This has slots (2) rather than plain round holes for the cortical screws (3) which are inserted eccentrically. When the screws are tightened (4) their heads (5) pinch the plate, causing the slight movement necessary to give fracture compression (6).

21. *Cancellous screws:* Screws designed to hold in cancellous (spongy) bone are generally in the shape of a coarse-pitch helix, of buttress or rectangular form. No preliminary tapping of bone is required. (Ill: tibio-fibular diastasis held with a cancellous screw in the spongy bone of the metaphysis. Note the washer supporting the head.)

22. *Screw and plate combinations:* In comminuted fractures it is sometimes necessary to use a combination of cancellous screws, cortical screws, and a plate to hold small fragments in line with one another and with the shaft of the bone. (Ill comminuted ankle fracture held in anatomical position with 3 cortical screws, 4 cancellous screws, and a T-shaped plate.

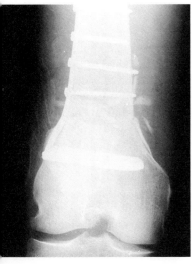

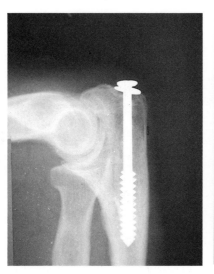

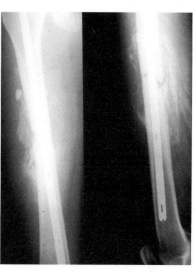

3. *Nail or blade-plates:* When a fracture as occurred close to the end of a long bone, he fragment carrying the articular surfaces nay sometimes be held best by a blade or ail passing through its cancellous mass. This is then held in alignment with the shaft sing a plate and screws. (Ill: supracondylar racture of the femur held with one-piece ail-plate. For many examples of hip nails nd nail plates, see Pelvis 85, 86.)

24. *Intra-medullary fixation* (1) The medullary cavity of a long bone may be used for fixation devices. At the elbow, a fracture of the olecranon may be held using a large diameter cancellous screw passed through the olecranon fragment into the medullary cavity of the ulnar shaft.

25. *Intra-medullary fixation* (2) Intramedullary nails are designed to lie within the medullary cavity and bridge the fracture. The commonest device is the Kuntscher nail for femoral shaft fractures. (Ill: note fracture callus.) To prevent axial rotation, the medullary canal may be reamed to allow the insertion of a close fitting nail. (See Femur 45–48.) Intramedullary nails have been developed for the other long bones. For other devices see Index and regions.

Internal fixation in compound injuries

The use of internal fixation devices in compound fractures is a controversial subject, but cases which pose real difficulty for the uncommitted are in practice rather uncommon. The following points should be noted:

1. In children, internal fixation seldom needs to be considered; in most fractures, if angulation and axial rotation are controlled, the remarkable powers of re-modelling can usually be relied upon, and an anatomical reduction is only occasionally required. It is useful to remember, as in the adult, that if the compounding is more than technical, that the opportunity should always be taken to inspect the fracture through the wound, and to reduce it under vision; a stable reduction is often attainable.

2. In the adult, where a fracture is undisplaced, conservative methods of treatment can generally be followed without difficulty; once skin healing has occurred, any secondary procedure can be carried out with comparative security.

3. Where a fracture is unstable, and is compound from within out with minimal contamination of the tissues (Grades 1 and 2) internal fixation may be carried out in reasonable safety once the wound has been adequately dealt with.

4. Where there has been extensive skin and soft tissue damage or loss, and the wound is badly contaminated, internal fixation should be avoided; the fracture should be supported by (i) plaster fixation alone, or if very unstable, with (ii) Steinman pins incorporated in the plaster or (iii) by an external skeletal fixation system.

Difficulty tends to occur in the handling of the unstable fracture where skin cover is perhaps poor and/or the risks of infection are appreciable but not certain. *Against* the use of internal fixation in these circumstances is (i) the risk of wider dissemination of infection into uncontaminated tissue by the greater exposure required for the insertion of an internal fixation device, (ii) the greater risks of wound break-down, and (iii) the greater difficulty in obtaining healing if infection becomes established, because of the presence of the fixation device acting as a foreign body. *In favour* of internal fixation are the following: (i) the chance of obtaining a good reduction, (ii) the possibility of holding that reduction for as long as required, and (iii) the better prospects of securing bone union. The eventual decision rests on the particular circumstances of the case, and the surgeon's individual assessment of the factors discussed.

5. Factors affecting healing; complications; pathological fractures

1. Factors affecting the rate of healing of a fracture

(1) Type of bone: *(a) Cancellous bone (spongy bone):* Healing in cancellous bone is generally well advanced 6 weeks from the time of the injury, and protection of the fracture can almost invariably be abandoned by that time. This applies to fractures of bones which are composed principally of cancellous tissue, and also to fractures involving the cancellous bone to be found at the ends of long bones. This rule is illustrated in the following examples:

(i) Weight bearing after a fracture of the calcaneus may be permitted after about 6 weeks.

(ii) A patient with a traumatic wedge fracture of a vertebral body may be allowed up after 6 weeks.

(iii) Plaster fixation may be discarded after 5–6 weeks following a Colles fracture.

(iv) Weight may be allowed through the leg 6 weeks after a fracture of the tibial table.

(v) Bed rest for 6 weeks is usually advised for any substantial fracture of the pelvis, etc.

(b) Cortical bone (Compact bone): Endosteal callus may take many months to become reasonably well established, and many uncomplicated long bone fractures may take 9–18 weeks to unite. In some cases, however, abundant external bridging callus may allow an earlier return of function. For example, (i) The average time to union of a fracture of the tibial shaft treated conservatively is 16 weeks. (ii) Fractures of the humeral shaft can often be left unsupported after 10 weeks. (iii) On the other hand, fractures of the metatarsals, metacarpals and phalanges, where external bridging callus is usually substantial, are usually quite firm in 4–5 weeks.

(2) The patient's age: In children, union of fractures is rapid. The speed of union decreases as age increases, until skeletal maturity is reached. There is then not a great deal of difference in the rate between young adults and the elderly. For example, in a child, union may be expected in a fractured femur a little after the number of weeks equivalent to its numerical age have passed: viz., a fractured femur in a child of 3 is usually united after 4 weeks: a fractured femur in a child of 8 is usually sound after 9 weeks. In contrast, a fracture of the femoral shaft in an adult may take 3–6 months to unite.

Apart from great rapidity of union it should be noted that children have remarkable powers of remodelling fractures. These powers are excellent as far as displacement is concerned, and are often good for slight to moderate angulation. Remodelling is poor in the case of axial rotation. The power to remodel decreases rapidly once adolescence is reached and epiphyseal fusion is imminent.

(3) Mobility at the fracture site: Excessive mobility persisting at the fracture site (due, for example, to poor fixation) may interfere with vascularisation of the fracture haematoma; it may lead to disruption of early bridging callus and may prevent endosteal new bone growth. One of the main aims of all forms of internal and external splintage is to reduce mobility at the fracture site, and hence encourage union. If splintage is inadequate, union may be delayed or prevented.

(4) Separation of the bone ends: Union will be delayed or prevented if the bone ends are separated, for this interferes with the normal mechanisms of healing. Separation may occur under several circumstances:

(a) Interposition of soft tissue between the bone ends: For example, in fractures of the femoral shaft, one of the bone ends may become isolated from the other by herniating through some of the surrounding muscle mass, thereby delaying or preventing union. Fractures of the medial malleolus may fail to unite due to infolding of a layer of periosteum between the fragments.

(b) Excessive traction: Excessive traction employed in the maintenance of a reduction may lead to separation of the bone ends and non-union. This may occur, for example, in femoral shaft fractures, particularly those treated by skeletal traction.

(c) Following internal fixation: In some situations where internal fixation is used to hold a fracture, resorption of bone may occur at the fracture site; the fixation device may continue to hold the bone fragments in such a way that they are prevented from coming together.

(5) Infection: Infection in the region of a fracture may delay or prevent union. This is especially the case if, in addition, movement is allowed to occur at the fracture. Infection of the fracture site is extremely rare in conservatively treated simple fractures: infection, if it occurs, follows either a compound injury or one treated by internal fixation. Where infection becomes well established in the presence of an internal fixation device, it is seldom possible to achieve healing without removal of the device which acts as a foreign body and a nidus for persisting infection. This is especially the case if there is breakdown of the overlying skin and the establishment of a sinus. If the internal fixation device is removed, it may not be possible to maintain adequate fixation of the fracture by external support, and the ensuing movement is almost invariably followed by non-union. Not infrequently the situation arises where the fracture is unlikely to unite if the fixation device is removed, and where infection is likely to remain if it is not. In these circumstances, it is usually wiser to retain the fixation device until union is reasonably well advanced; only then should its removal be undertaken, when healing may be achieved.

(6) Disturbance of blood supply: It is obvious that for the normal multiplication of bone cells and their precursors an adequate blood supply is required. Where the blood supply to an area is reduced, or where there is interference with the blood supply to both major fragments—e.g. in radio-necrosis of bone healing may be interfered with. On the other hand, reduction of the blood supply to one fragment, especially if cancellous bone is involved, may not interfere with union; indeed, in some situations it may apparently stimulate it. The most striking examples of this are fractures of the femoral neck and scaphoid, where the phenomenon of avascular necrosis is most frequently discovered in soundly united fractures. Interference with the blood supply to one fragment at the time of injury leads to immediate bone death: this is frequently followed by sound union of the fracture. Collapse of necrotic bone beyond the level of union is observed at a later date.

(7) **Properties of the bone involved:** Fracture healing is also affected by a number of imperfectly understood factors which lead to variations in the speed of union. The clavicle is a spectacular example: non-union is extremely rare, the time to clinical union is unexcelled by any other part of the skeleton, yet movement at the fracture site cannot be controlled with any efficiency. Union of the tibia is often slow to a degree that is difficult to explain even when the influence of its nutrient artery and fracture mobility are taken into account.

(8) **Joint involvement:** When a fracture involves a joint, union is occasionally delayed. This may be due to dilution of the fracture haematoma by synovial fluid.

(9) **Bone pathology:** Many of the commonest causes of pathological fracture do not seem to delay union in a material way. (Union may progress quite normally in, for example, osteoporosis, osteomalacia, Paget's disease and most simple bone tumours.) Some primary and secondary malignant bone tumours may delay or prevent union. (See pp. 72–3.)

2. The complications of fractures

Complications which may occur in a patient who has suffered a fracture or dislocation may be grouped in the following way:

(1) **The complications of any tissue damage:** These include (a) internal and external haemorrhage, oligaemic shock, etc. (b) infection (in compound injuries) (c) electrolyte shifts, protein breakdown and other metabolic responses of trauma.

(2) **The complications of prolonged recumbency:** These include (a) hypostatic pneumonia (b) pressure sores (c) deep venous thrombosis (d) muscle wasting (e) skeletal decalcification and formation of urinary tract calculi (f) urinary tract infections, etc.

(3) **The complications of anaesthesia and surgery:** These include (a) atelectasis and pneumonia (b) blood loss leading to anaemia or shock with their secondary effects (c) wound infection, mechanical failure of internal fixation devices, etc.

(4) **The complications peculiar to fractures:** These include (a) disorders involving the rate and quality of union (b) joint stiffness (c) Sudeck's atrophy (d) avascular necrosis (e) myositis ossificans (f) infections (g) neurological, vascular and visceral complications.

The last group will be considered in more detail.

(1) **Slow union:** In slow union, the fracture takes longer than usual to unite, but passes through the stages of healing without any departure from

normal clinically or radiologically.

(2) Delayed union: In delayed union, union fails to occur within the expected time. As distinct from slow union, radiographs of the part may show abnormal bone changes. Typically there is absorption of bone at the level of the fracture, with the production of a gap between the bone ends. External bridging callus may be restricted to a localised area and be of poor quality. There is, however, no sclerosis of the bone ends.

(3) Non-union: In non-union, the fracture has failed to unite, and there are radiological changes which indicate that this situation will be permanent—i.e. the fracture will never unite—unless there is some fundamental alteration in the line of treatment. Two types of non-union are recognised:

(a) In hypertrophic non-union the bone ends appear sclerotic, and are flared out so that the diameter of the bone fragments at the level of the fracture is increased ('elephant's foot' appearance). The fracture line is clearly visible, the gap being filled with cartilage and fibrous tissue cells. The increase in bone density is somewhat misleading, and conceals the fact that the blood supply is good.

(b) In atrophic non-union there is no evidence of cellular activity at the level of the fracture. The bone ends are narrow, rounded, and osteoporotic; they are frequently avascular.

Treatment: *(a) Slow union:* Assuming that the fracture is adequately supported, patience should ultimately be rewarded with sound bony union.

(b) Delayed union: The difficult problem in this field is to differentiate between delayed union which is going to proceed with proper encouragement to union, and delayed union which is going to go on to non-union. The only sure arbiter is time, but the disadvantage of delay is that it tends to encourage irreversible stiffness in those joints which are immobilised with the fracture (besides frequently creating problems from prolonged hospitalisation and absence from work).

If union has not occurred within the time normally required (or certainly if the fracture is un-united by 4 months) or if gross mobility is still present at 2 months, there should be a careful appraisal of the radiographs and the methods of fixation. As the commonest cause of delayed union is inadequate fixation, particular attention should be paid to this aspect of the case. If the radiographs show the changes of slow or delayed union, but none of the changes of non-union, and the fracture is well supported, immobilisation should be continued and the situation re-assessed, with further radiographs in 4—6 weeks. Improvement in the radiological appearance will then be an encouraging sign, suggesting that persistence in the established line of treatment will lead to union. If there is no change, or if there is deterioration this is an indication for more active treatment (e.g. rigid internal fixation).

(c) Hypertrophic non-union: If the fracture can be fixed with absolute rigidity by mechanical means (which substitute for the primary bridging callus which is wanting) the cartilaginous and fibrous tissue between the bone ends will mineralise and be converted to bone (by induction). In the femur, this may be accomplished by careful reaming of the medullary canal and the introduction of a stout, large-diameter intramedullary nail. The bone ends are not disturbed. In the tibia and the other long bones, rigid fixation

may usually be obtained by compression plating.

There is some evidence that the process of induction which results in the conversion of the tissue at the fracture into bone may also be stimulated by the creation of small electric currents in the gap between the bone ends. This may be achieved by embedding per-cutaneous electrodes in the fracture gap, or by placing field coils round the limb. Treatment by this method is lengthy (extending over several months) but can often be administered on an out-patient basis and is particularly indicated where it is desirable to avoid surgery (e.g. in the presence of continued infection).

(d) Atrophic non-union: Treatment for atrophic non-union is less easy or reliable, and involves 4 important aspects:

(i) The fracture must be held rigidly; this usually implies internal fixation (e.g. the use of a large diameter intramedullary nail or a rigid compression plate).

(ii) Fibrous tissue should be removed from between the bone ends which should be 'freshened' by a limited local trimming with an osteotome.

(iii) The bone ends should be de-corticated from the level of the fracture back to healthy bone; fine interrupted cuts are made in the outer surface of the bone cortex until it has a feathered or shingled appearance.

(iv) The area round the fracture is packed circumferentially with cancellous bone grafts.

(4) Mal-union: In theory the term mal-union could be applied to any fracture which has united in less than anatomical position. In practice, it is used in the following circumstances:

(a) Where a fracture has united in a position of persistent angulation or rotation which is of a degree that gives the limb a displeasing appearance or affects its function.

For example, mal-union in a Colles fracture may lead to undue prominence of the distal ulna. The cosmetic effect may cause the patient some distress, although functionally the result may be good. Again, persistent angulation in a fracture of the femur may not be particularly conspicuous, but will lead to impairment of function in the limb as a result of shortening and the effects of abnormal stresses on the knee and hip (leading possibly ultimately to secondary osteo-arthritis in these joints).

(b) Where a fracture has united with a little persistent deformity in a situation where even the slightest displacement or angulation is a potential source of trouble. This applies particularly to fractures involving joints. For example, slight persistent deformity in a Potts fracture of the ankle may pre-dispose to early secondary osteo-arthritis.

Treatment: In treating fractures, one of the main objectives is adequate reduction and avoidance of mal-union. Regrettably, mal-union is sometimes a sign of poor management.

If detected before union has become complete, angulation may sometimes be corrected by wedging of a plaster (see Tibia 20) or forcible manipulation under anaesthesia—i.e. manipulation which re-fractures the limb through the early callus. If union is already complete, an osteotomy may be considered if the deformity is particularly severe.

(5) Shortening: This is generally a sequel of mal-union. It occurs in transverse fractures which are off-ended, and often in spiral or oblique fractures which are displaced. It also results from marked angulation of a fracture.

In children, bone growth is always accelerated in the injured limb, presumably as a result of the epiphyses being stimulated by the increased blood supply. Any discrepancy in limb length is usually quickly made up. For example, a fracture of the femoral shaft in a child may heal with the fragments overlapping and with perhaps 3—4 cm of shortening. After a year the leg lengths may be equal—or the injured leg may even be a little longer than the other.

In adults, shortening in the lower limb is seen most frequently after fractures of the tibial shaft. It is also seen after fractures of the shaft of the femur, and of the femoral neck where there is persistent coxa vara.

Shortening of 1.5 cm is easily tolerated, being compensated for by tilting of the pelvis. Shortening in excess of this should be dealt with by alteration of the footwear: for example, 3.5 cm of shortening may be corrected by a 2 cm raise to the affected heel, some of which can be given by a cork lift within the shoe. Where shortening is due to severe, persistent angulation of fracture, a corrective osteotomy may be indicated, not only to correct the shortening but to reduce abnormal stresses on the related joints.

In the upper limb, shortening seldom causes any problem other than to the patient's tailor. (Note, however, that shortening of either the radius or the ulna, while leading to little overall shortening, may cause severe disability at the wrist or elbow.)

(6) Traumatic epiphyseal arrest: The epiphyseal plate may be damaged a a result of trauma. If the whole width of the plate is affected, then growth may be arrested at that level, leading to progressive shortening of the limb. The final discrepancy in limb lengths is dependent on the epiphysis affected and the child's age at the time of injury: obviously the younger the child, the greater the potential growth and potential shortening.

More commonly the epiphyseal plate is incompletely affected, so that growth continues more or less normally at one side, while at the other it ma be severely retarded or arrested. This irregularity of growth leads to some shortening of the limb, and to distortion of the associated joint which can only be partly corrected by re-modelling. In practice there may be progressive tilting of the axis of movement of the joint. For example, a supracondylar fracture may be followed by a cubitus varus deformity as a result of a degree of mal-union. This deformity may become more severe as (uneven) growth continues. Traumatic epiphyseal arrest also occurs after compound injuries, where the delicate epiphyseal plate is damaged, especially by friction. This is seen in road traffic accidents when a child is dragged along by a vehicle, sustaining skin loss and progressive abrasion of the deeper tissues by friction against the road surface.

In all cases of suspected epiphyseal damage a careful follow-up is necessary. The child should be seen every 6—12 months, and any residual deformity carefully assessed by clinical and radiological measurement. In the upper limb, if the deformity is progressive, it may produce an unsightly appearance and may be responsible for delayed neurological involvement. In the lower limb, abnormal stresses may be produced in the weight bearing joints giving rise to pain, stiffness, instability and often a rapidly progressive secondary osteo-arthritis. In these circumstances, a corrective osteotomy may be indicated.

(7) Joint stiffness: This is a common complication. It must be borne in mind at every stage of fracture treatment in order that its effects may be minimised. Stiffness may result from a combination of factors which include pathology (a) within the joint (b) close to the joint (c) remote from the joint.

Intra-articular causes of stiffness: (a) Intra-articular adhesions: Fibrous adhesions may form within a joint as a result of (i) organisation of a haemarthrosis or fracture haematoma, produced, for example, when a fracture runs into a joint (ii) damage to the articulating (cartilaginous) surfaces with subsequent organisation within the joint (iii) prolonged immobilisation leading to degenerative changes in articular cartilage.

(b) Mechanical restrictions: (i) The fracture may disrupt the joint to such an extent that there is mechanical restriction of movement—for example, bony fragments may block part of the range of movements in a joint. (ii) Movements may be restricted by the formation of loose bodies.

(c) Osteo-arthritis (osteo-arthrosis): Joint movements may be restricted as a result of (secondary) osteo-arthritis. This may be caused by (i) irregularity of the joint surfaces (caused, for example, by trauma to the articular cartilage or by displacement of a fracture which runs into a joint) (ii) avascular necrosis (produced as a result of damage to the blood supply of an intra-articular fragment of bone) (iii) mal-union of a fracture (leading to abnormal stresses on the joint from persistent angulation).

Peri-articular causes of stiffness: (a) Joint capsules and musculo-tendinous cuffs may become functionally impaired, leading to joint stiffness. There are many causes which include (i) fibrosis resulting from direct injury, passive stretching, or disuse (ii) oedema, often encouraged by dependency, disuse, or Sudeck's atrophy.

(b) Persistent displacement of a fracture lying close to a joint may lead to a mechanical block to movement.

(c) Persistent angulation of a fracture lying close to a joint may lead to loss of part of a range of movements (sometimes with a corresponding gain elsewhere). For example, persisting anterior angulation in a Colles fracture will result in loss of some palmar flexion. There is sometimes a corresponding gain in dorsiflexion.

(d) In a fracture lying close to a joint, movements may be restricted by adhesions forming between the fracture and overlying muscle or tendon. This leads to tethering of these structures with inevitable restriction of movements. As a general rule, the closer a fracture is to a joint, the greater the danger of movements being restricted in this way. Restriction of movements by tendon tethering is a particular problem in phalangeal fractures.

(e) Myositis ossificans, if present, will act as a mechanical block to movement.

Stiffness from causes remote from a joint: (a) Stiffness may result from tethering or entrapment of muscle by adhesions forming between a fracture and overlying muscle. This is commonly seen in fractures of the femoral shaft where the quadriceps muscle may become tethered to the bone; this effect may sometimes be aggravated by surgery, where exposure of the fracture requires further muscle division. This effect may be minimised by early mobilisation.

(b) Muscle ischaemia, followed by replacement fibrosis and contractures, may occur when there is a vascular injury accompanying the fracture. Deformity of the distal parts is common, and there may be restriction of passive as well as active movements. (For exmple, Volkmann's ischaemic contracture of the forearm or calf leading to restriction of movements in the hand and foot respectively.)

Avoidance of stiffness: Some of the basic principles in the avoidance of joint stiffness are as follows:

a. Accurate reduction of the fracture wherever possible.
b. Splintage of the minimal number of joints compatible with security.
c. Splintage of the fracture for the shortest time compatible with the relief of pain and fracture healing.
d. Urgent mobilisation of all unsplinted joints in the limb: for example, a patient with a Colles fracture should practise finger, elbow and shoulder movements from the day of injury.
e. Elevation of the injured part during the initial stages to decrease joint oedema.
f. Where applicable, supporting the joints in such a postion that restoration of movement on discarding splintage will be encouraged.
g. Where a fracture involves articular surfaces, early movement becomes particularly important if an adequate range is to be regained.
h. Where stiffness is present or anticipated, physiotherapy and where appropriate, occupational therapy should be started as early as possible.
i. Anticipate complications and avoid procrastination, especially with regard to non-union.
j. When internal fixation is being contemplated, there is some merit in selecting techniques and devices which will support the fracture to such an extent that the limb may be exercised without external support.

(8) Sudeck's atrophy: This fracture complication is seen most frequently after Colles fractures of the wrist. In most cases it is not recognised until removal of the plaster at the end of the normal 4–6 weeks' period of immobilisation. There is swelling of the hand and fingers, and the skin is warm, pink and glazed in appearance. There is striking restriction of movements in the fingers, and diffuse tenderness over the wrist and carpus. This tenderness may at first suggest that the fracture is un-united, but check radiographs will show that this is not the case. Typically the radiographs demonstrate union of the fracture, with diffuse, osteoporotic mottling of the carpus. Although seen most frequently after Colles fractures, Sudeck's atrophy may follow scaphoid fractures or indeed any injury about the wrist. The condition is also seen in the lower limb, the foot being similarly affected after, for example, a Potts fracture.

The cause of the condition is uncertain, but may be due to an atypical sympathetic response to trauma. It is self-limiting, the abnormalities of circulation and calcification usually resolving slowly over 4–12 months. Nevertheless, restriction of movements may be permanent; to minimise this, intensive physiotherapy is usually prescribed and continued to resolution. Analgesics may be required in the early stages.

(9) Avascular necrosis: Avascular necrosis is death of bone due to interference with its blood supply. It is an important and serious complication of certain fractures.

There is no doubt that in many comminuted fractures fragments of bone are often completely detached from their surrounding tissues and deprived of their blood supply. If the fragments are small, healing is usually uneventful. If the fragments are larger, healing may be delayed, but it is often difficult to attribute the relative effects of avascularity and the poorer immobilisation associated with comminution. It is not, however, with the shafts of long bones that this complication is most closely associated. Avascular necrosis is seen in the femoral head after some intracapsular fractures of the femoral neck or after dislocation of the hip. It is found in the scaphoid after certain fractures of the proximal half of that bone. It sometimes occurs in the talus after fractures or dislocations. In the lunate it may follow frank dislocations or apparently occur without any obvious previous trauma.

The importance of avascular necrosis is that the affected bone becomes soft and distorted in shape, leading to pain, stiffness, and secondary osteo-arthritis. The following points are of some importance:

(a) Interference with the blood supply to the bone is a direct result of the fracture: the fracture shears those blood vessels which are travelling within the bone towards its articular surface.

(b) As the fracture is responsible for the disruption of the blood supply, it follows that the disruption is attributable to the injury, and dates from the time of injury.

(c) Restoration of the microcirculation within the bone cannot be effected by treatment.

(d) The greater the displacement of the fracture, the greater the vessel disturbance and the greater the chance of this complication ensuing.

(e) When an injury has occurred at one of the high-risk sites, the chances are that any patent circulatory channels are highly vulnerable. Reduction should be carried out with minimal force and delay if there is to be any hope of avoiding this complication.

(f) Avascular necrosis is quite distinct from non-union. In the majority of femoral neck and scaphoid fractures with avascular necrosis, *the fracture has united.*

(g) Clear cut radiological evidence of this complication may be quite slow in appearing, especially in the case of the femoral head. Symptoms of pain and stiffness usually *precede* the radiological changes. In the case of femoral neck fractures it is common practice to look for avascular necrosis for up to three years after the injury.

Treatment: The natural course of avascular necrosis is for the slow revascularisation of necrotic bone from the periphery. This process takes 6–18 months, but in spite of it, secondary osteo-arthritic changes in the affected joints are inevitable. In the lower limb, deformity of the avascular bone may be minimised by the avoidance of weight bearing, and this is of some value at least in the case of the talus; otherwise treatment has little influence on the condition.

If symptoms are commanding and secondary osteo-arthritis is well established, surgery may be required (e.g. hip replacement in the case of femoral neck fractures—see under appropriate sections).

(10) Myositis ossificans: Myositis ossificans is a complication of trauma. In its commonest form, a calcified mass appears in the tissues near a joint, leading generally to considerable restriction of movements because of its mechanical effects.

The commonest site is the elbow. It may, for example, develop some weeks after a supracondylar fracture, especially where there has been difficulty in reduction and manipulation has been repeated. Myositis ossificans is also found in the elbow after dislocations, or fractures of the radial head. It is thought that these injuries result in haematoma formation in the brachialis muscle at the front of the joint, and that this is dealt with by the tissues in the same way as a fracture haematoma—that is by calcification and ossification.

The ensuing mass may be as large as a plum, and will greatly restrict flexion of the elbow. It is known that myositis ossificans can follow passive stretching of joints, and in the past it was frequently seen in cases where, in good faith, this treatment had been carried out to encourage movement after injury. The risks of this complication are so great, however, that passive stretching must never be practised round the elbow.

Myositis ossificans is also seen at other sites, especially the shoulder, hip and knee. It is found particularly frequently in patients suffering from head injuries or paraplegia. In some cases, especially where there is limb spasticity, routine passive joint movements may be a causal factor.

Treatment: Early excision of the mass gives bad results, being almost always followed by massive recurrence. Late excision (say after 6–12 months) is often successful in removing the mechanical obstruction to movement with less risk of recurrence.

(11) Osteitis: Infection in closed fractures (due to systemic spread of organisms) is rare and seldom diagnosed until infection is well established. is sometimes seen in patients suffering from rheumatoid arthritis who have been treated with anti-inflammatory preparations. Recurrent pyrexia, a raised sedimentation rate and white count, and unduly prolonged pain, local tenderness and swelling should arouse suspicion. Radiological changes may not be diagnostic and are slow in appearing.

Bone infection is a feared complication of open fractures, and is also seen on occasion after the internal fixation of closed fractures. The symptoms and signs are as detailed above. In addition, there will usually be a purulent wound discharge with staining of the plaster or dressings which become foul smelling.

Treatment: (a) The risk of this complication should always be kept in mind in the handling of compound injuries or when internal fixation is planned, so that the techniques practised may be above criticism.
(b) Once fairly established, bone infections are peculiarly resistant to treatment, and may become virtually incurable. Delay must therefore be avoided at all costs.
(c) If possible, a sample of pus should be obtained so that the bacteriology and antibiotic sensitivity may be firmly established. The appropriate antibiotic must then be administered in adequate dose for an adequate time.

(usually 4 weeks as a minimum). If a choice is available, preference should be given to an antibiotic which may achieve high concentration levels in bone. In patients being treated in plaster casts, access to the wound may be obtained by windowing of the plaster.

(d) Unless discovered early, drainage should be established, and regular dressings performed with aseptic precautions in an attempt to allow healing by granulation tissue.

(e) Although discharge from the wound may persist until any internal fixation device is removed, this should be delayed until fracture healing is well advanced.

(f) When infection is well established and unresponsive, more radical measures may be called for. These include:

(i) Saucerisation of the area, with radical excision of all infected bone and open packing of the wound.

(ii) Raising the local concentrate of antibiotics by the implantation of irrigation tubes, gentamycin beads or other devices.

(iii) Rarely, amputation may have to be considered where there is profound toxaemia with deterioration of the patient's general condition, uninfluenced by treatment or where there is widespread bone destruction or avascularity, poor control of the infection, and certain continued infection and non-union.

(12) Acute aterial arrest: The arterial blood flow distal to a fracture is occasionally interrupted, and assessment of the circulation in a fractured limb is an essential part of the examination. Arterial arrest results in loss of the distal pulses, pallor and coldness of the skin, loss of the capillary responses, severe pain in the limb, paraesthesiae and eventually muscle paralysis. The commonest cause is kinking of the main arterial trunks by the displacement of a fracture or dislocation. In these cases, the circulation is immediately restored by correction of the deformity, and this should always be carried out as expeditiously as possible. In closed fractures other arterial disturbances are found, but these are relatively uncommon. A ragged bone edge may cause arterial rupture, leading to the rapid formation of a large haematoma. A fracture may also give rise to profound arterial spasm, aneurysm, or intimal stripping. In compound injuries, arterial rupture often declares itself by the nature and extent of the accompanying haemorrhage.

Treatment: It is obvious that the survival of a useful limb is dependent on restoration of the circulation. Where this is not achieved by reduction of the fracture, exploration of the affected vessel is mandatory. Treatment is then dependent on the findings. If the artery is cleanly divided, an end-to-end anastomosis may be performed. In the presence of a deficit, an in-line reversed vein graft is often used. In either case, to prevent damage to the suture line, internal fixation of the fracture is an essential part of the procedure and is often performed first.

Most of those cases which appear to be due to arterial spasm are in fact associated with intimal damage. Opening of the vessel is necessary to elucidate this, although preliminary irrigation with papaverine is sometimes tried. If intimal damage is confirmed, resection of the affected segment with grafting may be required.

Arterial obstruction leading to muscle death and nerve palsy may also result from swelling within the muscle compartments of a limb. For example, in the anterior compartment of the leg, haemorrhage, or oedema muscles following trauma or overactivity, may lead to an inexorable rise of pressure beyond the systolic blood pressure. This will result in muscle necrosis, loss of conduction in the deep peroneal nerve, sensory disturbance in the foot and foot drop. Prompt splitting of the roof of the affected compartment may avert this complication.

(13) Immediate neurological disturbance: Neurological complications occurring immediately after fractures and dislocations are comparatively uncommon. Nevertheless, in certain situations a nerve may be stretched over a bone edge in a displaced fracture, or over a bone end in a dislocation. If prolonged this will lead to local ischaemia and interruption of nerve conduction. If stretching is more severe there may be rupture of axons or of neural tubes: actual nerve division is rare, being seen mainly in association with compound injuries (especially gunshot wounds). The commoner fractures and dislocations associated with nerve palsies include the following:

Dislocation of the shoulder	Axillary nerve palsy: rarely other brachial plexus lesions
Fracture of the shaft of the humerus	Radial nerve palsy
Dislocation of the elbow	Ulnar nerve palsy; sometimes median nerve affected
Fractures round the elbow	Median nerve palsy; less commonly, ulnar nerve, or posterior interosseous nerve
Dislocation of the hip	Sciatic nerve palsy
Dislocation of the knee or rupture of lateral ligament of the knee and fracture of medial tibial table	Common peroneal nerve palsy

Treatment: The majority of nerve lesions are in continuity. Assuming that the fracture or dislocation has been reduced, recovery often begins after 6 weeks, progressing quite rapidly thereafter. *The skin* must be protected during the recovery period against friction, burns and other trauma so long as sensation remains materially impaired. *The joints* should be exercised passively to avoid stiffness. *Deformity* due to over-activity of unaffected muscles should be prevented: this applies particularly to the drop wrist of radial palsy, and the drop foot where the sciatic or common peroneal nerve are involved. Lively splintage may be particularly helpful in these circumstances.

Where there is a nerve palsy accompanying a fracture which is going to be treated surgically, opportunity may be taken to inspect the affected nerve. This will often help in establishing a prognosis, and may also permit definitive treatment of the injury (for example, by removing any local pressure on the nerve).

When an expected recovery does not occur, electromyography and nerve conduction studies may be of occasional diagnostic value, but exploration often required.

In the case of nerve injury complicating a fresh injury, primary suture should be undertaken if the risks of infection are judged to be slight and facilities are good. Otherwise the nerve ends should be approximated with radio-opaque sutures or markers, and elective repair delayed until sound wound healing has been obtained. If nerve repair is not possible, reconstructive surgery or orthotic support of the paralysed part may be required.

(14) Delayed neurological disturbance: Sometimes a nerve palsy gradually develops long after a fracture has healed.

(a) Tardy ulnar nerve palsy is the most striking example of this process. In a typical case the patient gradually develops over a period of a few months an ulnar nerve palsy which may become complete. The injury responsible is usually a supracondylar fracture or a Monteggia fracture-dislocation. The striking feature is the interval between the fracture and the nerve palsy. It is usually in the order of several years, and indeed may be as much as 60.

In a number of these cases there is a cubitus valgus deformity, and the resultant stretching of the nerve is usually regarded as being responsible for the onset of the palsy. Nevertheless, tardy ulnar nerve palsy also occurs in the presence of cubitus varus, so that progressive ischaemia of the nerve has come to be considered as another possible factor.

Treatment: Tardy ulnar nerve palsy is usually treated by early transposition of the ulnar nerve. (The nerve is mobilised from its exposed position behind the medial epicondyle, brought round to the front of the elbow, and buried in the flexor muscles of the forearm just beyond their point of origin.)

(b) Median nerve palsy: Signs of median nerve compression may gradually develop a few months after a Colles fracture of the wrist. This is generally akin to the partial nerve lesions seen in the carpal tunnel syndrome. Some residual displacement of the fracture may reduce the space available in the carpal tunnel leading to pressure on the nerve and an incomplete palsy.

Treatment: Symptoms are usually relieved by carpal tunnel decompression (by dividing the flexor retinaculum).

(15) Delayed tendon rupture: This uncommon fracture complication is seen most frequently at the wrist where, after a Colles fracture, a patient loses the ability to extend the terminal joint of the thumb. This is due to rupture of the extensor pollicis longus tendon some weeks or months after the fracture. The rupture may result from the gradual fraying of the tendon as it rubs against the healing fracture; or it may be caused by traumatic or fibrotic interference with its arterial blood supply, resulting in local sloughing of the tendon.

Treatment: In the case of the thumb, the best results are obtained by transposition and suture of the tendon of extensor indicis to the distal segment of extensor pollicis longus. (But see Wrist and Hand 45.)

(16) Visceral complications: (i) Rupture of the urethra or bladder, and perforation of the rectal wall may complicate fractures of the pelvis.

(ii) Rupture of the spleen, kidney or liver may follow severe local trauma, abdominal compression or crushing (such as, for example, run-over injuries).

(iii) Rupture of the intestines or tearing of the mesenteric attachments may also follow abdominal compression.

(iv) *Paralytic ileus:* Paralytic ileus is occasionally seen following fracture of the pelvis and lumbar spine, the most likely cause being disturbance of the autonomic control of the bowel from retro-peritoneal haematoma. Distension of the abdomen, absent or faintly tympanitic bowel sounds and vomiting are the usual features. It is, of course, imperative to exclude the possibility of perforation, especially when there is a history of a run-over injury. The diagnosis may be made on the basis of the history and clinical findings, but plain radiographs of the abdomen, abdominal paracentesis, laparoscopy or laparotomy may be necessary where there is a history of direct injury.

Treatment: (a) Naso-gastric suction. (b) Intravenous fluids—the quantity and proportions being determined by the amount of aspirate and other losses, and serum electrolyte estimations. In the majority of cases, bowel sounds return within 36 hours, and intravenous fluids and suction may be discontinued shortly afterwards.

(v) *The cast syndrome:* Abdominal distension and vomiting sometimes occur in patients being treated in plaster jackets, hip spicas, or plaster beds, especially if the spine is hyperextended. When the onset is extremely rapid leading to shock and prostration, the superior mesenteric artery or cast syndrome may be suspected (i.e. there is a high intestinal obstruction due to duodenal compression by the superior mesenteric artery).

Treatment: (a) If a plaster jacket has been applied, it should be removed. A patient being nursed in a plaster bed should be transferred to an ordinary bed or a Stryker frame. (b) A large bore gastric tube should be passed. (c) Fluid replacement therapy may be required.

(17) Fat embolism: This complication is usually thought to be due to micro-particles of marrow fat escaping into the circulation from the region of the fracture. The pathology is by no means clear cut, and disturbance of lipid metabolism may account for certain features of the condition.

It occurs most frequently after fractures of the femoral shaft and pelvis. Excessive mobility at the fracture site may be a contributory factor. Commonly, there is an unexplained deterioration in the condition of a patient a few days after sustaining such an injury. There may be a slight pyrexia, petechial haemorrhages appear in the skin, the patient may become confused, aggressive or comatose, and there may be evidence of renal insufficiency. Radiographs of the chest often show mottling of the lung fields; these changes are generally considered to be due to fat embolisation of the lungs. The systemic effects on the brain, kidneys and skin are less easy to explain unless cardiac septal defects are more common than supposed.

Treatment: (i) Heparinisation of the patient may be followed by improvement. (ii) Routine supportive measures such as the administration of oxygen and the giving of intravenous fluids should be carried out.

(18) Osteo-arthritis: See under causes of joint stiffness.

3. Pathological fractures

A pathological fracture is one which has occurred in a bone which is abnormal or diseased.

In some cases the pathological process leads to progressive weakness of the bone so that fracture may occur spontaneously or after slight injury only. Fracture may occur as an inevitable event in some disease process—e.g. a fracture in the course of a destructive, chronic osteitis: always unwelcome, but causing no surprise. On the other hand, the disease process may be unknown to the patient and his practitioner, the trivial nature of the trauma giving concern to both.

Where bone strength is not materially impaired, the causal violence producing the fracture may not cause comment; in these circumstances the radiographs taken after the incident may give the first indication to anyone that something else is amiss. It follows that virtually any condition capable of being detected by radiographs of the skeleton may fall into this category—a limitless range of congenital, metabolic and neoplastic disease. Diagnosis as a result may be difficult, but fortunately there is one important point to take into consideration: where fracture is the presenting feature, the number of conditions commonly responsible is small. These include the following:

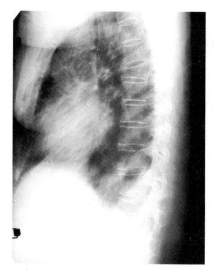

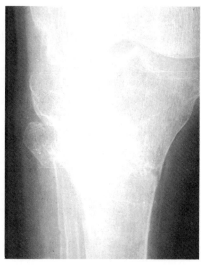

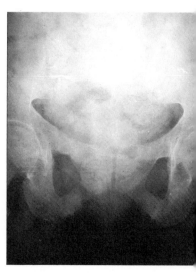

1. *Osteoporosis:* This is the commonest cause of pathological fracture, being especially important in the spine, the wrist, and the femoral neck. It is most frequently due to lowering of hormone levels in association with age or the menopause: less frequently it follows disuse, rheumatoid arthritis, or Vitamin C deficiency which lead to a failure of osteoid tissue formation, and the translucent appearance of bone on the radiographs. (Ill: fracture of D6.)

2. *Osteomalacia* (1) This is due to a failure in osteoid mineralisation and the radiographic appearances may be difficult to differentiate from osteoporosis. (Ill: fracture of tibia and fibula). It is usually secondary to an inability to utilise Vitamin D (adult rickets) but is also seen where calcium is deficient in the diet (or excreted in renal acidosis), where phosphate is excreted in excess (Fanconi syndrome) or where Vitamin D is not absorbed (e.g. steatorrhoea).

3. *Osteomalacia* (2) Stress fractures are common. Areas of bone translucency (Loosers zones) in the pelvis and long bones are characteristic. (Ill: note changes in ischium and pubic ramus fracture.) There are disturbances in the blood chemistry: the serum PO_4 is reduced, and the serum calcium normal or reduced. If the product of the serum calcium and phosphate is lower than 2.25 (using S.I. units) the diagnosis is confirmed.

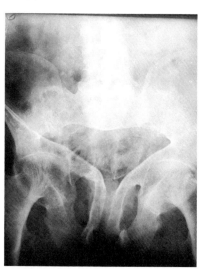

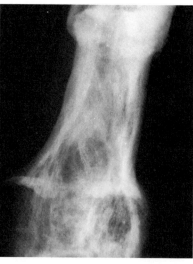

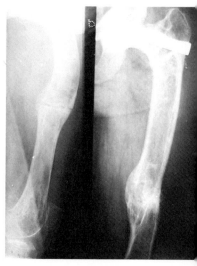

4. *Osteomalacia* (3) Occasionally a tri-radiate pelvis may be present and also be diagnostic. Osteomalacia may be treated with Calciferol 1.25 mg per day, and calcium gluconate 1–2 g per day. The serum calcium, phosphate and urea should be monitored at regular intervals. Osteoporosis is resistant to treatment although calcium and anabolic steroids are sometimes given. Fracture healing is not materially impaired in either condition.

5. *Paget's disease* (1) This common condition is frequently seen in association with fracture, particularly in the tibia and the femur. (Ill: two healing fractures of the femur.) The radiological picture is complex, with frequently cyst formation, bone thickening, increased bone density, and disturbances of bone texture. Stress fractures are common, and complete fractures are usually transverse.

6. *Paget's disease* (2) Increased bone density and deformity may in many situations make the use of internal fixation devices difficult. (Ill: femoral neck fracture pinned in coxa vara: healing fracture of shaft.) The rate of healing and the soundness of bone union is not, however, usually greatly affected. In many situations conservative methods may be employed with success.

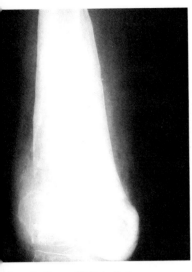

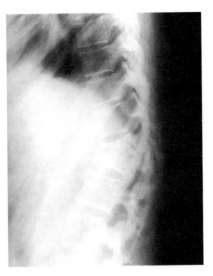

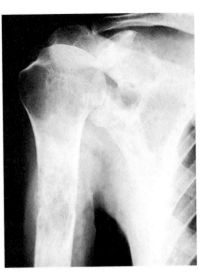

Paget's disease (3) Note that sarcomatous change (Ill.) in this condition may be followed by fracture as the cortical bone is eroded. Note, too, that the bone changes found in hyperparathyroidism and sometimes in metastatic disease may mimic Paget's disease.

8. *Osteitis:* Sudden collapse of bone secondary to infection is comparatively uncommon as a presenting feature, but is seen where the destructive processes are comparatively low grade. Thorough investigation and appropriate treatment is mandatory. (Ill: Tuberculosis at the thoraco-lumbar level.)

9. *Malignant bone tumours* (1) The commonest malignant bone tumour is the metastatic deposit. Secondaries in bone occur most frequently from primary growths in lung or bronchus (Ill.), breast, prostate or kidney. Any bone may be affected, but the spine, subtrochanteric region of the femur and the humeral shaft are amongst the commonest sites.

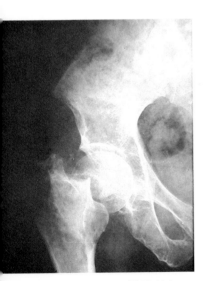

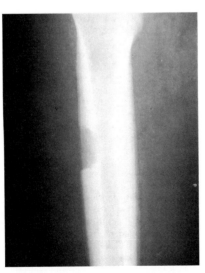

12. *Malignant bone tumours* (4) *Treatment:* Note the following points: (a) Without treatment, union of a fracture occurring at the site of a malignant bone tumour seldom occurs.
(b) If the tumour is responsive to local radiotherapy or to chemotherapy, healing may occur with appropriate splintage, but will be slow.
(c) In the case of metastatic disease, internal fixation has much to recommend it unless the patient is moribund. Acrylic cement is sometimes used to reinforce a bone defect.
(d) In the case of primary malignant bone tumours, the occurrence of fracture may be a factor in some circumstances in the advocation of amputation.

10. *Malignant bone tumours* (2) Multiple myeloma in the pelvis (Ill: with fracture of the femoral neck and a destructive lesion of the ilium) may sometimes be confused with secondary deposits from carcinoma of the prostate or other organs: full investigation is essential.

11. *Malignant bone tumours* (3) Primary malignant tumours of bone generally present with pain and swelling rather than fracture, but this is not always the case, especially perhaps in Ewing's tumour (Ill: radiograph prior to fracture) and osteosarcoma. The aggressive, locally malignant osteoclastoma again usually presents with pain and swelling rather than fracture.

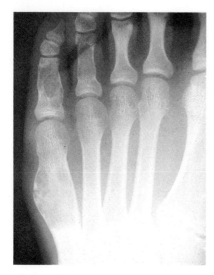

13. *Simple bone tumours and cysts* (1) In the metacarpals, metatarsals (Ill.) and phalanges (Ill.), enchondromata are frequently encountered as a cause of pathological fracture. These are generally best treated by exploration, curettage, and the packing of the resultant cavity in the bone with cancellous bone grafts.

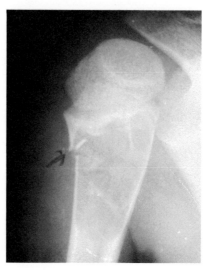

14. *Simple bone tumours and cysts* (2) In children between 5 and 15, unicameral bone cyst is one of the most frequent causes of pathological fracture, especially in the proximal humeral shaft. The bone cortex may be thinned, but expansion is rare. The fracture should be treated conservatively. (If the fracture fails to heal and the cyst disappear, curette and pack with bone grafts.)

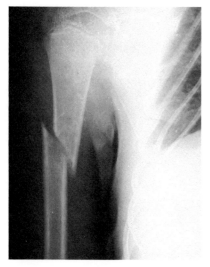

15. *Osteogenesis imperfecta:* This hereditary disorder (dominant transmission) is characterised by bone fragility leading to bowing of the long bones, deformities of modelling, pathological fractures and stunting of growth. (Ill. fracture of humerus: note deformities of ribs.) Deafness and blue sclerotics are commonly associated. The condition generally declares itself in infancy or childhood, but occasionally may not be diagnosed until skeletal de-mineralisation is noted later in life. Fracture healing is usually quite rapid, and most fractures may be treated successfully by conservative methods. Occasionally in the severer forms of this condition which present in childhood, internal fixation of the long bones by intramedullary nailing may be advocated as a prophylaxis against further fracture and to lessen bowing and other deformities of the legs.

Investigation of pathological fractures:
Investigation of a pathological fracture may require some or all of the following:
(a) A full personal and family history.
(b) Full clinical examination, including pelvic examination.
(c) Radiographs of the chest.
(d) Radiographs of the pelvis.
(e) Radiographs of the skull and skeletal survey.
(f) Estimation of the sedimentation rate.
(g) A full blood count, including a differential cell count.
(h) Estimation of the serum calcium, phosphate, alkaline phosphatase, and where appropriate, the acid phosphatase.
(i) Estimation of the serum proteins.
(j) Serum electrophoresis.
(k) Examination of the urine for Bence-Jones proteose.
(l) A bone scan.
(m) Marrow biopsy.
(n) Bone biopsy.
(o) Occasionally, radiographs of parents c sibs.

Section B:
Regional injuries

Section D

6. The shoulder girdle and humerus

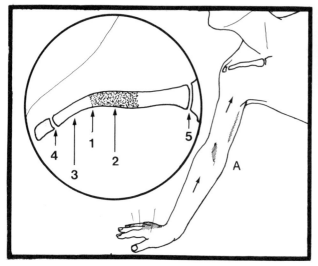

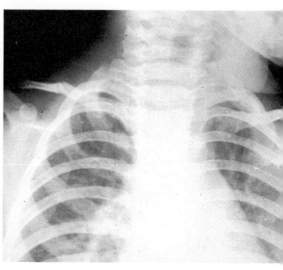

1. *Clavicular injuries: Mechanism of injury:* Most clavicular injuries result from a fall on the outstretched hand, force being transmitted up the arm to the clavicle (A); the clavicle may also be injured by falls or blows on the point of the shoulder, and by direct violence.

Fracture is commonest at the junction of the middle and outer thirds (1) but is also common throughout the middle third (2) and to a lesser extent the outer third (3). *Subluxations and dislocations* may involve the acromio-clavicular joint (4) and the sterno-clavicular joint (5).

2. *Common patterns of fracture* (1) Greenstick fractures are common, particularly at the junction between the middle and oute thirds. Fractures may not be particularly obvious on the radiographs and it is often helpful in children to have both shoulde included for comparison. The only abnormality visible in many cases is local kinking of the clavicular contours. (Fracture of right clavicle ill.) Healing of this type of fracture is *rapid*, and *reduction not required.*

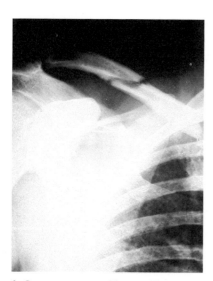

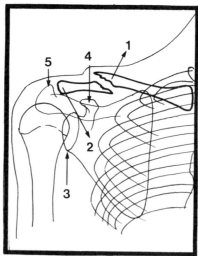

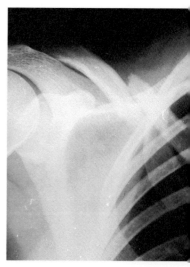

3. *Common patterns of fracture* (2) In the adult, undisplaced fractures are also common, and are comparatively stable injuries. Late slipping is rare. Symptoms settle rapidly and minimal treatment is required.

4. *Common patterns of fracture* (3) With greater violence, there is separation of the bone ends. The proximal end, under the pull of sternomastoid often becomes elevated (1). The shoulder loses the prop-like effect of the clavicle, so that it tends to sag downwards and forwards (2). Note (3) the glenoid, (4) the coracoid, (5) the acromion.

5. *Common patterns of fracture* (4) With greater displacement of the distal fragment there is overlapping and shortening. In spit of the off-ending, union is rapid, and re-modelling, even in the adult, is so effective that strenuous attempts at reduction are unnecessary. Pathological fracture may result from radio-necrosis (following radiotherapy for breast carcinoma) and ma be mistaken for local recurrence.

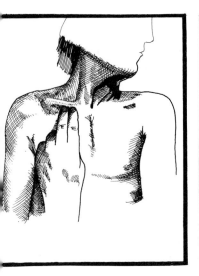

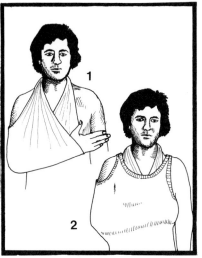

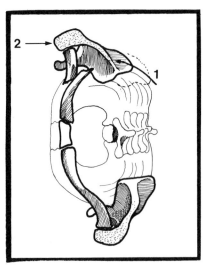

Diagnosis: Clinically there is tenderness the fracture site: sometimes there is ▸vious deformity with local swelling, and ▸e patient may support the injured limb ▸th the other hand. In cases seen some days ▸ter injury, local bruising is often a striking ▸ature. Diagnosis is confirmed by ▸ppropriate radiographs; a single A.P. ▸ojection of the shoulder is usually ▸equate in the adult.

7. *Treatment* (1) The most important aspect of treatment is to provide support for the weight of the arm which has lost its clavicular tie. As a rule this is best achieved with a broad-arm sling (1). Additional fixation may be obtained by wearing the sling under the clothes (2). No other treatment is needed in greenstick or undisplaced fractures.

8. *Treatment* (2) Where there is marked displacement of a clavicular fracture it is usual practice to attempt to correct the anterior drift of the scapula round the chest wall (1). There is no simple way of achieving this. All methods attempt to apply pressure on the front of the shoulder (2) and although they are comparatively ineffective in terms of reduction, are helpful in reducing pain.

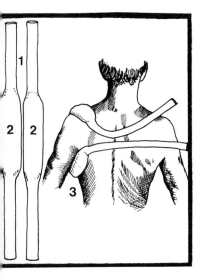

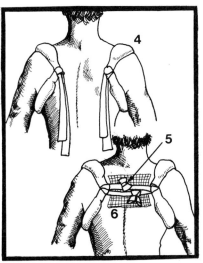

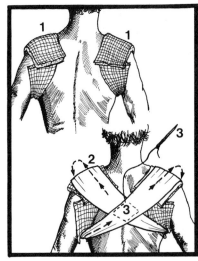

▸ *Treatment* (3) *Ring or Quoit method:* ▸arrow gauge stockingette is cut into two ▸ngths of about a metre each (1). The ▸ntral portions are stuffed with cotton ▸ool (2). One of the strips is taken and the ▸added area positioned over the front of the ▸houlder and tied firmly behind (3).

10. *Treatment* (4) The second strip is applied in a similar manner to the other shoulder (4). The patient is then advised to brace the shoulders back and the free ends of the ring pads are tied together (5). A pad of gamgee may be placed as a cushion beneath the knots (6).

11. *Treatment* (5) *Figure-of-8 bandage:* Pads of gamgee (gauze/cotton wool sandwich) or cotton wool alone are carefully positioned round both shoulders (1). The patient, who should be sitting on a stool, is asked to brace back the shoulders; a wool roll bandage is then applied in a figure-of-8 fashion (2). For added security the layers may be lightly stitched together at the cross-over (3).

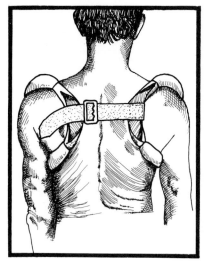

12. *Treatment* (6) Commercially available clavicle rings, covered with chamois leather, may be applied and secured with a web strap and buckle. With all these methods care must be taken to avoid pressure on the axillary structures and the additional support of a sling is desirable for the first 2 weeks or so. Note that elderly patients tolerate clavicular bracing methods poorly, and sling support only may be advisable.

13. *After care:* 1. Clavicular braces of all types require careful supervision and, at least initially, may require inspection and possible tightening every 2–4 days. 2. Where braces are used in conjunction with a sling, the sling may usually be discarded after 2 weeks. 3. All supports may be removed as soon as tenderness disappears from the fracture site. 4. Physiotherapy is seldom required except in the elderly patient who has developed shoulder stiffness. 5. A child's mother should always be advised that the prominent callous round the fracture is a normal occurrence, and that it will disappear in a few months with re-modelling.

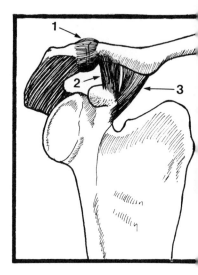

14. *Acromio-clavicular joint injuries:* Injury to the acromio-clavicular joint usually results from a fall in which the patient rolls onto the shoulder. Note that the clavicle is normally attached to the scapula by (1) acromio-clavicular (2) conoid and (3) trapezoid ligaments. The scapular component of shoulder abduction requires free acromio-clavicular movement.

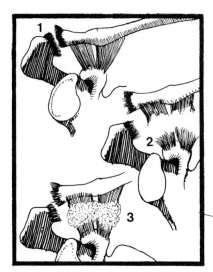

15. *Pathology:* Note that (1) in subluxations and sprains, damage is confined to the acromio-clavicular ligaments, and the clavicle preserves some contact with the acromion. In dislocations (2) the clavicle loses all connection with the scapula, the conoid and trapezoid ligaments tearing away from the inferior border of the clavicle. The displacement may be severe, and the ensuing haematoma may ossify (3).

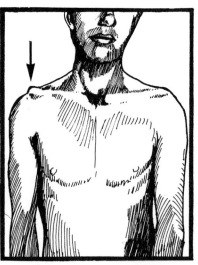

16. *Diagnosis* (1) The patient should be standing and the shoulders compared. The outer end of the clavicle will be prominent, and in cases of damage to the conoid and trapezoid ligaments, the prominence may be quite striking. Local tenderness is always present.

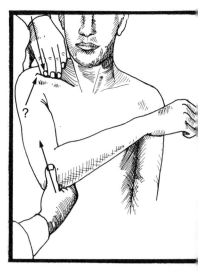

17. *Diagnosis* (2) Confirm any subluxation by supporting the elbow with one hand and gently pushing the clavicle down with the other. Improvement in the contour of the outer end of the clavicle will confirm the diagnosis of subluxation or dislocation.

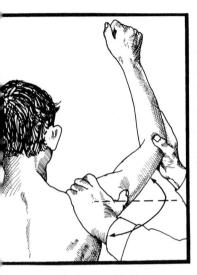

18. *Diagnosis* (3) Now stand behind the patient and abduct the arm to 90°. Flex and extend the shoulder while gently palpating the acromio-clavicular joint. *Failure of the outer end of the clavicle to accompany the acromion indicates rupture of the conoid and trapezoid ligaments.*

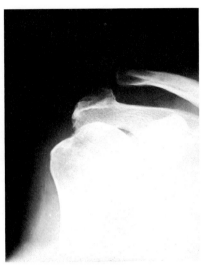

19. *Radiographs* (1) Displacement of the clavicle by a diameter or more relative to the acromion (illustrated) suggests rupture of the conoid and trapezoid ligaments. The radiographs however are often fallacious in indicating the severity of the injury (and indeed may not show it). The reason is that spontaneous reduction tends to occur in recumbency—the position in which A.P. radiographs are normally taken.

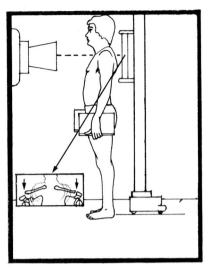

20. *Radiographs* (2) It must be clearly indicated on the radiograph request form that the acromio-clavicular joint is suspect. The radiographs should then be taken with the patient standing. The weight of the limb is often sufficient to show up the dislocation, but it is common practice to have the patient hold weights in both hands, and to include both shoulders for comparison.

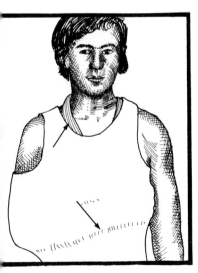

21. *Treatment* (1) If there is no gross instability, treat by the use of a broad arm sling under the clothes for 4–6 weeks. Physiotherapy is seldom required and an excellent result is the rule. *N.B.* Subluxations are easily reduced and held by adhesive strapping, but this treatment should *not* be employed as early skin reactions will always force abandonment.

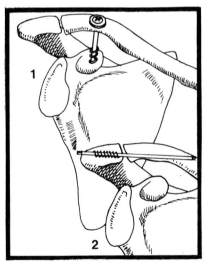

22. *Treatment* (2) Where there is gross instability, the clavicle must be re-aligned with the acromion and held there till healing is advanced. Methods include: (1) Coraco-clavicular screwing (care must be taken to avoid splitting the clavicle). (2) Use of a threaded pin across the joint. In the approach for either method, the associated rents in trapezius and deltoid should be repaired.

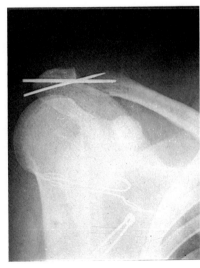

23. *Treatment* (3) Less satisfactory is the use of Kirschner wires across the joint, or figure-of-8 acromio-clavicular wiring. In all cases there is a strong tendency for the devices to cut out, and it is imperative that there is the additional support of a broad arm sling (under the clothes or with a body bandage). *Internal fixation devices must be removed at 6–8 weeks before full mobilisation.*

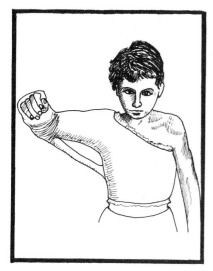

24. *Treatment* (4) If a dislocation reduces with the arm in abduction, a shoulder spica for 6–8 weeks may be used as an alternative to surgery. *Complications:* Symptoms from acromio-clavicular osteo-arthritis may be relieved by acromionectomy or excision of the outer 2 cm of the clavicle. (2) Fascial reconstruction of the coraco-clavicular ligaments can be used for persistent instability.

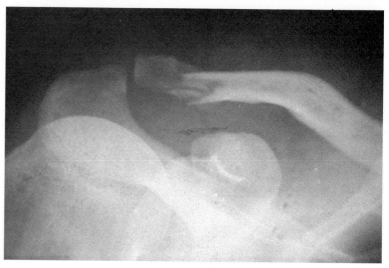

25. *Fractures of the outer third of the clavicle:* Displacement is generally minimal as the coraco-clavicular ligaments are not usually torn. When these ligaments are damaged, however, displacement may be marked and give rise (rarely) to non-union. These injuries should be treated along similar lines to acromio-clavicular joint injuries: clavicular bracing is valueless and a sling under the clothes for 4–5 weeks is usually quite adequate.

Complications of clavicular fractures: 1. Gleno-humeral joint stiffness in the elderly may require physiotherapy. 2. Even after normal re-modelling (which continues for many months) a persistent sharp clavicular spike may cause discomfort against the clothes, and require excision. 3. Non-union is extremely rare and is treated along conventional lines by internal fixation and bone grafting.

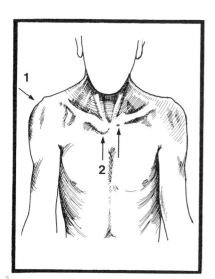

26. *Sterno-clavicular dislocation:* By far the commonest injury is a mild subluxation, caused by a fall or blow on the front of the shoulder (1) or fall on the outstretched hand. *There is asymmetry of the inner ends of the clavicles* (2) due to the clavicle on the affected side subluxing downwards and forwards. There is local tenderness. *The diagnosis is essentially a clinical one.*

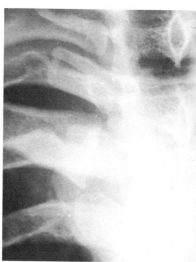

27. *Radiographs:* A.P. and oblique radiographs are difficult to interpret. They are of little help in the diagnosis of dislocations with minor displacement. Radiographs may be confirmatory in major dislocations when the inner end of the clavicle is displaced on to the sternum, or in the rare case (illustrated) where the clavicle passes *behind* the sternum, endangering the great vessels.

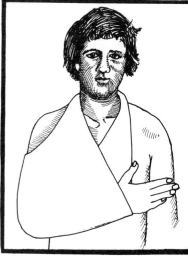

28. *Treatment* (1) Minor subluxations should be accepted. The clavicle stabilises in the subluxed position; some prominence of the inner end of the clavicle may persist, with some asymmetry of the supra-sternal notch, but a pain-free result is usual. The arm should be rested in a sling for 2–3 weeks until acute pain has settled.

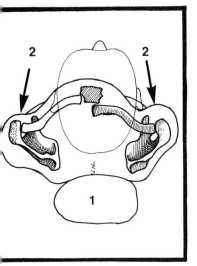

. *Treatment* (2) Gross displacements ould be reduced under general aesthesia. A sandbag (1) is placed tween the shoulders which are firmly essed backwards (2). Clavicular braces are en applied (see 8–12) along with a broad m sling for 4–5 weeks. Should the duction be extremely unstable, surgical pair with fascia lata slings should be nsidered.

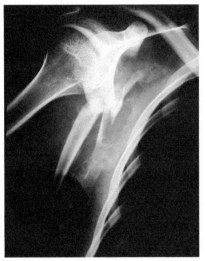

30. *Scapular fractures* (1) Fractures of the blade of the scapula are usually caused by direct violence. Even when comminuted and angled (illustrated) healing is usually extremely rapid and an excellent outcome the rule. Treatment is by use of a broad arm sling and analgesics. Mobilisation is commenced as soon as acute symptoms have settled, and is usually possible after 2 weeks.

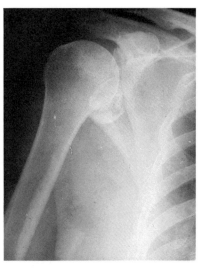

31. *Scapular fractures* (2) Fractures of the scapular neck are associated with much bruising and swelling. Comminution is common, sometimes with involvement of the gleno-humeral joint. If so, the position of the humeral head should be checked. In spite of frequently daunting radiographs, a good outcome is the rule, provided mobilisation is commenced as early as possible. (Treat as 30) Fractures of the spine or coracoid are dealt with similarly.

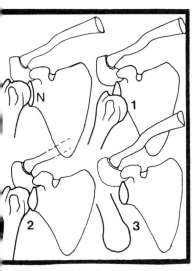

2. *Dislocation of the shoulder:* When the oulder dislocates, the head of the humerus ay come to lie *mainly* (1) in front of the enoid (anterior dislocation of the shoulder) (2) behind the glenoid (posterior slocation of the shoulder) or (3) beneath e glenoid (luxatio erecta). Anterior slocation if *by far* the commonest of these.

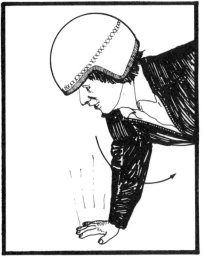

33. *Anterior dislocation* (1) This most commonly results from a fall leading to external rotation of the shoulder (e.g. the trunk internally rotating over a fixed hand). It is rare in children, common in the 18–25 age group (from motor cycle and athletic injuries) and again comparatively common in the elderly, where the stability of the shoulder may be impaired by muscle degeneration and where falls are common.

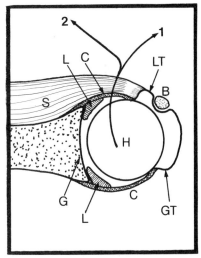

34. *Anterior dislocation* (2) The head of the humerous externally rotates out of the glenoid (1) and having become free, comes to lie medially in front of the scapula (2). B = biceps tendon; C = capsule; G = glenoid; GT = greater tuberosity; H = head of humerus; L = glenoid labrum; LT = lesser tuberosity; S = subscapularis.

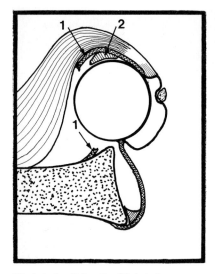

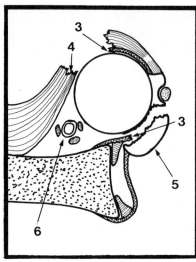

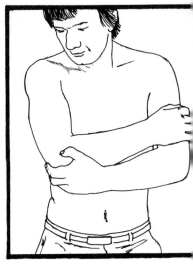

35. *Anterior dislocation* (3) Anterior dislocation is inevitably associated with damage to the anterior structures. Commonly the capsule is torn away from its attachment to the glenoid (1). This is the so-called Bankart lesion, although the frequent simultaneous displacement of the glenoid labrum (2) usually attracts this term.

36. *Anterior dislocation* (4) In the older patient especially, there may be tearing or stretching of the anterior capsule (3), sometimes with associated damage to the shoulder cuff, especially subscapularis (4). The greater tuberosity may fracture (5) and occasionally there is damage to the axillary artery or brachial plexus (6).

37. *Diagnosis* (1) The shoulder is very painful: the patient resents movement, and to prevent this, often holds the injured limb at the elbow with the other hand. The arm does not always lie into the side, appearing to be in slight abduction. The outer contour of the shoulder may appear to be slightly kinked due to the displacement of the humeral head.

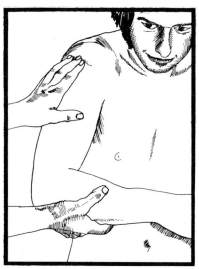

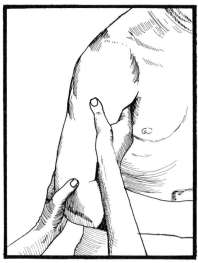

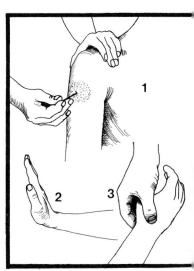

38. *Diagnosis* (2) Palpate under the edge of the acromion. The usual resistance offered by the humeral head will be absent. If in doubt, compare the two sides. The displaced humeral head may be palpable lying anteriorly.

39. *Diagnosis* (3) Nevertheless the acromion and clavicle make examination difficult. In the doubtful case, it may be helpful to try to assess the relative positions of the humeral head and glenoid by palpation in the axilla.

40. *Diagnosis* (4) Axillary (circumflex) nerve palsy is the commonest neurological complication. Test for integrity of the nerve by assessing sensation to pin prick (1) in its distribution over the 'regimental badge' area. (The shoulder is usually too painful to assess deltoid activity with certainty.) Look for other (rare) involvement of the radial portion of the posterior cord (2) and involvement of the axillary artery (3).

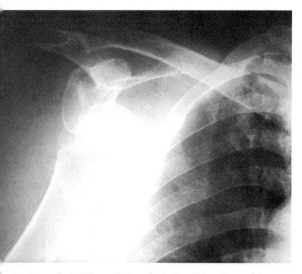

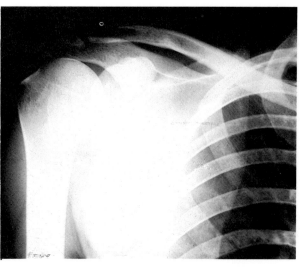

. *Radiographs* (1) The majority of anterior dislocations of the
ʃoulder show quite clearly on the standard A.P. radiographs of the
ʃoulder. The humeral head is displaced anteriorly and medially; in
ʃ final position it may be described as lying (a) pre-glenoid (b) sub-
ʃracoid (c) sub-clavicular. This classification is of little practical
ʃportance. The important diagnostic feature is the loss of
ʃngruity between the humeral head and the glenoid as illustrated.

42. *Radiographs* (2) This radiograph of a normal shoulder is
included for comparison. In both films you should be able to
identify the following features: (1) the glenoid (2) the humeral head
(3) the coracoid (4) the acromion and (5) the clavicle, (6) the
vertebral border of the scapula, and less clearly (7) the axillary
border of the scapula and (8) the spine of the scapula.

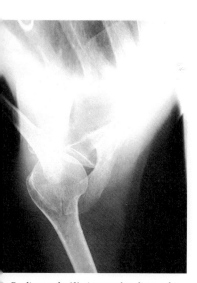

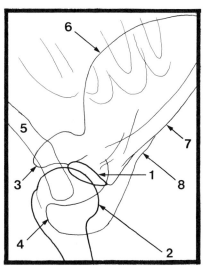

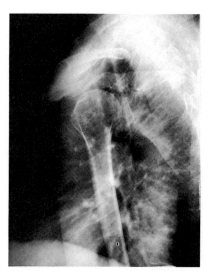

. *Radiographs* (3) *A second radiographic
ojection is essential if the diagnosis is in
ʃubt.* Note that if the humeral head has
ʃinimal medial displacement, the A.P. view
ʃay appear *normal.* (This is especially the
ʃse in posterior shoulder dislocations.) The
ʃost useful additional projection is the axial
ʃeral (sometimes called the tangential
ʃeral). The illustration shows the *normal
ʃpearances* in such films.

44. *Radiographs* (4) The axial lateral is
usually taken with the patient lying on his
back with the arm abducted to 90°. The X-
ray tube is adjusted so that it lies roughly
parallel to the trunk; the central ray passes
through the axilla to the plate which is
placed above the shoulder. The bony
features are easy to identify. (The numerical
key is the same as 42.)

45. *Radiographs* (5) Unfortunately the
shoulder may be too painful to allow an
axial lateral to be taken. Second best is the
trans-lateral which is often difficult to
interpret. Note that in the normal shoulder
(ill.) the posterior border of the humerus and
the axillary border of the scapula form a
shallow parabolic curve: this is disturbed in
any dislocation. (See for example 61.)

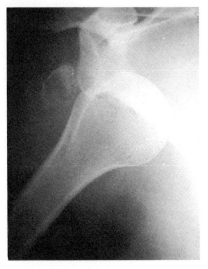

46. *Radiographs* (6) An associated fracture of the greater tuberosity is not uncommon (see 36 for mechanism). This does not influence the initial treatment of the dislocation by reduction, but may require subsequent attention (see 57). The radiographs of an acute dislocation may show evidence of previous episodes (for description, see 75).

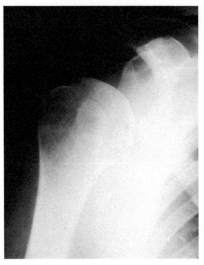

47. *Radiographs* (7) *Subluxation of the gleno-humeral joint:* Note that if any painful lesion of the arm is treated in a sling for several weeks, wasting in the shoulder girdle will commonly result in a minor subluxation: this is most obvious if the A.P. radiograph is taken with the patient erect; no active treatment is required, but frank dislocation should be excluded by a lateral projection.

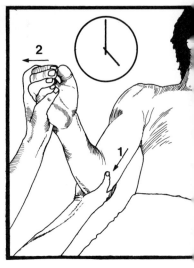

48. *Treatment: Reduction by Kocher's method* (1) This, the most popular of reduction methods, may often be successfully carried out in the older patient after the administration of intravenous diazepam, or in the younger patient, after a substantial dose of intra-muscular pethidine. Severe pain or a muscular patient are indications for general anaesthesia. Apply traction (1) and begin to rotate the arm externally (2).

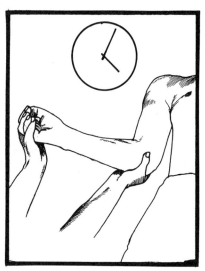

49. *Kocher's method* (2) Take plenty of time over external rotation. In the conscious patient, if muscle resistance is felt, stop for a moment and then continue, distracting the patient's attention with conversation. It should be possible to reach 90° of external rotation. (If severe pain and muscle spasm prevent rotation, general anaesthesia will be required.)

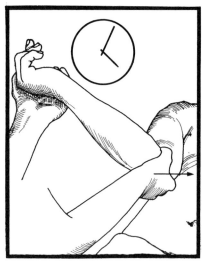

50. *Kocher's method* (3) The shoulder frequently reduces with a clear 'clunking' sensation during the external rotation procedure, but if this does not happen, adduct the shoulder so that the elbow starts to come across the chest. (This and the following movements may be carried out rapidly.)

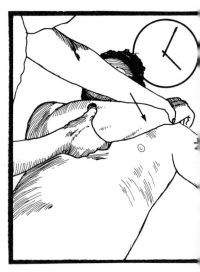

51. *Kocher's method* (4) Now internally rotate the shoulder, bringing the patient's hand towards the opposite shoulder. If reduction has not occurred, repeat all stages attempting to get more external rotation in stage 2. If doubt remains, repeat radiographs should be taken. Complete failure is rare under general anaesthesia. In the sedated patient, failure is an indication for general anaesthesia.

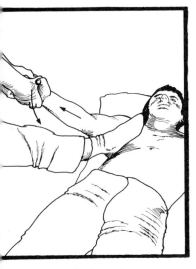

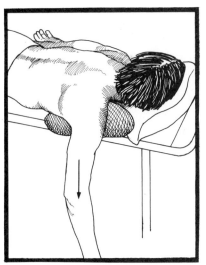

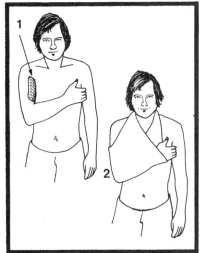

. *Alternative methods of reduction:* *Hippocratic method:* The principle is that traction is applied to the arm (1) and the head of the humerus is levered back into position. The stockinged heel (2) is placed against the chest (without being pressed hard into the axilla) to act as a fulcrum, while the arm is adducted (3).

53. *Gravitational traction:* The patient is given a generous dose of a powerful analgesic (e.g. 200 mg of pethidine in a fit athletic male). A sandbag is placed under the clavicle and the arm allowed to hang over the side of the couch. With muscle relaxation secondary to the analgesia, and the gravitational traction, the shoulder may reduce spontaneously within an hour. Failure is an indication for general anaesthesia.

54. *After care* (1) Check radiographs should be taken. This should be done before any anaesthetic is discontinued if there is doubt about the reduction. If the patient is a young adult with a first or second dislocation, the shoulder should be kept at rest for 4 weeks to lessen the risks of recurrent dislocation. Begin by placing a gamgee or wool pad in the axilla (for perspiration) (1) and apply a broad arm sling (2).

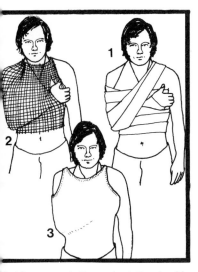

56. *After care* (2) If the shoulder has been dislocated several times before, prolonged fixation is valueless. An outside sling for a few days until the local symptoms have settled is all that is immediately necessary. If the shoulder has been dislocated four times or more, the patient should be considered to be suffering from recurrent dislocation, and be assessed for reconstructive surgery.

After care (3) In the elderly patient the risks of recurrent dislocation are minimal, but the risks of stiffness are great. A sling support under the clothes should be applied initially, and discarded as soon as pain will permit. Mobilisation of both the shoulder and the elbow may usually be started after 1–2 weeks. Referral for physiotherapy is advisable in nearly all cases of dislocation in the older patient.

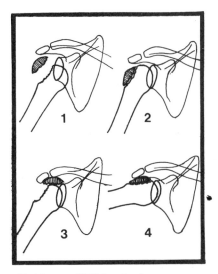

5. *After care ctd.:* External rotation should be prevented by a body bandage (1), stretchable net (Netelast) (2) or less securely by the outside clothes (3). The supports may require changing for the sake of hygiene from time to time until they are discarded at weeks. If there is some residual pain, an outside sling may be worn for a further week. Mobilisation is usually rapid without physiotherapy.

57. *After care* (4) If there has been an associated fracture of the greater tuberosity (1) this generally reduces adequately with the dislocation (2). Again, mobilisation should be commenced as soon as pain will permit (usually after 3–4 weeks). If the tuberosity remains seriously displaced—e.g. under the acromion (3)—and cannot be reduced by placing the arm in abduction (4) it should be openly replaced and fixed with a screw.

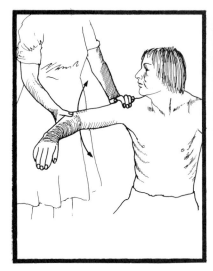

58. *After care* (5) Where there has been an axillary nerve palsy with loss of deltoid function, physiotherapy will be required. Although the lesion is usually in continuity and full recovery may occur, this may take several months and is not invariable. Assisted movements will be required—either normally, with the aid of slings and perhaps weights, or by hydrotherapy.

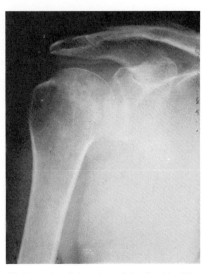

59. *Posterior dislocation of the shoulder* (1) This may result from a fall on the outstretched, internally rotated hand, or from a direct blow on the front of the shoulder. The head of the humerus is displaced directly backwards, and because of this, a single A.P. projection may show little or no abnormality as illustrated here. Nevertheless, clinically there is pain, deformity and local tenderness.

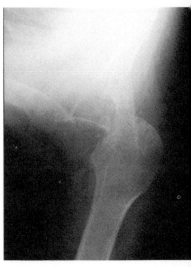

60. *Posterior dislocation* (2) The frequently apparently normal A.P. projection makes it essential for an additional lateral view to be obtained when there is any suspicion of posterior dislocation. Where pain is not severe (as for example if the dislocation occurs as a complication of a neurological disorder) a tangential lateral may show the humeral head lying clearly behind the glenoid. (Compare with 43.)

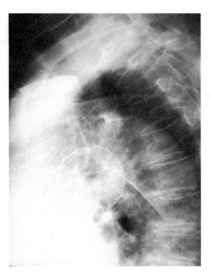

61. *Posterior dislocation* (3) Generally, however, pain will permit a trans-lateral projection only. The parabolic curve, shaped like the path of a comet, formed by the shaft of the humerus and the edge of the scapula will be broken, and further study will show the humeral head to lie behind the glenoid shadow. (Compare with 45)

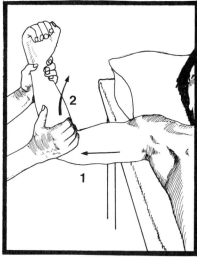

62. *Treatment* (1) Reduction is usually easily accomplished by applying traction to the arm in a position of 90° abduction (1) and then externally rotating the limb (2). If the reduction appears quite stable the arm should be rested in a sling as described for anterior dislocation of the shoulder.

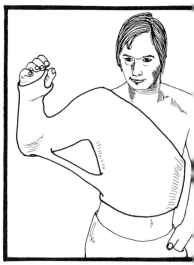

63. *Treatment* (2) If the reduction is unstable, it is essential that the arm be kept in 60° lateral rotation for four weeks to give the torn capsule and labrum a reasonable chance of healing. This can only be reasonably achieved by the application of a shoulder spica, with the shoulder abducted to about 40°, externally rotated 60°, and fully extended.

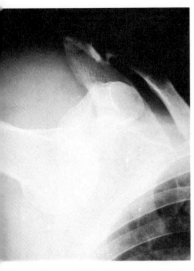

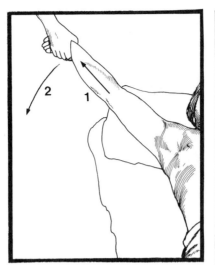

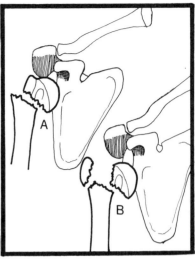

4. *Luxatio erecta* (1) In this comparatively rare type of shoulder dislocation, there is obvious deformity, with the arm being held in abduction. The radiographs pose no difficulty in interpretation. The patient should be carefully examined for evidence of neurological or vascular involvement, and reduction carried out without undue delay.

65. *Luxatio erecta* (2) Reduction is usually easily obtained by applying traction in abduction (the position in which the limb is lying) (1) and swinging the arm into adduction (2). The shoulder should be supported after reduction as for anterior dislocation.

66. *Fracture-dislocation of the shoulder* (1) These injuries result from severe violence (e.g. road traffic accidents, harness injuries in parachutists, etc.). The constant element is dislocation of the head of the humerus from the glenoid. In two-element fracture-dislocations there is a fracture through the surgical neck (A). In three-element injuries, there is an additional fracture of the greater tuberosity (B).

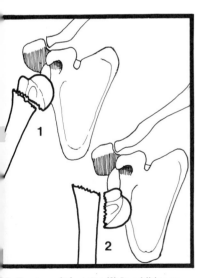

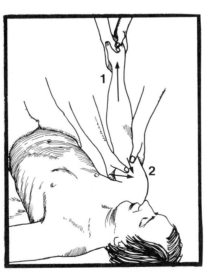

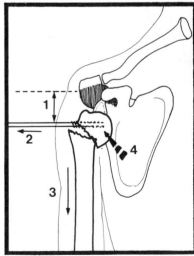

7. *Fracture-dislocation* (2) In addition to classifying these into two and three element injuries, the position of the humeral shaft in relation to the head is of importance. The shaft may remain related to the head (1) or there may be gross separation, often with the head rotated (2). Damage to the brachial plexus and axillary artery is more likely in such cases, and avascular necrosis almost inevitable.

68. *Treatment* (1) Unless the patient is too frail or elderly, reduction should be carried out. Open operation is generally required for type 2 injuries and if other methods fail for type 1 injuries: so cross matched blood and full theatre facilities should be available. *Closed reduction technique:* Apply strong traction in the neutral position or *slight* abduction (1) and pressure to the head via the axilla and front of the shoulder (2). Avoid hyperabduction.

69. *Treatment* (2) If the previous technique fails, pass a threaded pin into the humeral head: insert the pin from the lateral aspect of the shoulder 3 cms below the acromial arch (1). Apply lateral traction to the pin (2) with slight traction to the arm (3) and manual pressure over the humeral head (4). *After care* of these injuries is as for fractures of the neck of the humerus.

70. *Treatment* (3) Open reduction should be undertaken (a) if closed reduction fails or (b) if the humeral head is grossly displaced on to the medial axillary wall when tethering of the rough fracture surface within the muscle fibres of serratus anterior renders closed methods impossible. Exploration may also be advisable for inspection and possible repair where there is an extensive neurological deficit or circulatory impairment. In the latter case preliminary taping of the subclavian artery may be necessary.

Dislocation in fractures of the humeral neck: In severe abduction fractures, subsequent *adduction* of the arm may lead to subluxation or dislocation. In the elderly these injuries are best accepted, but in the young, open reduction may be considered if comminution is not great.

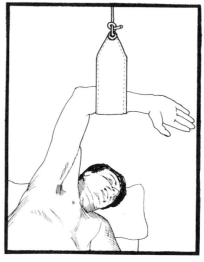

71. *Late diagnosed dislocation* (1) Anterior and posterior dislocations are sometimes discovered late; after 6 weeks, especially in the elderly, they should probably be left and re-assessed after a prolonged period of physiotherapy. Before 6 weeks, open reduction is often difficult and somewhat hazardous but closed reduction is often successful: under general anaesthesia the forearm is suspended by a canvas sling or bandage (e.g. from a ceiling hook).

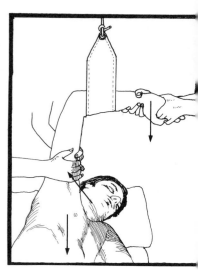

72. *Late diagnosed dislocation* (2) The patient should be on his side and the sling adjusted so that by using the arm as a lever, an assistant can exert considerable traction through the patient's body weight. The humeral head is then manipulated over the glenoid lip. An image intensifier may give considerable assistance. Mobilisation should be commenced at an early stage (say, one week).

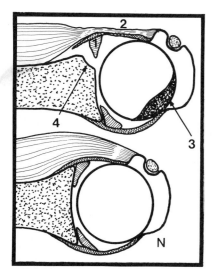

73. *Recurrent dislocation of the shoulder* (1) Even after early adequate treatment, re-dislocation of the shoulder may occur. Progressively less trauma is required on each occasion: eventually the patient may be able to reduce the dislocation voluntarily. Pathological features may include (1) a Bankart lesion (2) attrition of the anterior shoulder cuff (3) a defect, with flattening of the postero-lateral aspect of the head (4) rounding of the glenoid margin.

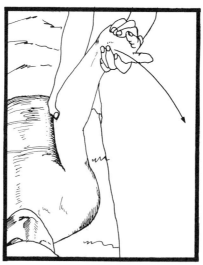

74. *Diagnosis* (1) The history is usually clear; clinically, external rotation of the shoulder may cause the patient considerable apprehension. Recurrent dislocation should be distinguished from habitual dislocation: in the latter condition the patients are frequently psychotic or suffer from joint laxity syndromes. They repeatedly dislocate the shoulder, often voluntarily and without pain, and the joint reduces easily and spontaneously.

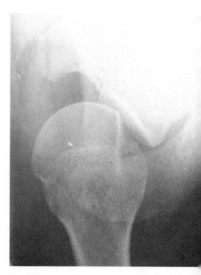

75. *Diagnosis* (2) An axial projection may clinch the diagnosis. Postero-lateral defects in the humeral head are often quite striking in recurrent dislocation (ill.). They do not occur in habitual dislocation. In the latter condition surgery frequently fails and should generally be avoided unless there are particularly strong indications and any underlying psychosis has been eliminated.

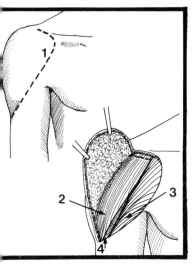
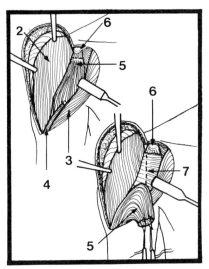
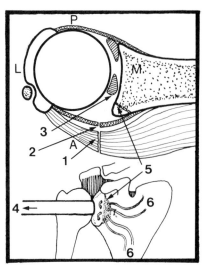

. *Treatment* (1) Two surgical repairs are
mmon: the Bankart and the Putti-Platt. In
oth, the anterior approach to the shoulder
usually employed. An incision is made
ong the line of the medial border of the
eltoid, turning laterally along the clavicle
). The groove between the deltoid (2) and
ectoralis major (3) is identified and opened
: the cephalic vein (4) may require
ation.

77. *Treatment* (2) The deltoid is turned back
by incising some of its fibres close to the
clavicle (2). The common tendon of the
coraco-brachialis and the short head of
biceps (5) is divided close to the coracoid (6)
and turned down, taking care to avoid the
musculo-cutaneous nerve. This reveals the
subscapularis (7).

78. *Treatment* (3) *Bankart repair* (1) The
shoulder joint is opened by dividing the
subscapularis (1) and the capsule (2). If the
glenoid labrum is loose and displaced into
the centre of the joint (3) it is excised; if not,
it is ignored. Access is improved by lateral
retraction of the humeral head (4). The
glenoid edge is rawed (5) and drilled
obliquely to take anchoring sutures (6).

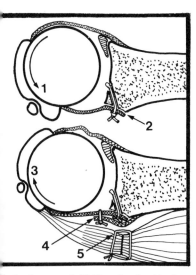
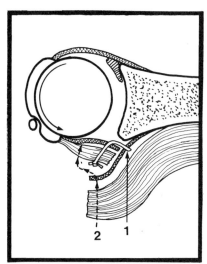
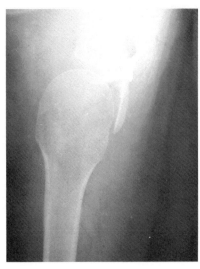

9. *Bankart repair* (2) Now the shoulder is
ternally rotated (1) and the sutures which
ave been passed through bone are used to
nchor the lateral part of the capsule to the
w edge of the glenoid (2). With the
oulder in neutral rotation (3) the medial
art of the capsule is sewn over the lateral
). The subscapularis is repaired (5)
llowed by layer closure. The arm is
andaged to the side for 4 weeks before
obilisation is commenced.

80. *Putti-Platt repair:* Strong mattress
sutures are inserted into periosteum, capsule
or other intact tissue on the scapular neck
(1) and used to anchor the lateral part of the
capsule and subscapularis. The medial parts
are sewn in front (2), deliberately restricting
external rotation, and forming a 4 layer
barrier of tissue in front of the joint. The arm
is kept in internal rotation for 4–6 weeks
before mobilisation. The failure rate with
either procedure is low (< 10%).

81. *Bone-Block repair:* In both anterior and
posterior (ill.) recurrent dislocation, a bone
graft fixed to the glenoid may be used to
buttress the joint mechanically. This
procedure is particularly indicated in the
rare (and generally unrewarding) case where
in spite of a joint laxity syndrome or
paralytic element to the dislocation, there is
some strong indication for attempted repair.

82. Late diagnosed posterior dislocation

On occasion posterior dislocation of the shoulder is not diagnosed until some weeks after the injury. If the delay is less than 6 weeks, closed reduction may be attempted, using the method described for late diagnosed anterior dislocation (71). If this fails, open reduction should be carried out.

If the delay in diagnosis exceeds 6 weeks, and the patient is elderly and frail, it may be wisest to accept the dislocation and advise prolonged physiotherapy. Generally pain subsides and scapular movement provides a fair, although restricted return of function in the shoulder.

If the delay in diagnosis exceeds 6 weeks, and the patient is young and fit open reduction should be carried out. If this is done from behind through a deltoid splitting incision, there is little risk of damage to the plexus or axillary vessels. As there is often initial instability after open reduction, a plaster should spica may be necessary for a few weeks before mobilisation.

Recurrent posterior dislocation

Surgery is advised for recurrent posterior dislocation, using similar criteria to those for recurrent anterior dislocation. The joint is exposed from behind After splitting the deltoid, the joint is opened by dividing infraspinatus with a vertical incision. Thereafter the joint may be stabilised by a Bankart-like procedure (by anchoring the lateral capsule to the glenoid and plicating the medial capsule) or by a repair similar to the Putti-Platt, (reducing internal rotation and forming a posterior buttress by securing the infraspinatus in a double-breasted, two-layer fashion behind the joint).

Shoulder cuff tears

With advancing years degenerative changes occur in the shoulder cuff. Minor trauma may then produce small tears which through impingement on the acromion give rise to a painful arc syndrome (principally pain in the shoulder over an arc of movement centred at about 90° abduction, with freedom from pain on movement outside the limits of that range). Osteo-arthritis of the acromio-clavicular joint gives superficially similar symptoms but local tenderness, palpable exostoses and crepitations, and characteristic radiographic changes permit easy distinction. Symptoms are often persistent, but local heat and infiltrations with hydrocortisone are often helpful. In some cases, as a last resort, the acromion may be excised.

More extensive tears may follow the sudden application of a traction force to the arm, and may give rise to difficulty in initiating abduction of the shoulder. If the patient is seen shortly after the incident, tenderness will be found under the acromial arch; a full range of passive movements will be present, but the shoulder is hunched when the patient attempts to abduct the arm. Later, even though the stabilising effect of supraspinatus remains lost, the patient may learn to abduct the arm by trick movements. The results of surgical repair in this condition are poor in the elderly; prolonged physiotherapy, commenced after the acute symptoms have settled, is usually followed by an adequate return of function in the joint. Repair is advocated for the rare occurrence of this lesion in the young patient.

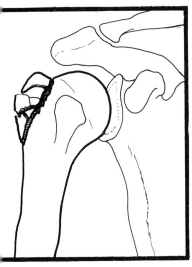

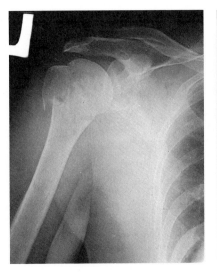

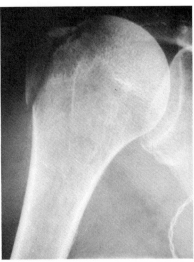

3. *Comminuted fracture of the greater
tberosity:* This injury usually results from
rect violence (such as a fall or blow on the
houlder). There is seldom any displacement,
nd a collar and cuff sling should be
rescribed until the acute symptoms have
ettled (say 1–2 weeks) when mobilisation
hould be commenced.

84. *Fracture of the greater tuberosity with
hair-line fracture of the neck of the
humerus:* This injury results from direct but
more severe local violence. Prolonged
immobilisation is not necessary; again a
collar and cuff sling should be worn until
pain has settled and shoulder mobilisation
may be started.

85. *Undisplaced segmental fracture of the
greater tuberosity:* This avulsion injury may
occur in isolation, or may accompany
dislocation of the shoulder (where it may be
missed, if as not uncommonly occurs, the
shoulder reduces spontaneously during the
radiographic examination). A good history
should clarify this point. (An isolated injury
should be treated as 83; accompanying a
dislocation, as 57.)

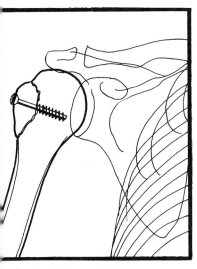

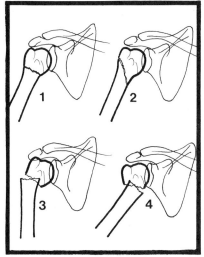

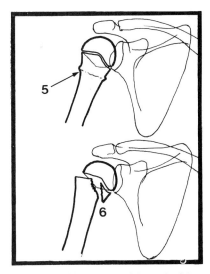

6. *Displaced fracture of the greater
tberosity:* If there is marked displacement
f the tuberosity, reduction should be
ndertaken, especially if the fragment comes
o lie under the arch of the acromion.
Manipulation of the arm in abduction using
n image intensifier (see 57) may succeed. If
his fails, open reduction with screw fixation
hould be carried out through a lateral
ncision.

87. *Fractures of the neck of the humerus:
Patterns* (1) In adults, the fracture line
passes through the surgical neck (fractures
through the anatomical neck are rare, but
are sometimes seen in fracture-dislocations
of the shoulder). *The majority are impacted*,
and the following patterns are common—
(1) undisplaced crack fracture
(2) undisplaced spiral (3) impacted
adduction (4) impacted abduction fracture.

88. *Patterns* (2) Fractures of the neck of the
humerus are common, particularly in the
middle aged, the elderly, and in children. In
children, the following comparatively stable
injuries are common, and correspond to the
impacted fractures of the adult:
(5) greenstick fracture, with or without
angulation (6) displaced humeral epiphysis
with slight to moderate displacement (Salter
and Harris Type 2).

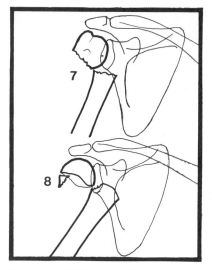

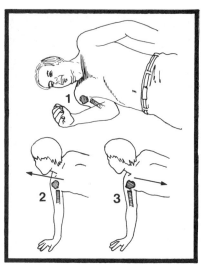

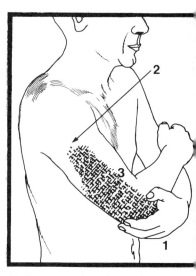

89. *Patterns* (3) The shaft of the humerus may be completely displaced in the more severe *unstable, unimpacted fractures of the humeral neck*. In both the adult (7) and in the child there may be damage to the axillary vessels or the brachial plexus. In children, epiphyseal displacement may occur (8) but the adult pattern of injury is also seen in children.

90. *Mechanisms of injury:* These fractures may be caused by a fall on the side or on the outstretched hand. Falls on the side tend to produce undisplaced or abduction fractures (1). The pattern of injury following a fall on the outstretched hand depends on the direction of motion of the trunk over the fixed hand. This may, for example, lead to abduction (2) or adduction (3) fractures.

91. *Diagnosis:* The patient tends to support the arm with the other hand (1). There is tenderness over the neck of the humerus (2) and in abduction fractures especially there may be obvious deformity. Later, gross bruising gravitating down the arm is an outstanding feature (3). (This may worry the patient unless its occurrence is predicted by the surgeon.)

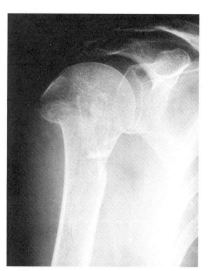

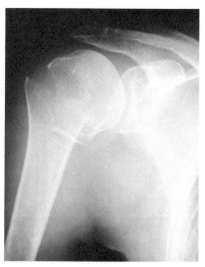

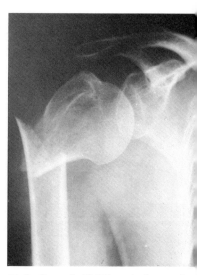

92. *Radiographs* (1) The diagnosis is established firmly by the radiographs. In a fair number of cases two features may be clear: namely, that the fracture involves the cancellous bone of the head and neck, and secondly, that there is impaction of the fragments. Both these factors contribute to the rapid healing associated with humeral neck fractures.

93. *Radiographs* (2) In many fractures the element of impaction is less clear. In the adduction fracture illustrated, the medial cortex of the neck is apparently engaged in the cancellous bone of the head. The nature of the surfaces in contact still ensures that healing will be rapid and that significant secondary displacement is unlikely *provided* the limb has some initial protection.

94. *Radiographs* (3) Where the fracture line lies distal as in this adduction fracture, cortical rather than cancellous bone is involved. As a result healing takes longer and a longer period of fixation is required. Note the severe angulation (50°). Nevertheless, deformities of this amount are usually treated without any attempt at manipulative reduction.

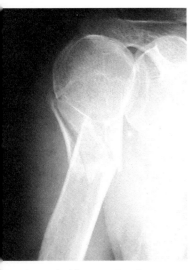

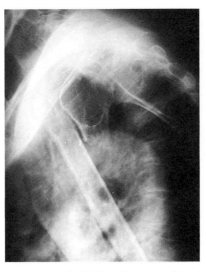

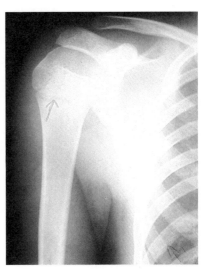

. *Radiographs* (4) Where there is a severe, ble abduction deformity of the type ustrated, gentle manipulative reduction is visable; if the deformity persists till union ere is risk of late subluxation of the oulder.

96. *Radiographs* (5) *Note that a second radiographic projection of the shoulder is desirable for a true assessment of these injuries.* Pain will generally allow a trans-lateral view only: nevertheless, this is generally clear enough to demonstrate the relationship between the two fragments (complete off-ending illustrated).

97. *Radiographs* (6) Note that in children the epiphyseal line is frequently mistaken for fracture. In many radiographic projections the epiphyseal plate lies obliquely, so that instead of appearing as a line, it is seen as an oval; as one part of this will be less distinct than the other (see arrow) it may be misinterpreted. (Ill: normal shoulder.)

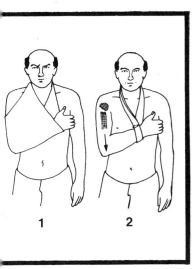

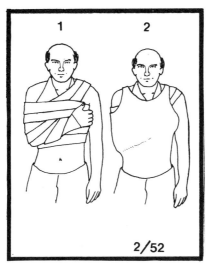

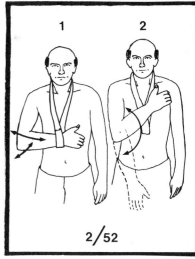

. *Treatment of impacted fractures:* atterns 1–6, frames 87–88) The arm is ld by a sling. Where disimpaction is an vious disadvantage (e.g. the impacted acture at 92) a broad arm sling is eferable (1). Where there is potential obility at the fracture site, with impaction ore implied than real (e.g. 94) then a collar d cuff sling (2) is more likely to lead to avitational correction of angulation.

99. *Treatment* (2) In addition, the arm should be protected from rotational stresses by a body bandage (e.g. of crepe bandages) (1) under the clothes (2). Alternatively, an expanding net support may be used (e.g. Netelast, 55) and this is certainly more comfortable in hot weather. Pain is often severe, and analgesics will be required in the first 1–2 weeks.

100. *Treatment* (3) After 2 weeks the body bandage may be discarded unless pain is commanding. The sling should be worn under the outer clothes. The patient is instructed to commence rocking movements of the shoulder (abduction, flexion (1)) and to remove the arm from the sling 3 or 4 times per day to flex and extend the elbow (2).

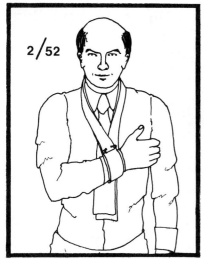

101. *Treatment* (4) At 4 weeks the sling can be placed outside the clothes. Gentle active movements should be practised throughout the day. Over the next 2 weeks the patient should be encouraged gradually to discard the use of the sling.

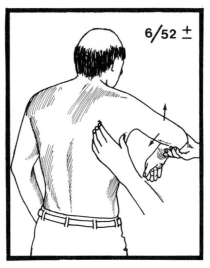

102. *Treatment* (5) At 6 weeks the patient should be referred for physiotherapy, if as usual, there is considerable restriction of movements. The range of movements (particularly gleno-humeral, ill.) should be recorded at fortnightly intervals, and physiotherapy discontinued when gains cease. Some permanent restriction of gleno-humeral movement is common, but seldom incapacitating.

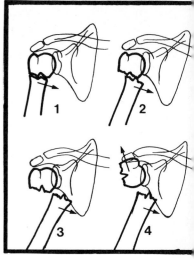

103. *Unimpacted fractures:* The majority of unimpacted fractures are primarily *abduction* injuries. With increasing violence the humeral shaft displaces until it escapes from under the head which may then rotate freely under the influence of the shoulder cuff, giving the appearance of an adduction injury. Always examine the patient carefully for evidence of neurological or vascular complications.

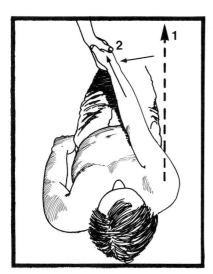

104. *Treatment* (A) In the very frail, elderly patient with an uncomplicated fracture, the displacement should be accepted and treated along the lines of an impacted fracture. (B) In all other cases, reduction should be attempted. Under general anaesthesia, apply traction in the line of the limb (1) and then swing the arm into *adduction* (2).

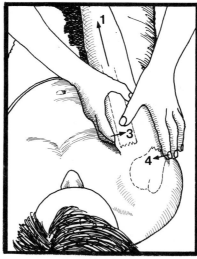

105. *Treatment* (B) An assistant maintains traction in adduction (1). Now apply pressure on the humeral shaft, pushing it laterally (3). At the same time, attempt to control the proximal fragment with the other hand, applying firm pressure beneath the acromion (4).

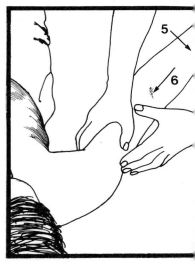

106. *Treatment* (C) If the medial edges of the fracture can be opposed, reduction may be completed by the assistant abducting the arm gently (5) and gradually releasing the traction (6). If closed methods fail, open reduction and internal fixation (e.g. by Rush pinning) should be considered. (After care as for impacted fractures.)

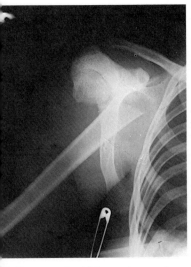

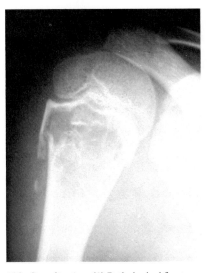

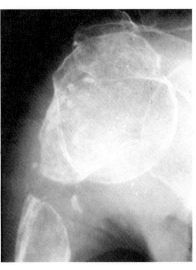

7. *Treatment:* In children, unimpacted ractures may be of adult pattern lustrated) or Group 2 epiphyseal injuries. *en reduction should be avoided.* anipulate as described, but if the deformity curs on bringing the arm to the side, apply shoulder spica in abduction. Bony position should be obtained, but persisting gulation in excess of 30° should not duce pessimism as rapid recovery of nction through re-modelling is the rule.

108. *Complications* (1) Pathological fracture from simple bone cyst is common in the proximal humeral shaft in children. The injury should be treated as an uncomplicated fracture. Healing usually proceeds normally, often with spontaneous disappearance of the cyst. Only rarely (following repeated fracture or cyst expansion) is curettage and packing with bone chips indicated.

109. *Complications* (2) Radionecrosis may follow radiation therapy for breast carcinoma, leading to pathological fracture. Active treatment is difficult due to local fibrosis and vascular change, but joint replacement might be considered in the selected case. (3) Arterial obstruction generally responds to reduction of the fracture; if exploration is required, preliminary exposure and taping of the subclavian trunk at the root of the neck must be anticipated.

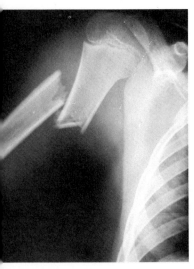

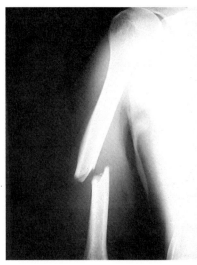

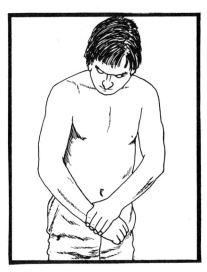

10. *Fractures of the humeral shaft:* athology (1) (a) Fractures of the humeral aft may result from indirect violence (e.g. fall on the outstretched hand) or from rect violence (e.g. a fall on the side or blow n the arm). (b) In fractures involving the pper third (ill.) the proximal fragment tends be pulled into adduction by the nopposed action of pectoralis major.

111. *Pathology* (2) (c) In fractures involving the mid third, the proximal fragment tends to be abducted due to deltoid pull. (d) Radial nerve palsy, non-union, and compounding are commonest in *middle third* fractures.

112. *Diagnosis* (1) The arm is flail and the patient usually supports it with the other hand. Obvious mobility at the fracture site leaves little doubt regarding the diagnosis. Confirmation is obtained by radiographs which seldom give difficulty in interpretation.

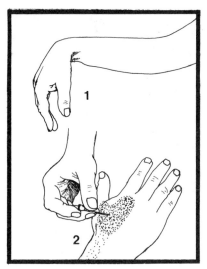

113. *Diagnosis* (2) In all cases, look for evidence of radial nerve palsy—drop wrist (1), sensory impairment dorsum of hand (2). This is in fact an uncommon complication, as a slip of brachialis lies beneath the nerve; this generally prevents it from coming in contact with the musculo-spiral groove or the fractured bone ends. If, however, radial nerve palsy accompanies a compound fracture, exploration is mandatory.

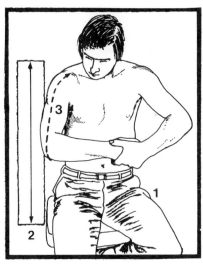

114. *Treatment* (1) *U-slab method:* Simple, single fractures may be treated by the application of a U-plaster. If angulation is slight, no anaesthetic is required. The patient should be seated (1) and a plaster slab prepared of about 8 thicknesses of 6″ (15 cm) plaster bandage (2). The length should be such as to allow it to stretch from the inside of the arm round the elbow and over the point of the shoulder (3).

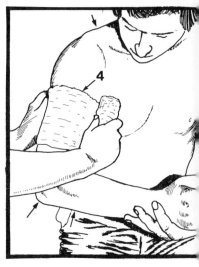

115. *Treatment* (2) Wool roll is then applied to the arm (4). Particular attention is paid to the elbow. The padding should extend from the shoulder to a third of the way down the forearm.

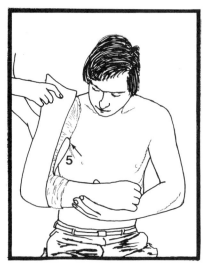

116. *Treatment* (3) The slab is now wetted and applied to the arm, starting on the medial side at the axillary fold (5), and then bringing it round the elbow up to the shoulder. The slab should be carefully smoothed down. Overlapping of the edges of the slab anteriorly or posteriorly is of little consequence.

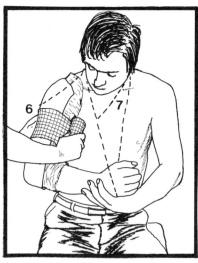

117. *Treatment* (4) The plaster is secured with a wet open weave cotton bandage (6). During the setting of the slab, the fracture may be gently moulded and slight angulation corrected. Thereafter the arm should be supported in a sling (7) which should be worn under the clothes.

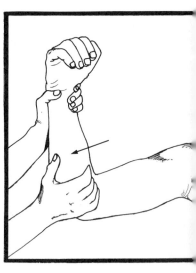

118. *Treatment* (5) If the fracture is badly displaced, heavy sedation or general anaesthesia is desirable. An assistant should apply light traction to the arm. A U-slab is applied as before, with careful moulding of the fracture as the plaster sets. A sling is worn under the clothes for additional support.

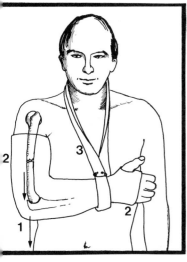

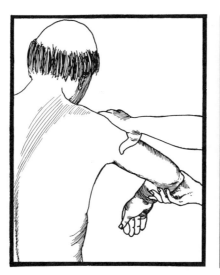

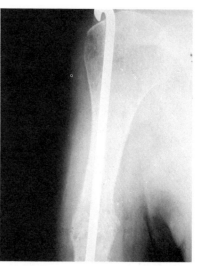

9. *Treatment* (6) *Hanging cast method:*
e principle of this form of treatment is
t the weight of the limb plus the plaster
luce the fracture and maintain reduction
. A long arm plaster (2) is applied along
h a *collar and cuff sling* (3). The patient
st be ambulant for this line of treatment
succeed, and it is claimed that there may
a higher rate of non-union from
casional distraction.

120. *Treatment* (7) In adults, union
commonly occurs in from 6–9 weeks. The
plaster should be removed at that time and
the fracture assessed for union clinically and
radiologically. If judged sound, a sling may
be worn as an additional precaution for 2
weeks, but exercises to the shoulder and
elbow should be commenced. Depending on
progress, the patient should be assessed for
physiotherapy.

121. *Treatment* (8) Internal fixation should
be considered when (a) the patient is bed-
ridden, especially with fractures in both
arms (b) there are 2 or more fractures in one
limb (c) there is a radial nerve palsy in a
'clean' compound fracture (d) radial nerve
palsy follows manipulation. Methods include
(1) Rush pinning (ill.) or Kuntscher nailing
from above (2) Rush pinning from the
olecranon fossa (3) plating.

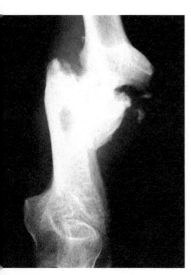

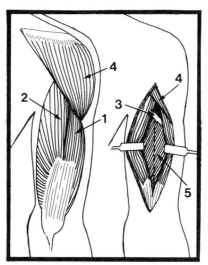

124. *Complications* (2) *Radial nerve palsy:*
This is generally a lesion in continuity, and
recovery often commences 6–8 weeks after
the initial injury. If there is no indication for
initial exploration (as for example the
presence of a radial palsy in a compound
fracture of the humerus) then the patient
should be treated expectantly.

The patient should be provided with a
drop wrist splint, preferably of lively type as
soon as possible, and he should attend the
physiotherapy department so that he can be
encouraged in active and passive movements
of the fingers, thumb and wrist. If there is no
evidence of recovery in 8 weeks an
electromyogram should be taken. If this
shows no sign of recovery, exploration of the
radial nerve should be undertaken.

2. *Complications* (1) *Non-union* (1) This is
n most frequently in middle third
ctures, especially in the obese patient
ere support of the fracture may be
ficult or where gravitational distraction of
fracture occurs. Rigid internal fixation
ell fitting Kuntscher nail, compression
ting, etc.) and often bone grafting are
vised, with post-operative fixation in a
ster shoulder spica.

123. *Non-union* (2) Visualisation of the
radial nerve is essential to avoid damage,
and a posterior approach is frequently used.
A midline posterior incision gives access to
the lateral (1) and long heads (2) of triceps,
which are separated. The nerve (3) lies close
to the deltoid margin (4) and should be
identified. The medial head of triceps (5) is
split to give access to the humeral shaft.

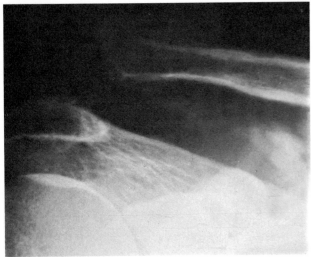

125. What injury and what sequel to injury is shown in this localised radiograph of the shoulder?

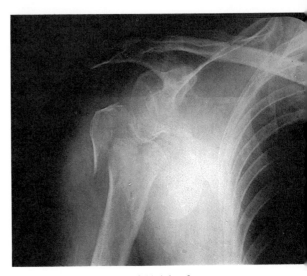

126. What is your analysis of this injury?

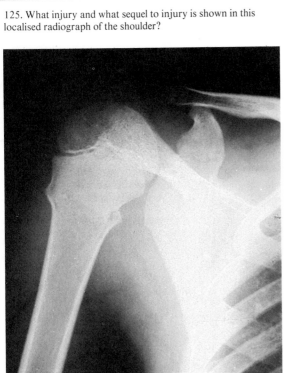

127. Classify this injury and comment on the position.

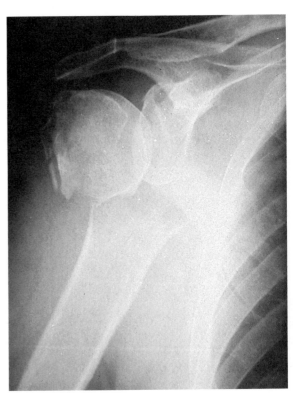

128. Describe this injury: what complication might you suspect?

25. Acromio-clavicular dislocation with massive calcification in the acromio-clavicular ligaments (no active treatment is likely to be required apart from physiotherapy).

26. The radiograph is of a three-element fracture dislocation of the shoulder. The faint shadow of the humeral head is in medial wall of the axilla, and there is a separate fracture of the greater tuberosity.

127. Greenstick fracture of the neck of the humerus: there is no apparent angulation, but a second projection would be necessary to make certain of this.

128. Fracture of the neck of the humerus; the fracture is of the unstable type and the shaft is displaced medially so that it has lost contact with the head. The axillary artery and the brachial plexus are at risk.

7. Injuries about the elbow

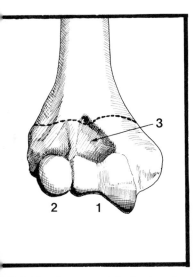

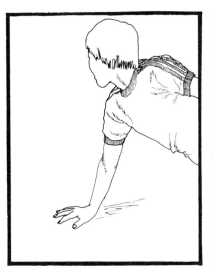

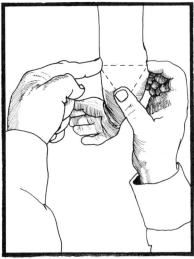

Definition: A supracondylar fracture of the humerus is a fracture which occurs in the distal third of the bone. The fracture line lies just proximal to the bone masses of the trochlea (1) and capitulum (capitellum) (2) and often runs through the apices of the coronoid (3) and olecranon fossae. The fracture line is generally transverse.

2. *Occurrence:* The supracondylar fracture is a common fracture of childhood; its incidence reaches a peak about the age of 8 years. It generally results from a fall on the outstretched hand, and should always be suspected when a child complains of pain in the elbow after such an injury.

3. *Diagnosis (1)* The olecranon and medial and lateral epicondyles preserve their normal equilateral triangular relationship (unlike dislocation of the elbow, also common in children). There is tenderness over the distal humerus, there may be marked swelling and deformity, and the child generally resists examination. Radiography is mandatory, but interpretation requires care.

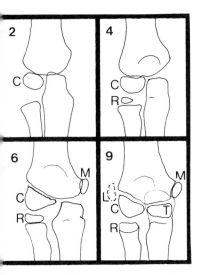

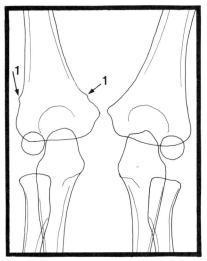

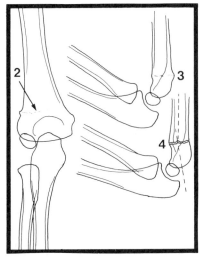

4. *Radiographs (1)* The interpretation of radiographs is made difficult by the changing complexities of the epiphyses. Typical appearances at age 2, 4, 6 and 9 are shown.

Note: C = Capitulum—present usually within the first year of life.
R = Radial head—appears 3–5.
M = *Medial epicondyle—present by 6.*
T = Trochlea—appears 7–9.
L = Lateral epicondyle—11–14.
(Olecranon—8–11 years.)

5. *Radiographs (2)* Variations in appearances occur, and if there is any difficulty in interpreting the radiographs, there should be no hesitation in having films taken of the other side for direct comparison. These may for example draw attention to (1) the slight cortical irregularity of a minor greenstick fracture.

6. *Radiographs (3)* In fractures associated with more violence, the next detectable sign may be a hairline crack, visible in the A.P. view only (2). With more violence, the fracture line will be detectable in the lateral projection as well (3). Next, the distal fragment is tilted in a backward direction (4).

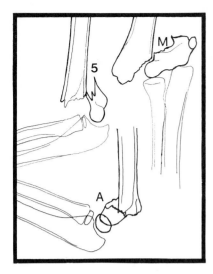

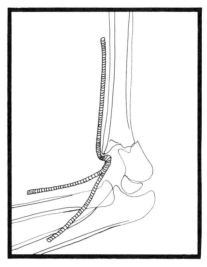

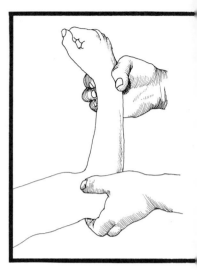

7. *Radiographs (4)* With still greater violence there is backward displacement (5), often leading to loss of bony contact. In the A.P. view there is often medial or lateral shift of the epiphyseal complex (M). The complex may also be rotated relative to the humeral shaft (generally lateral rotation). Rarely, as a result of other mechanisms the distal fragment is displaced and tilted anteriorly (A).

8. *Vascular complications (1)* Where there is appreciable displacement of the fracture, the brachial artery may be affected by the proximal fragment. In the majority of cases this is no more than a kinking of the vessel, but occasionally structural damage to the wall may occur.

9. *Vascular complications (2)* In every case the circulation should be assessed and recorded prior to any manipulation. Note if the radial pulse is absent; and seek other evidence of arterial obstruction (pallor and coldness of the limb, pain and paraesthesiae in the forearm, progressive weakness and paralysis of the forearm muscles). Look for excessive swelling and bruising round the elbow.

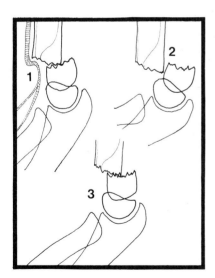

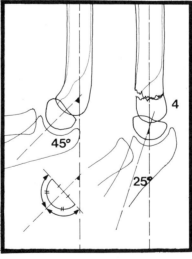

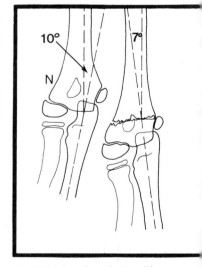

10. *Indications for reduction (1)*
Manipulation of the fracture should be undertaken (other things being equal) under the following circumstances:
1. If there is evidence of arterial obstruction and the fracture is displaced and/or angulated.
2. If there is off-ending of the fracture.
3. Ideally if there is 50 per cent or less of bony contact.

11. *Indications for reduction (2)*
4. If there is backward tilting (anterior angulation) of the distal fragment by 15° or more. Note that in the normal elbow that the articular surfaces of the distal humerus lie at 45° to the axis of the humerus. (The construction is shown and the actual deformity is 20° (45°–25°).) Persistent angulation leads to loss of flexion and does not re-model well.

12. *Indications for reduction (3)*
5. If there is lateral or medial tilting of 10° or more. Note that the normal 'carrying angle' of the elbow is about 10°. Illustrated is a cubitus varus deformity of 17° (10°+7°). Cubitus varus or cubitus valgus do not re-model well.

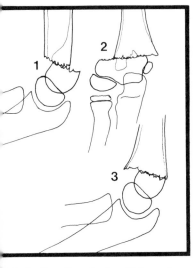

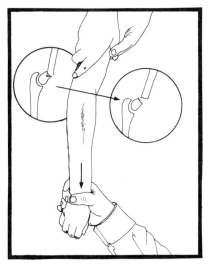

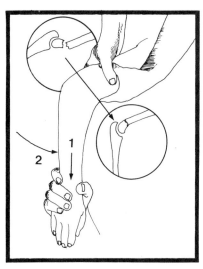

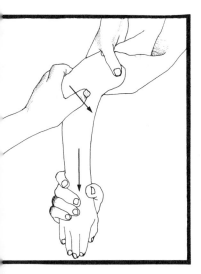

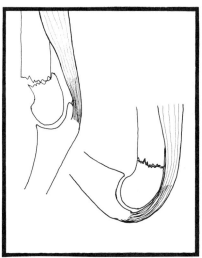

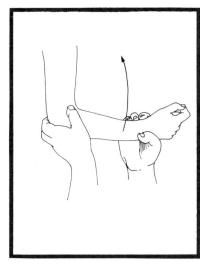

3. *Indications for reduction (4)* Assuming that no vascular complications are present, are posterior displacement (1) lateral displacement (2) or medial displacement of 0 per cent or less *may be accepted as re-modelling is generally rapid and effective.* Severe torsional deformity (axial rotation) 3) should be corrected by manipulation.

14. *Manipulation techniques (1)* The arm should be manipulated under general anaesthesia. Gentle/moderate traction is applied at about 20° of flexion while an assistant applies counter-traction. This leads to disimpaction of the fracture. Some surgeons advise that this and the following stages should be carried out with the arm in supination.

15. Manipulation (2) Now maintaining traction and counter-traction (1) flex the elbow to 80° (2). This lifts the distal fragment thereby reducing any posterior displacement and correcting any backward tilting (anterior angulation).

6. *Manipulation (3)* During this manoeuvre, the epiphyseal complex may be further coaxed into position by grasping it in the free hand. The thumb can be used to steady the proximal humeral shaft. Lateral displacement and torsional deformity (axial rotation) may also be corrected in this way.

17. *Fixation (1)* After reduction, the fracture must be maintained in a stable position. Flexion of the elbow stretches the triceps over the fracture, often splinting it most efficiently. *The aim should be to flex the elbow as far as the state of the circulation will permit.*

18. *Fixation (2)* Assuming that at 80° a pulse is present (if present before the manipulation, it should still be there; and if absent it will have hopefully been restored) continue flexion of the elbow until the pulse disappears (due to the elbow flexure crease along with the swelling compressing the brachial artery).

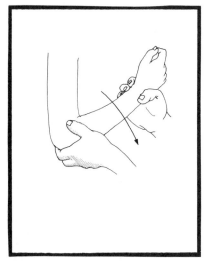

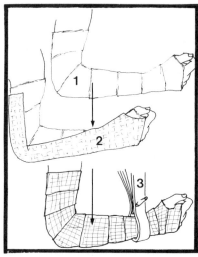

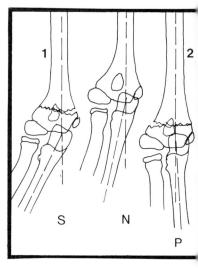

19. *Fixation (3)* Now extend the elbow slowly till the pulse just returns. *This is the position in which the arm should be maintained.* If 110°–120° or more of flexion can be preserved, a sling and body bandage, well secured with adhesive strapping, may suffice for fixation.

20. *Fixation (4)* Unfortunately further extension of the elbow may be required to restore the circulation. In such cases, apply a generous layer of wool (1) followed by a long arm plaster slab (2) secured with bandages and a sling (3). *Many surgeons favour this in every case. Warning:* never apply a *complete* plaster because of the risks of swelling.

21. *Fixation (5)* While the slab is being applied, the risks of recurrence of valgus or varus deformity may be reduced by careful positioning of the forearm: viz: If there has been valgus deformity (lateral tilting, medial angulation) (1) place the arm in supination. With varus (2) place the arm in pronation. With insignificant angulation the neutral position may be employed.

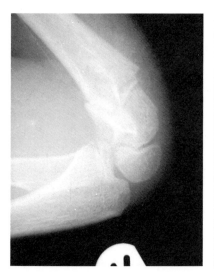

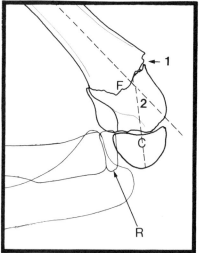

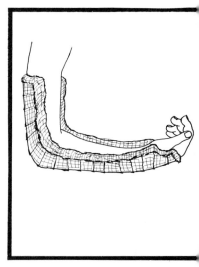

22. *Check radiographs:* Check radiographs must now be taken in 2 planes. (For interpretation of A.P. radiographs, see later.) In the lateral projection illustrated there has been a good reduction. Note how all posterior displacement has been corrected (1) and the normal angulation of the epiphyseal complex has been largely restored (2). (F = fracture line; C = capitellum; R = radial head.) If a good reduction has been achieved, (1) The anaesthetic can be discontinued; (2) The child should be admitted for overnight observation; (3) The arm should be elevated in a roller towel or similar device; (4) Access should be made in the dressings for observation of the pulse and circulation in the fingers.

23. *Late development of ischaemia:* If while under observation the pulse disappears, and especially if there are other signs of ischaemia, *all* encircling bandages should be cut, and *all* wool in front of the elbow teased out. If this does not lead to improvement, the elbow should be placed in a more extended position (e.g. by cracking the slab and slackening the sling).

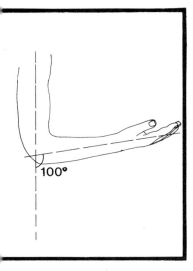

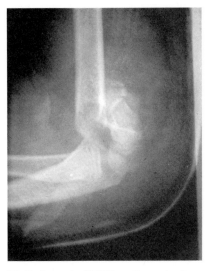

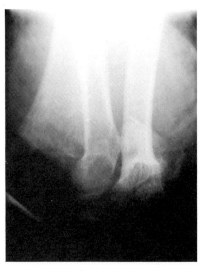

. *Absent pulse after manipulation:* :turning to Fig. 18: If after manipulation e pulse is *not* palpable, the elbow should be xed to *not more than 100°*, and aintained in that position with a sling and a ck slab (applied over wool and held with a htly applied bandage). The anaesthetic ould be continued while check diographs are taken.

25. *Radiographs (1)* If the radiographs show a poor reduction, then two further attempts at manipulation may be permitted under the same anaesthetic. The illustration shows a typical unsatisfactory lateral projection where the distal fragment is completely off-ended and also displaced proximally. (Compare with Fig. 23.)

26. *Radiographs (2)* An A.P. projection should also be taken and checked in every case, although errors in correcting the appearances seen in the lateral are more usual in causing circulatory impairment. As the A.P. view cannot be taken with the elbow straight, superimposition of the radius, ulna and humerus make interpretation difficult. (See next frame.)

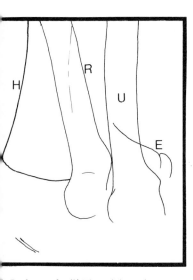

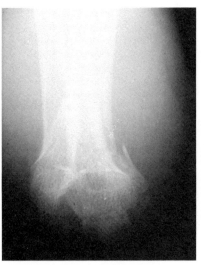

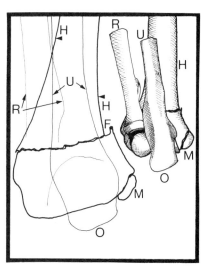

. *Radiographs (3)* The epiphyseal mplex preserves its relationship with the dius and ulna. In turn, with a good duction, the radius and ulna regain their gnment with the humerus. Note in this satisfactory reduction the radius (R) ulna) and epiphyseal complex (E) are splaced medially in relationship to the merus (H).

28. *Radiographs (4)* The preceding case with vascular impairment was re-manipulated and the above correction obtained. This is a good reduction, and was accompanied by restoration of the pulse at the wrist. (See next frame for interpretation.)

29. *Radiographs (5)* A line drawing of the preceding radiograph is shown along with a sketch of the forearm bones drawn in roughly the same position. (Compare also with 26.) R = radius, U = ulna, H = humerus, F = fracture, O = olecranon, M = medial epicondyle.

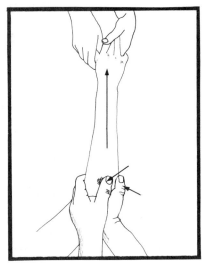

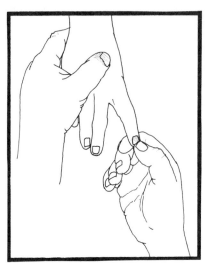

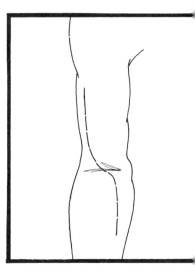

30. *Re-manipulation:* If a poor reduction has been obtained and re-manipulation is necessary, the preceding technique may be repeated; alternatively, while an assistant applies light traction to the forearm, the distal fragment is pushed forwards with the thumb while the fingers control the proximal fragment. Plaster fixation may be applied as described before.

31. *Absent pulse, adequate circulation:* If a good reduction has been obtained and the pulse remains absent, the circulation should be checked more critically. If the hand is warm and pink, with good capillary return in the nails, there is no immediate indication for further intervention. *Admission, elevation and close observation for 24 hours is essential.* (Generally the pulse returns spontaneously over 2–3 days.)

32. *Absent pulse, ischaemia:* If there are incontrovertible signs of gross ischaemia, either in the face of a good reduction or a failed reduction, *exploration of the brachial artery* must now be undertaken. Exposure of the artery is straightforward. (a) A lazy S incision may be used, following the lateral edge of biceps and crossing the elbow near the fold.

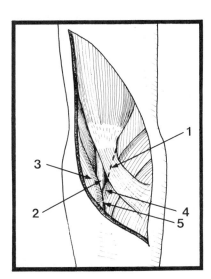

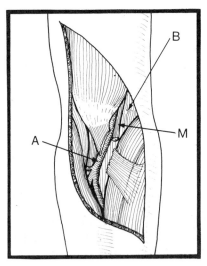

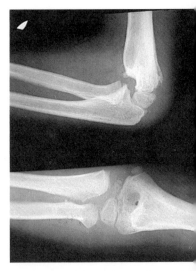

33. *Exploration of brachial artery ctd.* (b) The skin edges are reflected and the bicipital aponeurosis (1) divided close to the tendon (2). (c) The arm is put in full pronation and the space (5) between brachio-radialis laterally (3) and pronator teres medially (4) opened up with the finger tips.

34. *Exploration brachial artery ctd.* (d) The brachial artery (A) is found lying close to the biceps tendon. The median nerve (M) lies on its medial side. The fracture lies deep to the brachialis (B) in the floor of the wound. In some cases relief of local pressure on the vessel (e.g. from the fracture) may restore the circulation, but other measures, requiring experience in vascular surgery, may be necessary.

35. *Reduction failure with satisfactory circulation (A)* It is unwise to repeat manipulation beyond the third attempt due to the risks of increasing swelling. In these circumstances, marked displacement (but not angulation) may be accepted, relying on later re-modelling. The fracture illustrated was off-ended in the lateral: after a year, considerable re-modelling has occurred, with loss of 15° only of flexion.

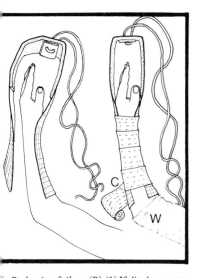

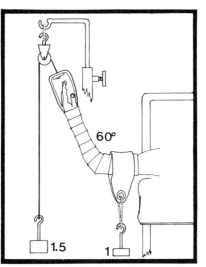

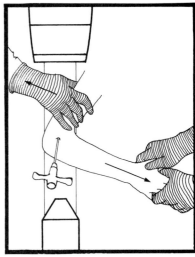

. *Reduction failure (B) (1)* If displacement
d angulation are outside acceptable limits,
en reduction is not recommended.
stead, continuous traction may be
nployed (Dunlop traction). This is
pecially indicated where there is minimal
rculatory impairment, and the elbow
nnot be flexed, but brachial artery
ploration is not indicated. Traction tapes
e applied to the limb. W = wool:
= *lightly* applied crepe bandage.

37. *Reduction failure (B) (2)* The arm is
abducted at the shoulder and traction of
$1\frac{1}{2}$ kg applied with the elbow at 60° flexion.
Counter-traction of 1 kg is applied directly
with a canvas sling. After swelling subsides
the situation may be re-appraised, or the
traction discontinued and a plaster slab
substituted at 2–3 weeks.

38. *Reduction failure (C) (1)* Reduction
failure may be avoided in a number of cases
if image intensification is available. With this
facility the problem may often be seen to be
due to excessive instability of the fracture.
Under these circumstances reduction may
be held by Kirschner wires inserted
percutaneously. (Reduction is effected by
traction as described.)

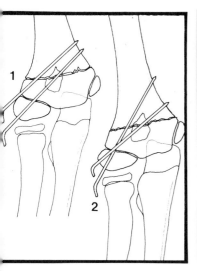

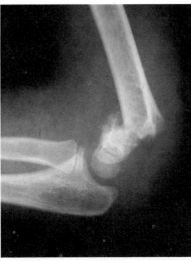

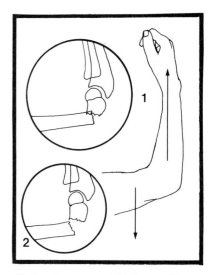

. *Reduction failure (C) (2)* Two wires
ust be used, either parallel (1) or
ossed (2). The wires are cut short, the ends
nt (to avoid migration) and slipped under
e skin. A plaster slab is used as additional
pport for about 4 weeks. The wires are
moved at 3 weeks.

40. *The anterior (reversed) supracondylar
fracture (1)* Supracondylar fractures in
which the distal fragment is displaced
anteriorly are comparatively uncommon.
The normal angle (45°) between the
epiphyseal complex and the shaft is
increased. *This deformity is aggravated by
flexion of the elbow.*

41. *Anterior supracondylar fracture (2)* An
uncommon, but related injury is the more
distally situated traumatic separation of the
epiphyseal complex (Salter and Harris Type
1 or 2) in which the displacement is identical.
To reduce either of these injuries, traction is
applied to the elbow in the flexed
position (1). This disimpacts the fracture (2).

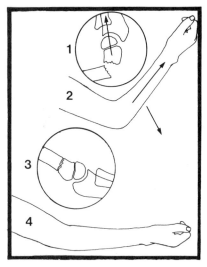

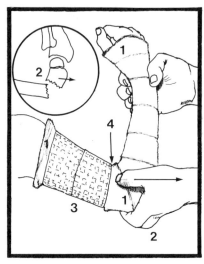

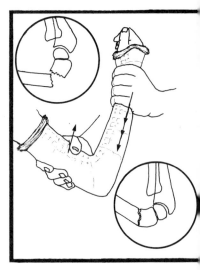

42. *Anterior supracondylar fracture (3)* Continuing the traction (1) the elbow is slowly extended (2), reducing the angulation (3). The arm is put in a plaster back slab in a position of 10° flexion. *This position should not be maintained for more than 3 weeks*. At that stage the elbow should be gently flexed (usually about 70°–80° can be achieved) and supported either with a sling or further slab till union.

43. Anterior supracondylar fracture (4) An alternative technique is to apply wool to the limb (1) and disimpact the distal fragment by direct traction on the epiphyseal complex (2). A plaster cuff (3) is then applied by an assistant and allowed to set. Care must be taken to avoid ridging at the distal end (4).

44. *Anterior supracondylar fracture (5)* The rest of the plaster is quickly applied, and while it is still soft flex to 110° or less and exert pressure on the distal fragment through the forearm: the position is held till the plaster has set. Check radiographs are taken and fixation continued as for a normal supracondylar fracture.

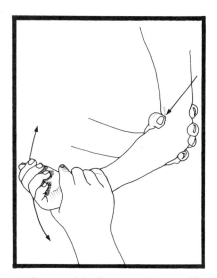

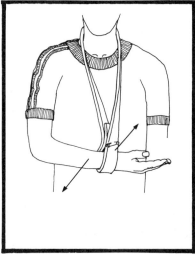

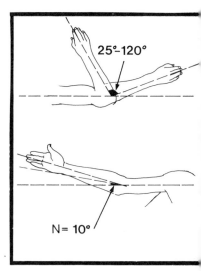

45. *Supracondylar fractures: After care (1)* Assess union about 3–4 weeks for a child of four, and about 4–5 weeks for a child of 8 by radiographs and fracture site tenderness. A further useful test is to place your thumb over the biceps tendon, and then flex and extend the elbow through a total range of 20°. Spasm of the biceps indicates that the elbow is not yet ready for mobilisation.

46. *Supracondylar fractures: After care (2)* Mobilisation may be commenced from a sling (i.e. the arm is removed from the sling for 10 minutes' active exercises 3–4 times per day). The sling is discarded as soon as any discomfort has settled. This procedure may also be used where there is a *little* residual fracture tenderness. Physiotherapy is indicated if after 2 weeks mobilisation there is still gross restriction.

47. *Supracondylar fractures: After care (3)* The range should be recorded at every clinic attendance; physiotherapy can be safely stopped when a range of 25°–120° is reached. (Normal 0°–145°.) On no account should passive movements be allowed, and *the parents* should be warned against this. If any cubitus varus or valgus is present it should be recorded and the child assessed yearly regarding deterioration and the need for corrective osteotomy.

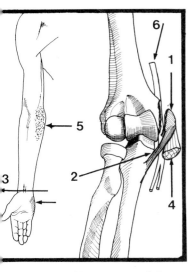

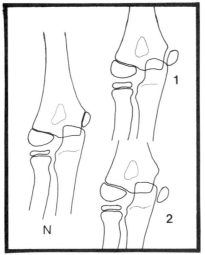

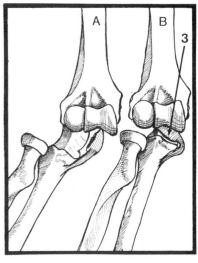

. *Medial epicondylar injuries: Pathology*
The medial epicondyle (1) may be pulled
by the ulnar collateral ligament (2) when
elbow is forcibly abducted (3). It may be
ured by direct violence, and possibly
ulsed by sudden contraction of the
earm flexors which are attached to it (4).
spect if there is medial bruising (5) and
vays test the integrity of the ulnar
rve (6).

49. *Pathology (2)* The most minor degrees of
violence result in slight separation of the
medial epicondylar epiphysis (1).
Comparison films may be helpful in
diagnosis. With greater violence the
epiphysis is separated and displaced slightly
in a distal direction (2). Injuries of these
types may be treated by immobilisation in a
long arm padded plaster for 2–3 weeks.

50. *Pathology (3) The potentially most
serious injury is when the medial epicondyle
is trapped in the elbow joint.* This may
follow dislocation of the elbow (A) which
must always be accompanied by rupture of
the ulnar collateral ligament or avulsion of
the medial epicondyle. In the latter case,
when the elbow is reduced (B), the
epicondyle may be trapped in the joint (3).

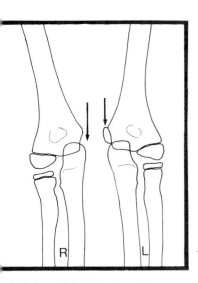

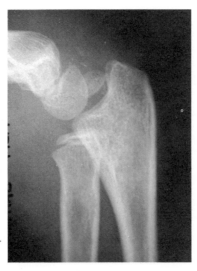

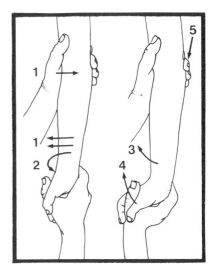

. *Pathology (4)* A further hazard in
agnosis is when the medial epicondyle is
apped in an elbow which has been
omentarily dislocated but has reduced
ontaneously. Note: (1) If the child is over
and the medial epicondylar epiphysis
nnot be seen in the A.P. view, it is
obably in the joint. (2) If there is any
ubt comparison films should be taken.

52. *Pathology (5)* (3) In the normal lateral
projection, the medial epicondyle cannot be
seen: if it can, as in the case here, it is lying
in the joint. The rules are quite clear: (a)
Should the medial epicondyle be visible? (i.e.
what is the child's age.) (b) Does it show in
the A.P. view? (c) Is it visible in the lateral?

53. *Treatment of trapped medial epicondyle
(1)* Removal by manipulation is often
successful. Under general anaesthesia,
increase valgus (1), supinate (2), extend
elbow (3) and jerk wrist into dorsiflexion (4). A finger placed over the medial
side of the elbow (5) may detect the medial
epicondyle slipping out of the joint. (After
care as 49.)

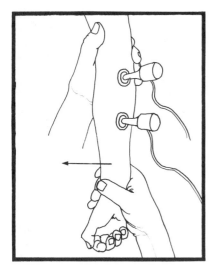

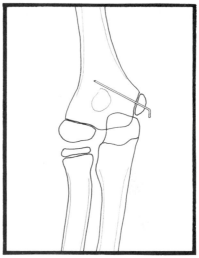

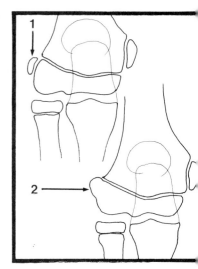

54. Trapped medial epicondyle (2) If the previous method fails, the medial epicondyle may be brought out by electrically stimulating the flexor mass. General anaesthesia is required, the elbow *must* be strongly abducted, and a good muscle contraction must be obtained. The necessary equipment and expertise in its use may be available through the physiotherapy department.

55. Trapped medial epicondyle (3) If both measures fail the medial epicondyle must be extracted through a small antero-medial incision and held in position either by a Kirschner wire (retained for 3 weeks) or soft-tissue suture.

The majority of ulnar nerve palsies found in association with medial epicondylar injuries are lesions of continuity: commencement of recovery can be expected in 3–6 weeks.

56. Lateral epicondylar injuries in children The epiphysis for the lateral epicondyle is inconstant, but usually appears about 11, fusing with the main epiphysis 2–3 years later (1). It may, however, ossify by direct extension from the capitellum (2). Detachment may follow adduction stress: rarely it may become trapped in the joint after a dislocation. Treat as for medial epicondyle.

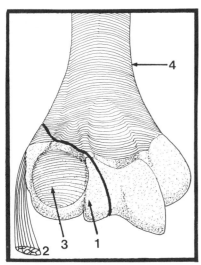

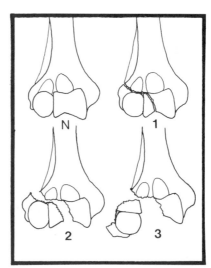

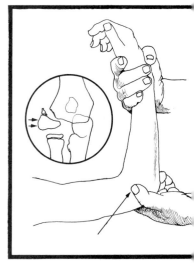

57. Lateral condylar injuries (1) Pathology (1) The common pattern of injury involves the *whole of the capitellum and nearly half the trochlea* (1). This large fragment may be displaced by the forearm extensors (2) or the lateral ligament. As the capitellar epiphysis (3) and the shaft (4) may be the only structures visible on the radiographs, *their relationship may be the only clue to injury*.

58. Lateral condylar injuries (2) Pathology (2) Fractures of the lateral condyle may be (1) undisplaced (2) laterally displaced (3) rotated. *Treatment (1) Undisplaced fractures* should be treated conservatively by a long-arm padded back-shell and sling for 3–4 weeks. As it is important to make sure no late slip occurs *radiographs should be taken at weekly intervals*.

59. Lateral condylar injuries (3) Treatment (2) Where there is slight to moderate lateral shift of the complex, close reduction may be attempted by applying local pressure (under general anaesthesia). reduction is successful, a long arm padded back shell should be applied and retained with a sling for 3–4 weeks. Again it is vital to detect any early slipping by weekly radiographs.

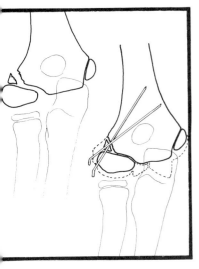

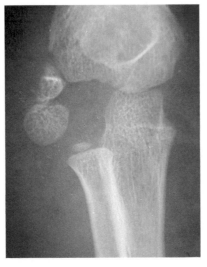

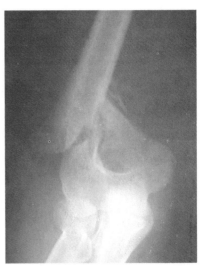

0. *Lateral condylar injuries (4) Treatment (3)* Where there is lateral displacement which is unstable or late ipping occurs, Kirschner wire fixation is dicated. Where image intensification is vailable, it may be possible to do this ithout open operation, but in many cases nis is necessary. Two wires must be used, ollowed by a plaster shell and sling. The vires may be removed after 2–3 weeks and nobilisation commenced at 4 weeks.

61. *Lateral condylar injuries: Treatment (4)* In injuries where there is rotation of the complex such as illustrated here, closed methods are unlikely to give a satisfactory reduction, so that there is risk of non-union, growth disturbance and progressive cubitus valgus. Open reduction and Kirschner wire fixation is therefore indicated. (After care as above.)

62. *Adult fractures: Supracondylar fractures (1)* In adults, the fracture line tends to lie a little more proximal than in children; comminution, obliquity or spiralling and medial or lateral tilting are common. Nevertheless, most may be treated successfully as in children by manipulation and plaster fixation. 6–8 weeks' immobilisation is usually required.

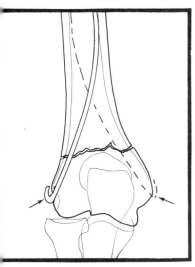

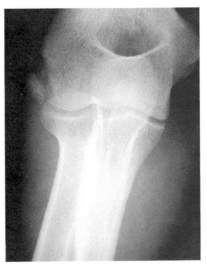

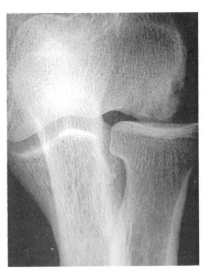

3. *Supracondylar fractures (2)* If instability s a serious problem and a good reduction :annot be obtained or held, open reduction with some form of stabilisation may be required. Wide exposure may run the risk of ost-operative stiffness and myositis ssificans; an alignment device such as a Rush pin(s) along with plaster fixation may give a good result provided there is early nobilisation.

64. *Medial and lateral epicondylar fractures:* Displacement of these fractures is seldom severe and although potential instability of the joint may be present, symptomatic treatment only is usually required. A crepe bandage applied over wool to limit swelling and a sling for 3–4 weeks is usually adequate. A short period in a long arm plaster is indicated if pain is severe.

65. *Fractures of the capitellum (1)* The cartilaginous and bony surfaces of the capitellum may be damaged by force transmitted up the radius from a fall on the outstretched hand, often in association with radial head injuries. There may be late osteochondritis dissecans and osteo-arthritis. *Treatment:* Initially symptomatic: later, excise loose bodies and drill the capitellum to encourage re-vascularisation.

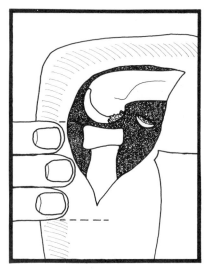

66. *Fractures of the capitellum (2)* A small flake may be detached from the capitellum as a result of force transmitted up the radius; it may come to lie in the front of the joint. It should be treated as a loose body and excised. This may be carried out safely through a small lateral incision (which must not extend as far as three finger breadths below the joint line to avoid damage to the posterior interosseous nerve).

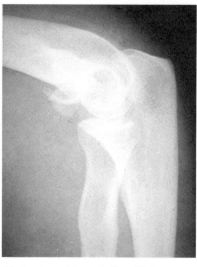

67. *Fracture of the capitellum (3)* A more serious fracture involves the major portion of the anterior half of the articular surface of the capitellum. Generally the corresponding part of the trochlea is involved. Severe disability will result if this is not accurately reduced, and generally exposure through an anterior approach will be necessary. Smillie pins may be used for fixation.

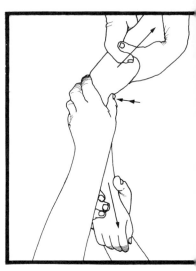

68. *Fractures of the capitellum (4)* Occasionally reduction may be achieved by pressure over the fragment while traction is applied to the arm. An imperfect reduction should not be accepted. After reduction, a long arm padded plaster should be retained for approximately 5 weeks before commencement of mobilisation.

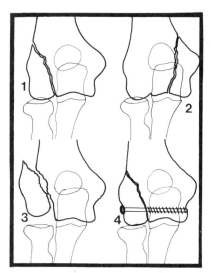

69. *Fracture of a single condyle (1)* Fracture of the lateral condyle (1) or medial condyle (2) may be caused by the same mechanisms responsible for the more severe Y-fractures. Displacement may be slight or marked (3). Where displacement is marked, best results are generally obtained by open reduction and cross screwing (4).

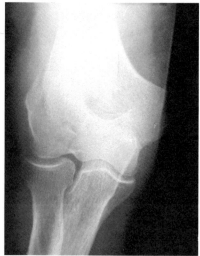

70. *Fracture of a single condyle (2)* If displacement is minimal, as illustrated, or the patient elderly and frail, apply a long arm plaster (over wool) and a sling. The plaster may usually be discarded safely after 4–5 weeks, and mobilisation commenced from the sling. Physiotherapy may be started shortly thereafter.

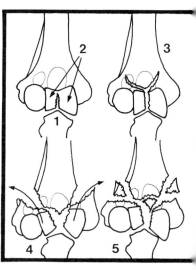

71. *Intercondylar, Y or T fracture (1)* This potentially serious injury is caused by the coronoid (1) being driven like a wedge between the two halves of the trochlea (2), often by a fall or blow on the elbow. The vertical split bifurcates (3) and with further violence the two main fragments may part and rotate (4). Comminution (5) is often a further problem.

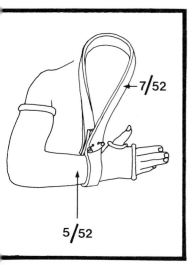

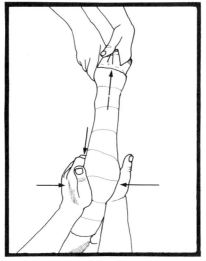

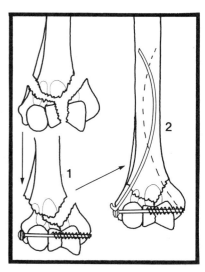

. *Intercondylar fracture (2)* Many riations of these fractures occur, and eatment is often difficult. If there is no wide paration of the fragments, or if there is oderate displacement and the patient frail, ply a long arm plaster over wool. This ould be discarded as soon as possible for obilisation (which may be started from the ng). Physiotherapy is essential.

73. *Intercondylar fractures (3)* If there is separation of the fragments and comminution, *surgery should not be attempted* (often impossibly difficult with risks of insurmountable post-operative stiffness). Instead apply a long arm plaster over copious wool: before the plaster sets apply traction and at the same time compress the main fragments together with the heels of the hands. (After care as above.)

74. *Intercondylar fractures (4)* Where there is no comminution, the two main fragments may be opposed with a cross-screw (1). This converts the injury into the equivalent of a supracondylar fracture. Thereafter, if required, further alignment may be achieved with a Rush pin(s) or similar device (2). External plaster fixation will also be required: again, early mobilisation is essential.

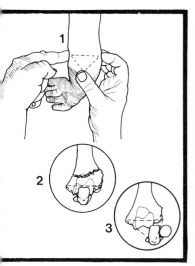

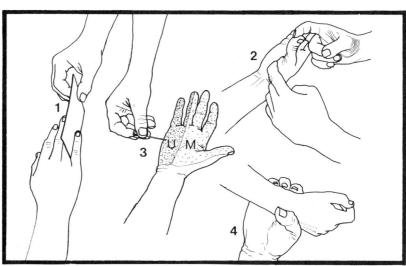

. *Dislocation of the elbow (1)* Dislocation the elbow is common both in children and ults and generally results from a fall on e outstretched hand. It is sometimes nfused with a supracondylar fracture. The o may be distinguished clinically by arching for the equilateral triangle formed the olecranon and epicondyles (1). This is disturbed in supracondylar fractures (2) t distorted in elbow dislocations (3).

76. *Dislocation of the elbow (2)* Damage to the ulnar nerve, median nerve or brachial artery is uncommon, but nevertheless should always be sought.

A number of motor tests may be used to assess function in both nerves. *In the case of the ulnar nerve* the ability to grip a sheet of paper between the ring and little finger (1) may be used to assess good interosseous muscle function. It is important that the fingers are not allowed to flex at the M.P. joints. *In the case of the median nerve* contraction and power in abductor pollicis may be assessed by feeling the muscle (2) while the patient attempts to resist the thumb being pressed from a vertical position into the plane of the palm. Sensory function in the areas supplied by the median and ulnar nerves should also be quickly tested (3). *In the case of the brachial artery* the quickest assessment is of course by identification of the radial pulse (4).

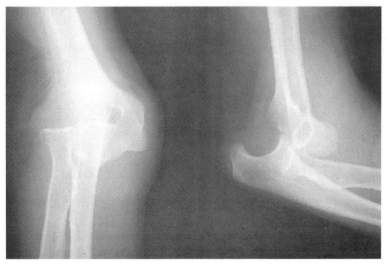

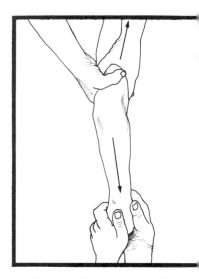

77. *Radiographs:* These radiographs show a typical dislocation of the elbow. Note how the radius and ulna are displaced posteriorly and laterally relative to the humerus. This is by far the commonest displacement ('postero-lateral dislocation of the elbow'). Fractures accompanying dislocation of the elbow are comparatively uncommon. Nevertheless, in adults in particular, fractures of the coronoid process and of the radial head should be looked for. In children, the epicondyles or the lateral condyle may be involved.

78. *Treatment (1)* Reduction should be carried out under general anaesthesia. A fair amount of force is often required, although the use of a muscle relaxant will reduce thi Apply strong traction in the line of the lim and if necessary slightly flex the elbow whi maintaining traction. Success is usually accompanied with a characteristic reductio 'clunk'.

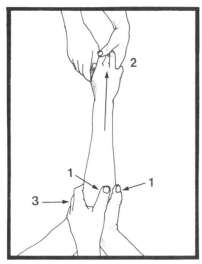

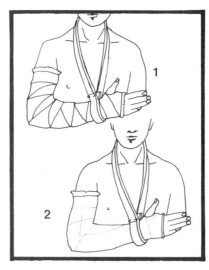

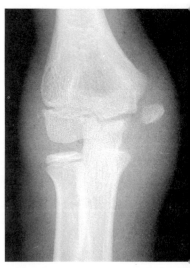

79. *Treatment (2)* If the last manoeuvre is not successful, clasp the humerus from behind and push the olecranon forwards (and medially) (1) while an assistant applies traction in the moderately flexed position (2). (The fingers apply counter-traction (3).) Check radiographs should always be taken.

80. *Treatment (3)* If a good reduction has been obtained, a padded crepe bandage may be applied and worn with a sling for a minimum of two weeks (1). Alternatively, a plaster back slab with the elbow in 90° flexion may be used with a sling (2). Too early or too vigorous mobilisation runs the risks of myositis ossificans, and passive movements must be avoided.

81. *Associated injuries:* (1) In children, the medial epicondylar epiphysis may be detached. *On reduction of the elbow,* it will generally be restored to an acceptable position (1 or 2 as in *49*) (2 ill.). A plaster slab and a sling are advised for 4 weeks. (2) *The medial epicondyle may be retained in the joint:* this must always be excluded (see 48 et seq.).

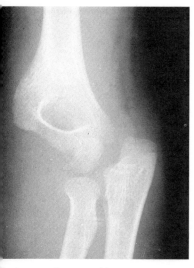

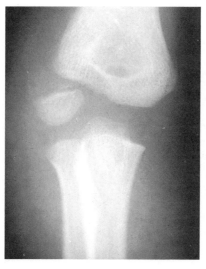

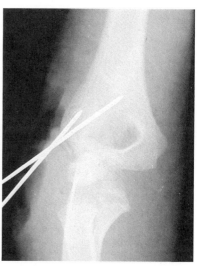

2. *Associated injuries:* (3) *Lateral condylar jury:* Note the following points. (a) The pitellar epiphysis (along with half the rtilaginous trochlea) has been carried edially by the radius, and is slightly tated. (b) The medial epicondylar iphysis has just appeared and is not splaced. (c) The unusual *medial* slocation of the elbow.

83. *Associated injuries: Lateral condylar injuries ctd.* The preceding injury was treated by manipulative reduction; the lateral condylar complex remained displaced. (Reduction could be achieved by firm local pressure, but displacement occurred in this unstable injury as soon as pressure was released.)

84. *Associated injuries: Lateral condylar injuries ctd.* Open reduction was therefore carried out and the condylar mass held in position with two Kirschner wires. Note how these pass through the cartilaginous epicondylar region. Note the small bone fragment from the shaft (Salter/Harris Type 2 injury). Fixation was complimented by a long arm plaster back shell for 4 weeks.

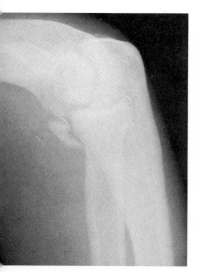

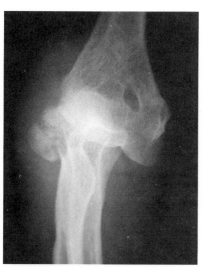

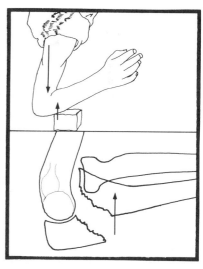

. *Associated injuries:* (4) *Fracture of the* *ronoid:* Small fractures of the coronoid .) may be unimportant, but certainly with rge fragments there is risk of recurrent slocation of the elbow (rare). Two extra ecautions are advised: (i) Plaster fixation r 6 weeks before mobilisation. (ii) Weekly diographs to detect any early subluxation. tablished recurrent dislocation may be ated by bone block reconstruction of the ronoid or repair of the capsule and medial ament.

86. *Associated injuries:* (5) *Fracture of the radial head* (a) If there is a highly comminuted fracture of the radial head (ill.) reduce the elbow dislocation and *delay excision of the radial head for at least 4 weeks* to lessen the risks of myositis ossificans. (b) Minor fractures of the radial head should not affect treatment.
(c) Fracture of the radial neck: reduce the elbow and proceed as for this injury (115).

87. *Anterior dislocation of the elbow (1)* This is an uncommon injury, but may follow a fall on the elbow which results in the forearm bones being pushed forwards. For dislocation to occur, the olecranon must fracture, and this becomes a potentially very unstable injury.

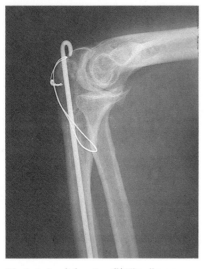

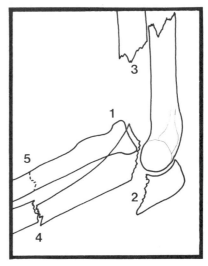

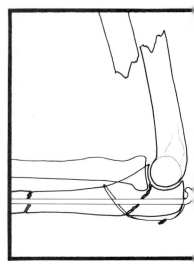

88. *Anterior dislocation (2)* The elbow may be reduced by applying traction and extending the joint. If the reduction is stable, it may then be treated by plaster fixation for a limited period in extension as in an anterior supracondylar fracture. Nevertheless, there is appreciable risk of late subluxation and difficulty in elbow mobilisation, so that on the whole, internal fixation is recommended for this injury (ill.).

89. *Anterior dislocation (3)* A more complex form of anterior dislocation is seen in the side swipe injury ('baby car fracture'). This occurs when a driver rests his elbow on his car's window ledge, and he is struck by a passing vehicle. Typically the elements of this injury include (1) anterior dislocation of the elbow with fractures of (2) the olecranon (3) the humerus (4) the ulna and sometimes (5) the radius.

90. *Anterior dislocation (4)* It is vital to reduce the dislocation immediately, and thi may be held by immediate internal fixation (ill.) or plaster fixation in extension for 2–3 weeks prior to delayed internal fixation of the olecranon. The other injuries may be treated with less urgency conservatively or surgically. It is not often possible or wise to attempt immediate fixation of all the elements of this severe injury.

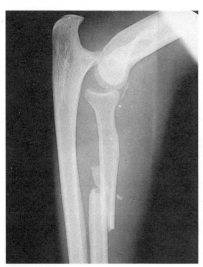

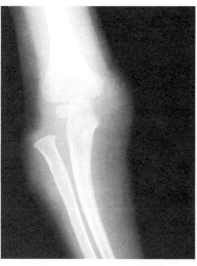

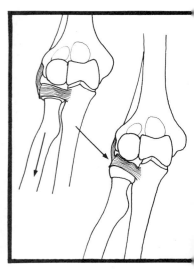

91. *Isolated dislocation of the ulna:* Dislocation of the ulna may occur in association with a fracture of the radial shaft. As such fractures may be quite distal, it is important that adequate radiographs of the forearm are taken. This double injury may be treated by manipulative reduction of the elbow followed by a long arm plaster until union of the radius (assuming a satisfactory reduction). Alternatively, internal fixation of the radius may permit earlier mobilisation.

92. *Isolated dislocation of the radius:* Lateral, anterior or posterior dislocation of the proximal end of the radius is almost invariably part of a Monteggia lesion (but see also forearm injuries) sometimes concealed because the ulnar fracture is of greenstick pattern (ill.). Great care must be taken in the assessment and treatment of these injuries which is dealt with separately. (See Monteggia fracture dislocations.)

93. *Pulled elbow (1)* This condition is due t the radial head stretching the orbicular (annular) ligament and slipping out from under its cover. It occurs in children in the 2–6 age group, and is normally caused by parent suddenly pulling on the child's arm (e.g. to prevent it running on to a road). It also said to occur in wrestlers.

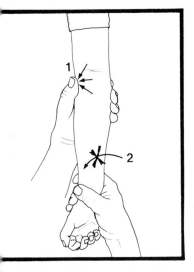

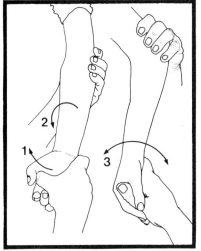

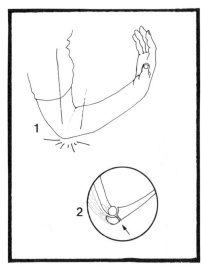

. *Pulled elbow (2) Diagnosis:* In addition
having the appropriate history of sudden
action on the arm, the child will be found
be fretful. There is tenderness over the
teral aspect of the joint (1), and supination
limited (2). Radiographs are usually
rmal, there being seldom any detectable
crease in the radio-humeral joint space
en with comparison films.

95. *Pulled elbow (3) Treatment:* In most
cases reduction can be achieved by either
(a) placing the wrist in full radial
deviation (1) and forcibly supinating the
arm (2) or (b) rapidly alternately pronating
and supinating the forearm (3).

If these measures fail, the arm should be
rested in a sling, when spontaneous
reduction usually occurs within 48 hours.

96. *Fractures of the olecranon (1)* The
olecranon may be fractured as a result of a
fall on the point of the elbow (1). Such
fractures may be displaced as a result of
triceps contraction (2). The olecranon may
also be fractured as a direct result of triceps
contraction.

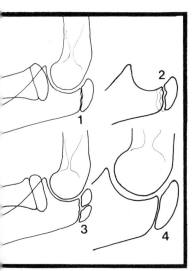

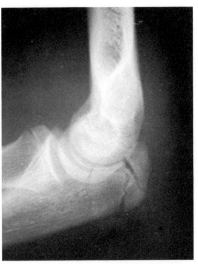

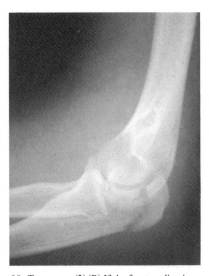

7. *Fracture of the olecranon (2)* Diagnosis
usually straightforward, but beware of the
llowing fallacies: (1) the normal epiphyseal
ne (2) duplication of the normal line due to
bliquity of the projection (3) normal bifid
ecranon epiphysis (the epiphyses appear
etween the ages of 8 and 11 and fuse at 14
ears) (4) patella cubiti, due to ossification in
e triceps tendon (note rounded edges).

98. *Treatment (1)* (A) *If the fracture is hair-
line and undisplaced,* it may be treated by
*immobilisation of the arm in a long arm
plaster* (3–4 weeks in a child, 6–8 weeks in
an adult). Note in the radiograph the three
lines running through the olecranon: the
most distal is a fracture; the middle, the
epiphyseal line; the most proximal either a
bifid epiphysis or a fracture of the epiphysis
(differentiate by looking for tenderness).

99. *Treatment (2)* (B) If the fracture line is
pronounced, but still undisplaced, it may be
treated in the same way, but radiographs
should be taken at weekly intervals during
the first 3 weeks in case of (unlikely) late
displacement.

(C) Minor epiphyseal separations may
also be treated conservatively in a similar
manner.

(D) Slight to moderate displacement may
be accepted in the frail elderly.

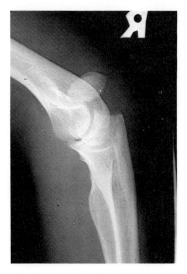

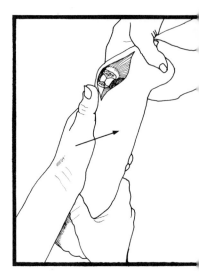

100. *Treatment (3)* (E) In the young adult, where the olecranon fragment is small (a third or less of the articular surface) and significantly displaced (by triceps pull) surgical excision gives excellent results. *Operation:* The operation is performed under a general anaesthetic using a pneumatic tourniquet to obtain a clear bloodless field. The fragment is exposed through a vertical posterior incision and excised. The tear in the triceps insertion is then carefully repaired with horizontal mattress sutures and the wound closed in layers. A pressure bandage (crepe over wool) and a collar and cuff sling are applied (or a plaster back shell and sling may be employed). The elbow may be mobilised after 2 weeks.

101. *Treatment (4)* If there is any doubt regarding the stability of the elbow (i.e. if the olecranon fragment is fairly substantial) this should be tested on the table by attempting to produce an anterior dislocation with the elbow flexed at 90°. If the elbow can in any way be subluxed, the olecranon must be retained.

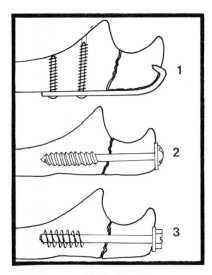

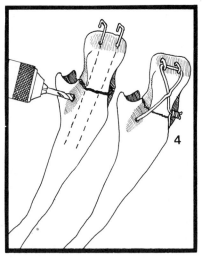

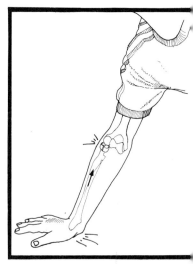

102. *Treatment (5)* (F) If the olecranon fragment is substantial it must be reduced and held by some form of internal fixation. The methods available include (1) a Zuelzer hooked plate and screws (2) a Croll olecranon screw (3) a lag screw. During the final tightening of a Croll or lag screw it is important to check that elbow movements are not prevented by a calliper-like action.

103. *Treatment (6)* (4) Tension band wiring: the Kirschner wires control alignment and rotation, which the stainless steel wire when twisted compresses the fragments together. The ends of the Kirschner wires are bent over and hammered home. A Rush pin may be used instead. The security of fixation dictates the need for any external fixation and when mobilisation may be safely commenced.

104. *Fractures of the radial head: Mechanics of injury (1)* Although the radial head may be fractured by direct violence, such as a fall or blow on the side of the elbow, injury frequently results from indirect violence. (ill.) A fall on the outstretched hand results in force being transmitted up the radius, with the radial head striking the capitellum (capitulum).

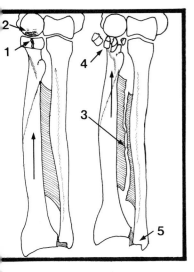

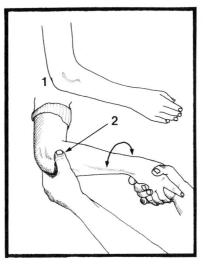

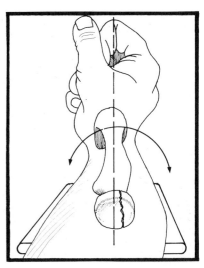

105. *Mechanics of injury (2)* The radial head fractures (1) but may also damage the articular surface of the capitellum (2) prolonging recovery. In some cases, where violence is severe, the interosseous membrane tears (3) severe comminution of the head occurs (4) and there is *subluxation of the distal end of the ulna (5)* due to proximal migration of the radial shaft. (Essex-Lopresti fracture-dislocation.)

106. *Diagnosis (1)* There is complaint of pain in the elbow and there may be local bruising and swelling (1). In *minor fractures*, tenderness may not be apparent until the damaged portion of the head is rotated under the examining thumb (gently pronate and supinate while palpating the radial head) (2). The range of pronation and supination is often full, but elbow *extension* is usually restricted.

107. *Diagnosis (2) Radiographs:* Most radial head fractures will show in the standard lateral and (supination) A.P. projections, but if there is clinical evidence of fracture and negative radiographs, *additional* A.P. projections should be taken in the mid prone and full pronation positions, so that all portions of the radial head will be visualised in profile.

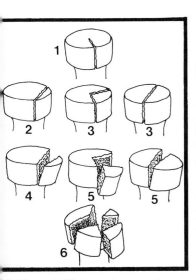

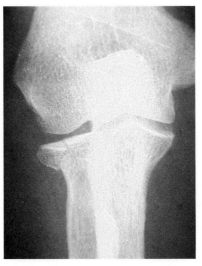

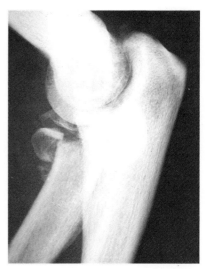

108. *Diagnosis (3)* Assess the type and severity of the fracture from the radiographs.
(1) Hairline (2) Undisplaced marginal
(3) Undisplaced segmental (2 types)
(4) Displaced marginal (5) Displaced segmental (6) Comminuted.
Always examine the forearm and wrist to exclude an Essex-Lopresti fracture-dislocation.

109. *Treatment (1)* Non-displaced fractures (1–3) should be treated with a light compression bandage and a sling before mobilisation from the sling is commenced after 2–3 weeks. The sling alone may be worn for a further 2 weeks. If pain is very severe initially, a plaster back slab may be used. An excellent outcome is usual, but note that many months may elapse before full *extension* is regained.

110. *Treatment (2)* Severely comminuted fractures (6) should be treated by immediate excision of the radial head. This may be carried out through a lateral incision (see 66) with care to avoid the posterior interosseous nerve. All fragments must be removed. The arm is then rested in a sling for 2–3 weeks before mobilisation.

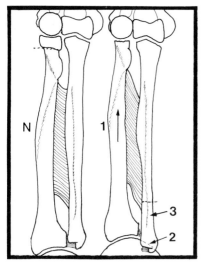

111. *Treatment (3)* Sometimes excision of the radial head is followed by proximal drift of the radius (1) so that the distal end of the ulna becomes prominent and painful (2). This in turn may be treated by excision of the distal end of the ulna, albeit with some weakening of the grip. Proximal drift is a feature of the Essex-Lopresti lesion, and may be minimised by delaying radial head excision for 6 weeks. In either case, prosthetic replacement is sometimes undertaken.

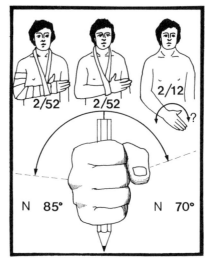

112. *Treatment (4)* Displaced marginal and segmental fractures (4 and 5) should be treated conservatively and re-assessed after 2–3 months. If pronation, supination and extension are severely restricted, *late excision* of the radial head should be considered. *Note well:* In any case of fracture, excision of the radial head should be performed *either* within the first 48 hours *or* after union (between carries the risk of myositis ossificans). *Late diagnosed injuries should be left till union.*

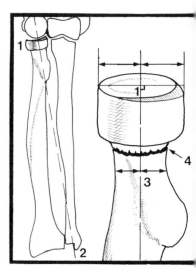

113. *Fractures of the radial neck (1)* The axis of rotation of the radio-ulnar joints passes through the centre of the radial head (1) and the attachment of the triangular fibrocartilage (2). The axis passes through the centre of the neck (3) and lies at right angles to the plane of the head. Fractures through the neck (4) have the potential to disturb this relationship between the head and the neck.

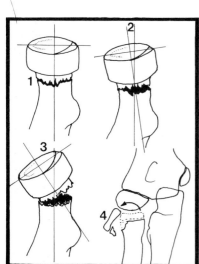

114. *Fractures of the radial neck (2)* Fractures of the radial neck may result from the same mechanisms as those causing fractures of the radial head, and diagnosis is also similar. Patterns: The fractures may be hair-line and undisplaced (1) or result in slight (2) or gross tilting (3). In children, the epiphysis of the head may be completely separated and widely displaced (4).

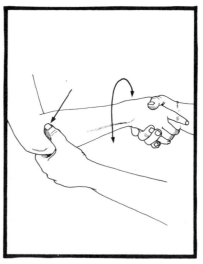

115. *Treatment* (a) With slight or no tilting (1 and 2) and up to 30° in children treat conservatively (as 109). (b) With marked tilting (3) (20° or more in adults) manipulate; do so by applying traction and gently pronate and supinate, feeling for the prominent part of the radial head to present: then apply pressure when the head is at its zenith. (Thereafter treat as 109.) Open reduction is indicated if closed methods fail.

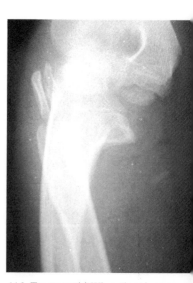

116. *Treatment* (c) Where there is gross epiphyseal displacement, operative reduction is indicated. On reduction, the fragments may be found to lock in a stable position. If not, a Kirschner wire may be used for 2–3 weeks to achieve stability.

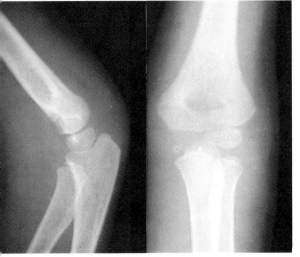

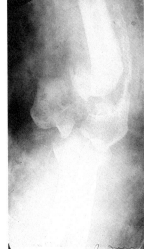

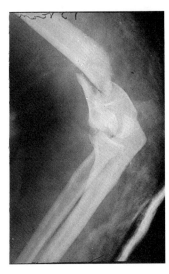

7. Diagnose and suggest treatment.

118. What is this injury? Comment on the position.

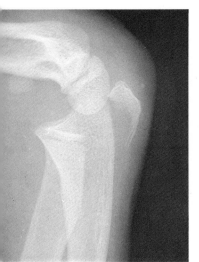

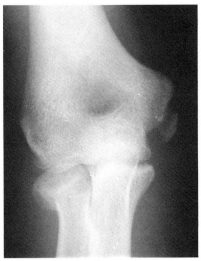

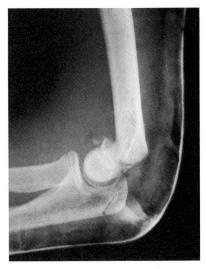

9. Diagnose and suggest treatment.

120. Comment on this A.P. radiograph of the elbow. What force has been responsible for the injury?

121. Comment on this supracondylar fracture which has been manipulated and put in plaster.

117. The radiographs show an undisplaced supracondylar fracture of the humerus in a child. Assuming there were no circulatory problems, a collar and cuff sling under the clothes should suffice for initial treatment.

118. T or Y-fracture of the humerus. Although the position on the lateral projection is good, there is still considerable separation of the two distal components and re-manipulation with side-to-side compression might lead to improvement in the position. The degree of comminution is a factor against open reduction.

119. Dislocation of the elbow with fracture of the olecranon. The elbow should be reduced and check radiographs taken. Moderate residual displacement of the olecranon should be accepted and it is unlikely that open reduction would be required. Note that the ossification centres for the olecranon have not yet appeared and this really represents a Salter/Harris type 2 injury.

120. There is a double injury—avulsion of the medial epicondyle and fracture of the radial neck, almost certainly both due to an abduction (valgus) injury.

121. This has been an anterior supracondylar fracture and the reduction is unacceptable.

8. Injuries to the forearm bones

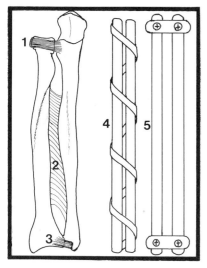

1. *Anatomical features:* The radius and ulna are bound together by (1) the annular (orbicular) ligament (2) the interosseous membrane (3) the radio-ulnar ligaments and the triangular fibro-cartilage. This gives the radius and ulna some of the features of (4) a bundle of sticks and of (5) a linked parallelogram.

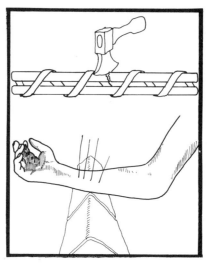

2. *Direct violence:* With direct violence it is possible to fracture either of the forearm bones in isolation. These injuries are comparatively uncommon, but do occur, especially in the ulna when in a fall the shaft strikes a hard edge. They may also occur when the ulna is struck by a weapon as the victim attempts to protect his head with his arms.

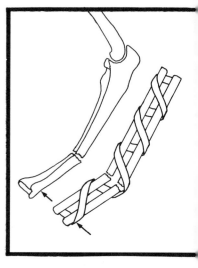

3. *Indirect violence:* More commonly the forearm is injured as the result of indirect violence, such as a fall on the back or the front of the outstretched hand. The force of impact on the hand stresses the forearm bones: the most common occurrence is for both to fracture.

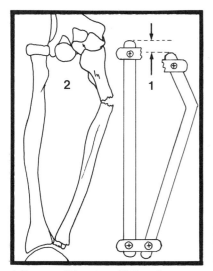

4. *Fracture dislocations (1)* If *one* forearm bone is seen to be fractured and angled, it has inevitably become relatively shorter (1). If its attachments to the wrist and humerus are intact, the other forearm bone *must* be dislocated. The commonest fracture-dislocation of this type is a fracture of the ulna with a dislocation of the radial head. (Monteggia injury) (2).

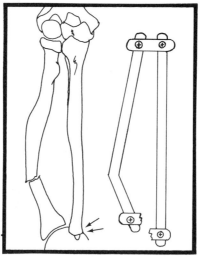

5. *Fracture dislocation (2)* The same pattern of injury occurs in the Galeazzi fracture-dislocation when a dislocation of the distal ulna accompanies a shaft fracture of the radius. *Never accept a single forearm bone fracture as an entity until a Monteggia or Galeazzi injury has been eliminated.*

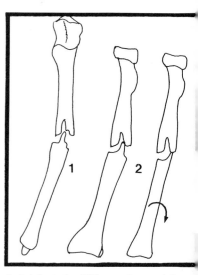

6. *Axial rotation (1)* In any forearm injury, when the ulna fractures it may angulate or displace like any other bone (1). When the radius fractures, however, *in addition* to angulation one fragment may rotate relative to the other (axial rotation) (2).

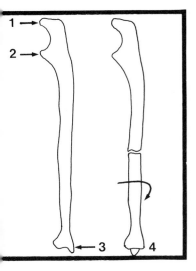

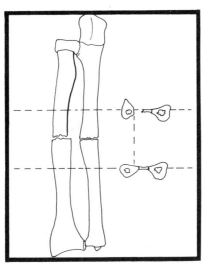

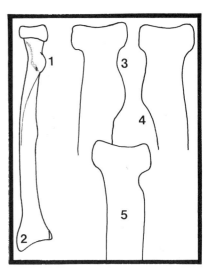

Axial rotation (2) Axial rotation of the ulna is rare, but always check to see that it is not present. To do so, note that in the lateral projection the olecranon (1) coronoid (2) and styloid process (3) should be clearly visible. This relationship is lost in the presence of axial rotation (4).

8. *Axial rotation (3)* In the case of the radius, note any discrepancy in the widths of the fragments at fracture level. A difference as illustrated indicates the presence of axial rotation.

9. *Axial rotation (4)* Note also the normal relationship between the radial tubercle (1) and the styloid process (2) in this A-P view of the radius in full supination. In *full supination* the radial tubercle lies *medially* (3). In *pronation* it lies *laterally* (4). In the mid position it is concealed (5). The position of the radial styloid should always correspond.

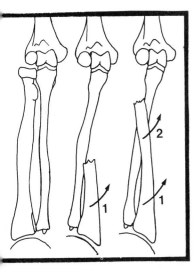

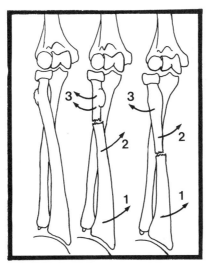

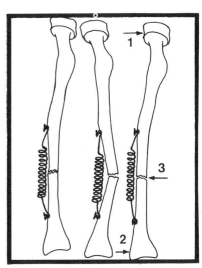

10. *Axial rotation (5) Forces responsible (a)* In all radial shaft fractures, pronator quadratus tends to pronate the distal fragment (1). In all upper (proximal) third fractures, pronator teres helps to pronate the distal fragment (2), assisting pronator quadratus in this movement.

11. *Axial rotation (6) Forces responsible (b)* In upper third fractures, the proximal fragment is fully supinated by biceps (3) while the distal fragment is fully pronated by pronators teres and quadratus (1, 2), (i.e. there is a maximal tendency to axial rotation). In fractures distal to the mid third, biceps is opposed, so the proximal fragment tends to lie in the mid position.

12. *Fracture slipping (1) Greenstick fractures:* In children's greenstick fractures any intact periosteum on the original concave surface of the fracture exerts a constant, springy force which may cause recurrence of angulation if the plaster slackens, impairing 3-point fixation. *Frequent check films may be essential in any conservatively treated fracture.*

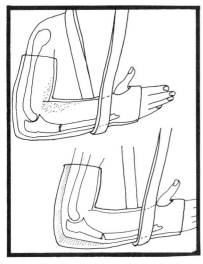

13. *Fracture slipping (2)* Another contributory cause of fracture slipping is when muscle wasting occurs in a patient in a full arm plaster wearing a collar and cuff sling. Loss of brachialis and brachio-radialis bulk leads to plaster slackening and angulatory deformity. (Note soft tissue shadow 26.) *Patients with conservatively treated fractures should be given broad-arm slings.*

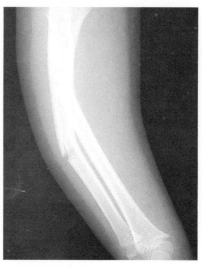

14. *Fracture of both bones of the forearm in children: Patterns (1)* Most fractures are greenstick in pattern as illustrated. The radiographs show fractures of the radius and ulna in the middle thirds. The distal fragments are tilted anteriorly (posterior angulation) but there is no displacement. An extensive, intact posterior hinge can be assumed and reduction of such a fracture involves correction of the angulation only.

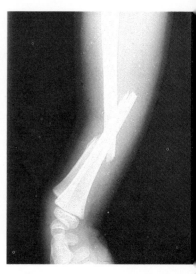

15. *Patterns (2)* When there is off-ending of one or both bones there is potential instability. Shortening and angulation are more likely, and axial rotation may occur; reduction may therefore be more difficult.

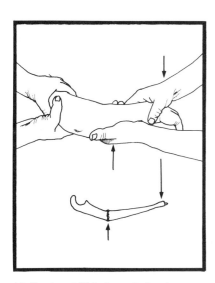

16. *Treatment (1)* In the undisplaced angulated greenstick fracture, the child should be given a general anaesthetic and the angulation corrected. One hand applies a little traction and the corrective force, while the other acts as a fulcrum under the fracture.

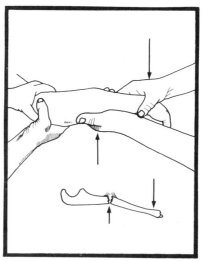

17. *Treatment (2)* If the fracture is over-corrected, the periosteum on the initially concave side of the fracture will be felt to snap. This will immediately give the fracture more mobility: this has the advantage of reducing the risks of late angulation, but has the disadvantage of requiring greater care with respect to the initial positioning in plaster.

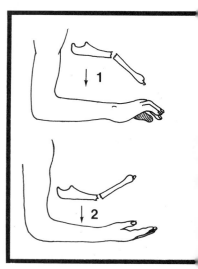

18. *Treatment (3)* In the undisplaced greenstick fracture where there is no axial rotation (torsional deformity) of any of the fragments, the position of the forearm is important in preventing re-angulation while in plaster. *Fractures with posterior tilting* (anterior angulation) (1) should be placed in full pronation. *The commonest fractures with anterior tilting* (posterior angulation) (2) should be placed in full supination.

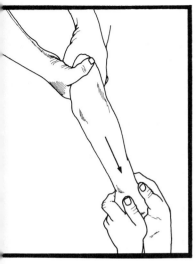

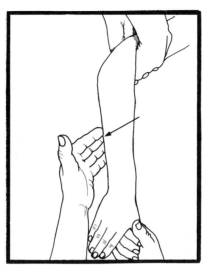

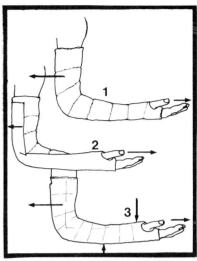

9. *Treatment (4) Displaced fractures:* When the fracture is displaced, axial rotation of the fragments should be looked for and the appropriate position in the pronation/supination range evaluated. The forearm is then placed in that position, and strong traction is applied for a quarter of a minute or so, with the patient well relaxed under a general anaesthetic. The elbow is flexed at a right angle for counter traction.

20. *Treatment (5) Displaced fractures ctd.:* Assessment of reduction is difficult, but often residual displacement may be detected by feeling the subcutaneous surface of the ulna in the region of the fracture. In the difficult case it is sometimes possible to gain bony apposition by applying traction and *increasing* the deformity before finally correcting it. Only rarely is open reduction and internal fixation indicated.

21. *Treatment (6) Fixation:* To lessen the risks of ischaemia, apply a plaster back shell (rather than a complete plaster). Try to maintain traction while this is done. Wool (1) is followed by the shell (2), held by cotton bandages. Just before the plaster sets, give it a final corrective moulding (3). (Posterior angulation fracture illustrated.) Check radiographs should be reviewed before discontinuing the anaesthetic.

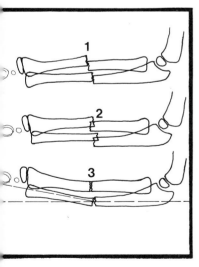

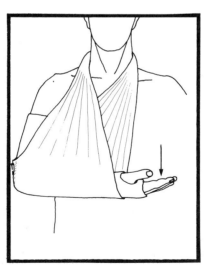

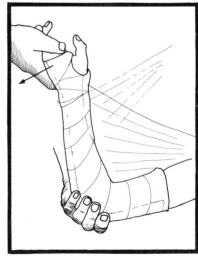

22. *Radiographs:* (1) Persistent displacement without angulation may be readily accepted. (2) Complete off-ending without angulation: re-manipulate, but accept if no improvement can be gained. Careful surveillance to detect early angulation is essential. (3) Slight angulation (10° or less) while undesirable *will* correct with remodelling in the younger child, and should be accepted. Marked angulation requires re-manipulation.

23. *Treatment (7)* A broad arm sling, keeping the arm well elevated, should be employed, and the fingers exposed. If there is much swelling, or the reduction has been difficult, the patient should be admitted for elevation of the arm and circulatory observation: otherwise the child must be seen within 24 hours of the application of the plaster and the parents given the usual warnings.

24. *Treatment (8)* On review, the fingers should be checked for swelling, colour and active movements. If there is some doubt, slowly and gently extend the fingers—if this produces excessive pain, it is suggestive of ischaemia. If ischaemia is present, the encircling bandages must be split and the situation carefully re-assessed after a short interval. If the circulation is perfect, the plaster may be completed.

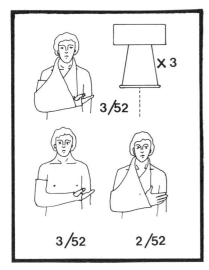

25. *Treatment (9)* In the unstable injury, check the plaster and the position of the fracture at weekly intervals for 3–4 weeks; if satisfactory, the sling may then be discarded. The plaster is maintained till union (usually after a further 3–4 weeks in a child of 10, and a further 1–2 weeks in a child of 4). In stable injuries, fortnightly checks will usually suffice. Mobilisation may be commenced from a sling.

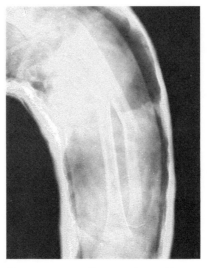

26. *Management of late angulation (1)* (Detected by progress radiographs) (1) Slight angulation of up to 10° may be accepted, especially under the age of 10, but a slack plaster must be changed to prevent *further* angulation. (2) Where angulation is more severe and has been detected before callus has appeared (ill.) the plaster should be changed under general anaesthesia and the angulation corrected by manipulation.

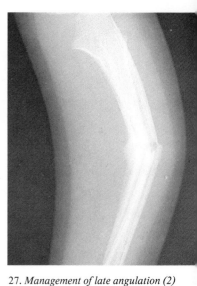

27. *Management of late angulation (2)* (3) In a young child, if callus has appeared, accept any angulation unless gross (20° or more).
(4) In the older child, say 10 or over, if angulation is marked, re-manipulation should be considered even in the presence of callus (ill.), as the powers of re-modelling are less good. Union after re-manipulation is usually rapid.

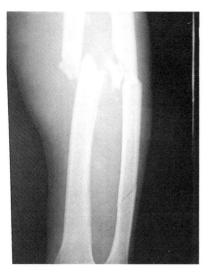

28. *Adult fractures:* Displacement is often marked (ill.), rotational deformities frequently occur, reduction is difficult, and late recurrence of deformity if treated in plaster is common. Consequently in the fit adult who suffers displaced fractures of the forearm bones, open reduction and internal fixation is now almost routine.

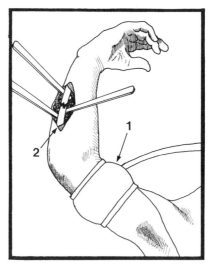

29. *Treatment (1)* The operation is performed under a tourniquet (1). The ulna is subcutaneous along its posterior border; a longitudinal posterior incision, followed by exposure and cleaning of the bone ends, usually permits easy reduction (2). Plating is usually carried out to stabilise the fracture; intramedullary nailing may not always control any (slight) tendency to axial rotation.

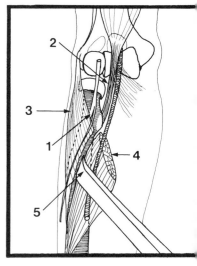

30. *Treatment (2)* Unless the radial fracture is in the distal third, a formal (Henry) exposure is required to avoid damage to the posterior interosseous nerve (1). The biceps tendon (2) is followed down to the tubercle, and the plane between the supinator (3) and the pronator teres (4) located. The supinator is reflected laterally (5) carrying the nerve away from danger. The rest of the shaft may then be exposed safely for reduction and plating.

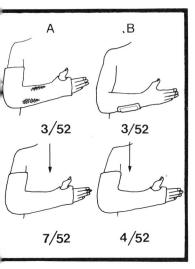

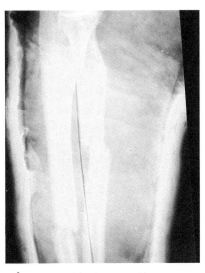

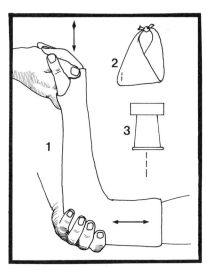

1. *Treatment (3)* Post-operatively, (A) plaster fixation is maintained till union occurs (circa 10 weeks) with a plaster change for removal of stitches. (B) If internal fixation is strong, after a few days with a crepe support the arm may be mobilised fully and a plaster support provided for a short period after discharge from hospital. (C) In some cases, no external support may be required.

32. *Treatment (4)* It is reasonable to treat fractures of the forearm bones in the adult conservatively (ill.) (a) if the fractures are undisplaced (b) in the elderly, or in the patient suffering from multiple injuries where the duration of anaesthesia required for open reduction and internal fixation is considered hazardous. If manipulation is required, proceed as 19, with attention to axial rotation.

33. *Treatment (5)* If internal fixation is not employed, the following precautions must be taken. (1) The plaster should be checked weekly for slackness, and changed if necessary. (A complete plaster, applied over wool, should be used in an adult.) (2) Only a broad arm sling should be used. (3) Weekly radiographs are necessary to detect and allow correction of early slipping.

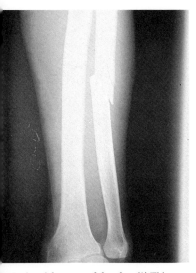

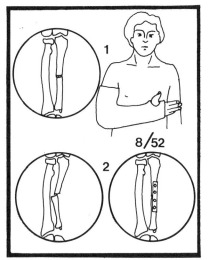

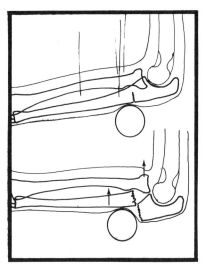

4. *Isolated fracture of the ulna (1)* This injury may result from direct violence (e.g. in warding off a blow from a stick or falling object, or by striking the arm against the sharp edge of, for example, a machine or a step). In all cases, however, the *whole* of the radial shaft should be visualised to exclude in particular an associated dislocation of the radial head.

35. *Isolated fracture of the ulna (2)* Treatment: Displacement is generally slight, and if this is the case, a long arm plaster should be applied with the hand in mid pronation (1). Beware of late slipping. The plaster is retained until union is advancing (usually about 8 weeks). If angulation is marked, then open reduction and internal fixation will have to be considered (2).

36. *The Monteggia fracture dislocation and related injuries: Mechanisms (1)* Severe angulation of a forearm bone is normally accompanied by fracture or dislocation of the other (see 4). In the Monteggia fracture-dislocation, fracture of the ulna is associated with dislocation of the radial head. The most easily understood mechanism is when a violent fall or blow on the arm fractures the ulna and displaces the radial head anteriorly.

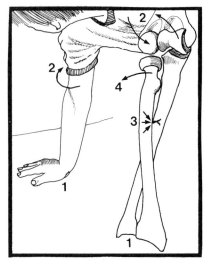

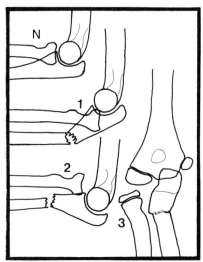

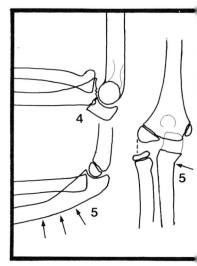

37. *Mechanisms (2)* More commonly the injury results from forced pronation. A fall on the outstretched, fully pronated arm (1) is followed by further pronation as the trunk continues to turn over the fixed hand (2). The radius is forced against the ulna, fracturing it (3) and in turn is levered away from the capitellum (4). Rarely the radial head may dislocate without damage to the ulna: *supination* of the arm is needed for reduction.

38. *Patterns (1)* (1) The radial head may dislocate backwards accompanied by fracture and posterior angulation of the ulna (posterior Monteggia) or (2) The radial head may dislocate anteriorly, with anterior angulation of the ulna (anterior Monteggia) or (3) The radial head may dislocate laterally, accompanied by lateral angulation of the ulna (lateral Monteggia).

39. *Patterns (2)* (4) The radial head may dislocate anteriorly and be associated with fracture of the olecranon (Hume fracture). (5) Greenstick fractures of the ulna, often difficult to detect, partly account for the fact that Monteggia lesions are frequently overlooked in children. *Always* check the position of the radial head in both views, and *always* look for distortion and kinking of the ulna.

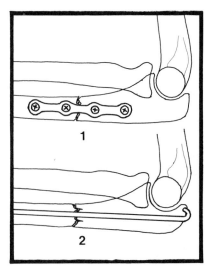

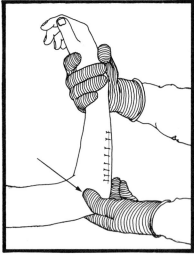

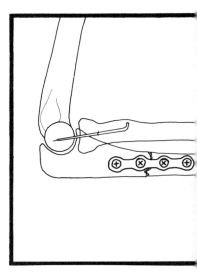

40. *Treatment (1)* The key to successful management of this potentially difficult injury is accurate reduction of the ulnar fracture. In the adult, and in children with displaced fractures, this is best achieved by open reduction and internal fixation. The fracture is easily approached through a posterior incision, and the reduction may be held with a plate and screws (1) or a Rush pin (2).

41. *Treatment (2)* Thereafter the elbow should be placed in right-angled flexion. The position of the radial head should be checked by palpation and by radiographs. Full supination may be required to maintain reduction, but generally the neutral position will be satisfactory in maintaining stability after the ulna has been fixed.

42. *Treatment (3)* If the radial head is unstable, it may be anchored with a per-cutaneous Kirschner wire which should be retained for three weeks before removal. On rare occasions preliminary exposure of the radial head through a small lateral incision may be necessary to achieve reduction. The normal precautions must be taken to avoid damage to the posterior interosseous nerve.

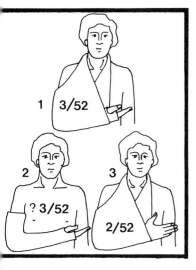

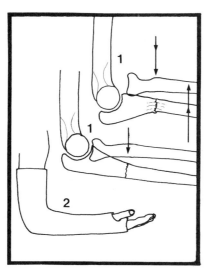

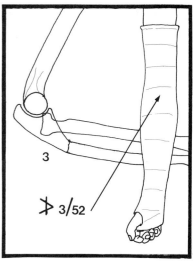

3. *Treatment (4)* After care (1) The plaster
changed at 3 weeks and the stitches and
ny Kirschner wires removed. (2) Plaster is
nally discarded when on your assessment
ere is adequate stability. Your opinion will
e based on the type of fixation, its technical
dequacy, callus formation, etc. In practice,
obilisation from a sling (3) may often be
arted about 6 weeks. Physiotherapy is
ften required.

44. *Treatment (5) Monteggia fractures in
children* (A) Any greenstick angulation of
the ulna should be corrected by
manipulation (1). Anterior Monteggia
fractures should be put up in a position of
90° flexion at the elbow and in
supination (2).

45. *Treatment (6) Monteggia fractures in
children* (B) Posterior Monteggia
fractures (3) are often stable in full extension
and may be fixed for not more than three
weeks in this position; the elbow should be
brought into a more flexed position for the
remainder of the time in plaster. The position
of the radial head must be confirmed by
weekly radiographs: if there is any evidence
of incongruity, per-cutaneous Kirschner
wiring should be carried out without delay.

6. *Late diagnosed Monteggia lesions:*
) In the adult, some restriction of elbow
ovements may be the only complaint.
xcision of the radial head may give
mporary relief, but is often followed by
roximal drift of the radius and troublesome
bluxation of the ulna at the wrist.
) Tardy ulnar nerve palsy may be the
atient's first complaint: transposition of the
lnar nerve is often effective in arresting the
rogress of this condition. (3) In children,
xcision of the radial head is contra-
dicated (it would lead to growth
sturbance). In some cases late
anipulation and Kirschner wire
abilisation may be possible, depending on
e delay. In late cases, good results have
ccasionally followed annular ligament
pair using palmaris longus.

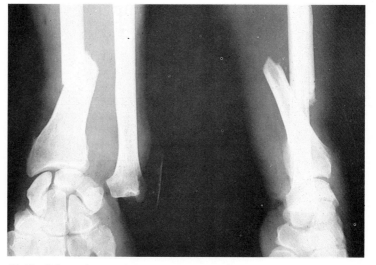

47. *The Galeazzi fracture-dislocation:* This is a fracture of the radius associated with a
dislocation of the inferior radio-ulnar joint. Note that in the normal wrist that the distal end of
the ulna (excluding the styloid process) lies just proximal to the articular surface of the
radius, the space between being occupied by the triangular fibro-cartilage. If the radius is
fractured, always look for subluxation of the ulna.

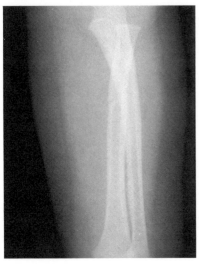

48. *Isolated fracture of the radius:* Fracture of the radius can occur without initial involvement of the inferior radio-ulnar joint. This comparatively uncommon situation may follow direct injury to the radius which results in an undisplaced fracture. Nevertheless, late subluxation of the inferior radio-ulnar joint may appear when, as is frequent, late angulation of the fracture occurs.

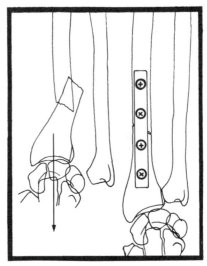

49. *Galeazzi fracture:* Treatment (1) In the adult, open reduction and plating of the radius through an anterior incision eliminates the risks of late slipping. Reduction of the radius is followed by spontaneous reduction of the ulnar subluxation, and the inferior radio-ulnar joint does not require opening. With stable internal fixation and an intact ulna, there is less need for additional external fixation.

50. (2) In the adult, isolated fractures of the radius with no significant angulatory or rotational deformity may be treated in plaster with the arm in supination. Slight axial rotation may be controlled by careful positioning of the forearm; in all cases careful surveillance is vital to detect early slipping, an indication for operative intervention. (3) In children, isolated fractures of the radius should also be treated conservatively. Galeazzi fracture-dislocations should be manipulated and put up in plaster in supination. Open reduction is seldom required. (4) *Late diagnosed Galeazzi lesions:* Prominence of the ulna with pain in the wrist is the commonest complaint, and excision of the distal ulna may give relief. (5) Non-union of the radius may be treated by internal fixation and bone grafting.

Self test

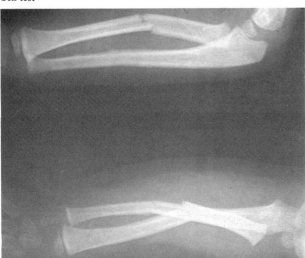

51. Describe this fracture. What treatment would you advocate?

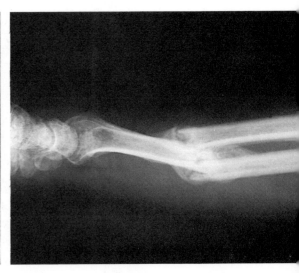

52. Interpret this radiograph. How might this appearance be avoided?

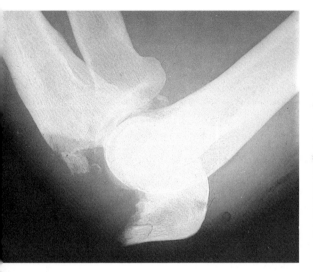

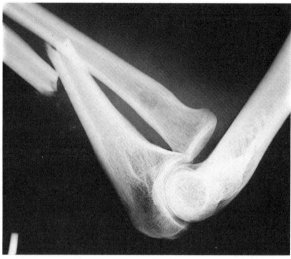

53. What is this injury?

54. Describe this injury. How would you treat it?

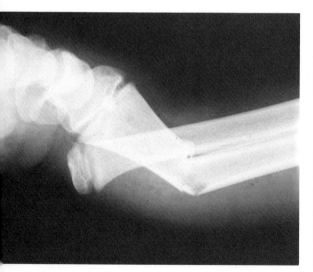

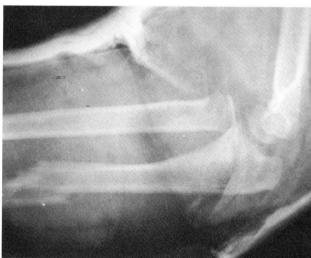

55. Describe this injury. What treatment would you carry out?

56. Comment on this radiograph.

51. Greenstick fractures of the radius and ulna, with anterior angulation. Treat by manipulation under general anaesthesia and the application of a long arm plaster slab.

52. Cross-union has occurred in this fracture of the radius and ulna. The distal fragments have rotated 90° relative to the proximal fragments (mal-union). No pronation or supination will be possible. This would be avoided by open reduction and internal fixation through separate incisions.

53. Hume fracture. (Anterior Monteggia fracture-dislocation where the ulnar fracture is one of the olecranon.)

54. Adult anterior Monteggia fracture-dislocation, with a fracture of the ulna in the upper middle third, with anterior angulation; the radial head is dislocated anteriorly. Treatment would be by open reduction and internal fixation of the ulna; reduction of the radial head would then have to be confirmed.

55. Galeazzi fracture-dislocation in a child: there is a greenstick fracture of the radius with anterior angulation. The distal end of the ulna is dislocated anteriorly.

56. The radiograph is of an arm in plaster; there is a fracture of the ulna, apparently in reasonable alignment in this single view, but the radial head is dislocated anteriorly: i.e. this is an anterior Monteggia fracture-dislocation which has not been satisfactorily reduced. The arm appears to be in the mid-prone position, and reduction of the radial head might have been achieved if the arm had been placed in supination. Further treatment here is imperative (e.g. reduction and internal fixation of the ulnar fracture, correct positioning of the forearm, and if necessary, Kirschner wire stabilisation of the radial head).

9. The wrist and hand

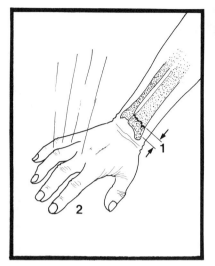

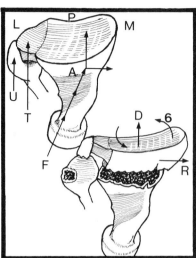

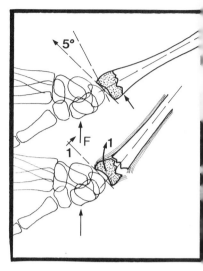

1. *Colles fracture:* A Colles fracture is a fracture of the radius within 2.5 cm of the wrist (1), with a characteristic deformity if displaced. It is the commonest of all fractures. It is seen mainly in middle aged and elderly women, and osteoporosis is a frequent contributory factor. It generally results from a fall on the outstretched hand (2).

2. *Displacements (1)* The *six* characteristic features of a displaced Colles fracture (see later for details) are shown in this foreshortened view of the pronated right arm, viewed from below. The slight obliquity of impact (F) produces the two most striking features of *dorsal and radial displacement* (D & R) of the distal fragment. (T = triangular fibro-cartilage: U = ulnar styloid)

3. *Displacements (2)* The deformity can be followed by studying the wrist in the two planes in which the radiographs are usually taken. The impact (F) fractures the radius through the cancellous bone of the metaphysis. With greater violence the anterior periosteum tears, and the distal fragment tilts into *anterior angulation (1)* with loss of the 5° forward tilt of the joint surface.

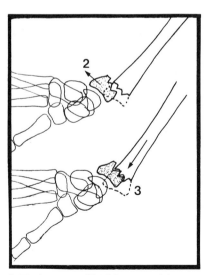

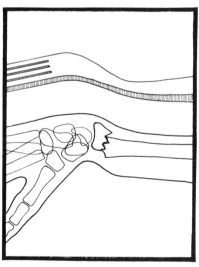

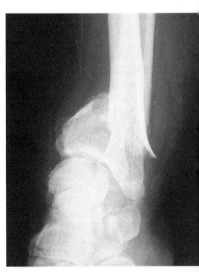

4. *Displacements (3)* With greater violence there is *dorsal displacement of the distal fragment (2).* The shaft of the radius is driven into the distal fragment leading to impaction (3). (The dotted lines indicate the position of the distal fragment prior to any displacement.)

5. *Displacements (4)* The altered contour of the wrist in a badly displaced Colles fracture is striking, and is referred to as a 'dinner fork deformity'. When viewed from the side, the wrist has the same curvature as a fork, with the tines resembling the fingers.

6. *Displacements (5)* This radiograph shows a typical displaced Colles fracture. The anterior angulation, dorsal displacement, and impaction are obvious. (Deformities 1, 2, 3.)

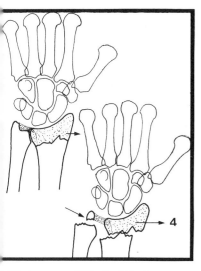

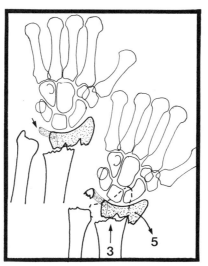

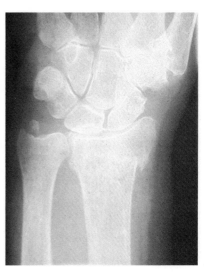

. *Displacements (6)* In the A.P. plane, a
mall lateral component of the force of
mpact causes *lateral (radial) displacement
f the distal fragment (4)*. The distal
ragment is attached to the ulnar styloid by
ne triangular fibro-cartilage, and generally
nis leads to avulsion of the ulnar styloid.

8. *Displacements (7)* Sometimes the
triangular fibro-cartilage is torn: in either
case there is disruption of the inferior radio-
ulnar joint. The distal fragment tilts laterally
into *ulnar angulation* (5) and impacts. The
sixth feature is a rotational or torsional
deformity (6) (see 2) not obvious in either
A.P. or lateral projections.

9. *Displacements (8)* In this A.P. radiograph
of a Colles fracture, note the features just
mentioned, i.e. radial deviation, ulnar
angulation and impaction of the distal
fragment.

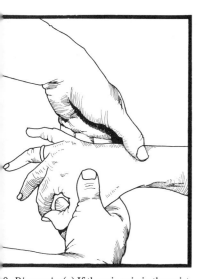

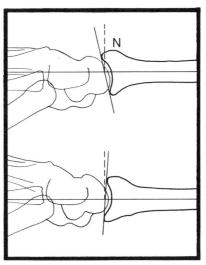

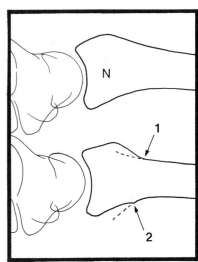

0. *Diagnosis:* (a) If there is pain in the wrist
nd tenderness over the distal end of the
adius after a fall, radiographs must be taken
n every case. The site of maximum
enderness will help to differentiate fracture
f the scaphoid (but see scaphoid fractures).
b) Where there is marked displacement the
linical appearance is so characteristic that
iagnosis presents no difficulty.

11. *Radiographs (1)* In the majority of cases
the fracture is easily identified.
(2) Sometimes it may be missed because
impaction has rendered the fracture line
inconspicuous. If in doubt, look at the angle
between the distal end of the radius and the
shaft in the lateral radiograph. Decrease to
less than 0° is suggestive of fracture (but
enquire about previous injury).

12. *Radiographs (3)* The minimally
displaced fracture will also reveal itself in the
lateral projection by an increase in the
posterior radial concavity, often with local
kinking (1) or by a separate or
accompanying break in the smooth curve of
the anterior surface of the radius (2).

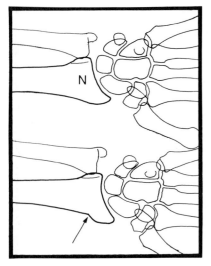

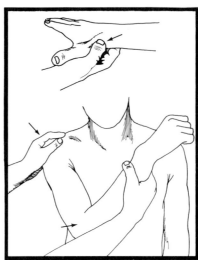

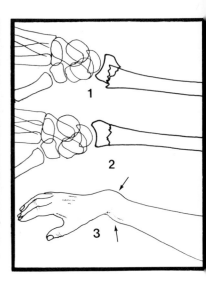

13. *Radiographs (4)* In the A.P. view of the wrist, look for any irregularity in the smooth lateral aspect of the radius.

If there is any doubtful radiographic feature suggesting fracture, return to the patient *and confirm whether there is any localised tenderness over the suspect area.*

14. *Diagnosis ctd.* A Colles fracture is generally caused by a fall on the outstretched hand—a mechanism common to many upper limb fractures. Although other injuries in the arm occurring in association with Colles fracture are *uncommon*, clinically the scaphoid, elbow and shoulder should be examined, and on the radiographs the scaphoid should be scrutinised. (Special views required if directly suspect.)

15. *Treatment: Does the fracture require manipulation? (1)* If the fracture is grossly displaced, it obviously should be reduced (1) If undisplaced, no manipulation is needed (2). Between these extremes, the following additional factors may be considered: if there is a readily appreciated naked eye deformity (3) manipulation should be carried out (but distinguish between *swelling* and *deformity*).

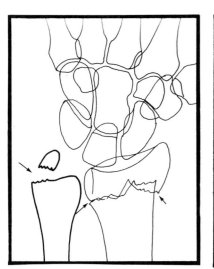

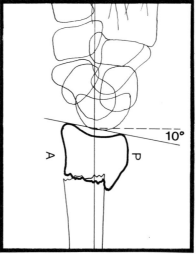

18. *Reduction technique (1)* Anaesthesia is necessary for the reduction of this fracture, and either a general anaesthetic or intravenous regional anaesthesia (Bier block) may be used with success. Although the latter has a good safety record, it should not be employed unless facilities for resuscitation are freely available. Where there is a preference for general anaesthesia but the patient attends late at night with a history of recent intake of food or drink, it is permissible and often safer to apply a temporary plaster back shell and an arm sling, and delay reduction of the fracture till morning.

16. *Does the fracture require manipulation? (2)* If there is displacement of the ulnar styloid, this indicates *serious disruption of the inferior radio-ulnar joint.* (Acute ulnar angulation of the distal fragment is also evidence of this.) An attempt at correction should be made *irrespective of other appearances.*

17. *Does the fracture require manipulation? (3)* If the joint line in the lateral projection is tilted 10° or more posteriorly rather than anteriorly, the fracture should be manipulated: but in the very old, frail patient somewhat greater degrees of deformity may be accepted.

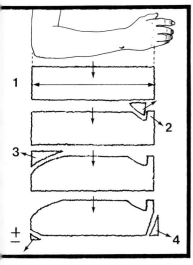

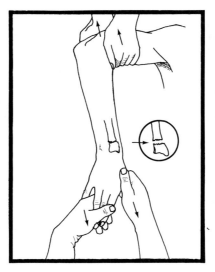

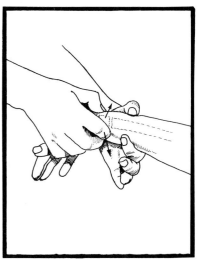

9. *Reduction technique (2)* Before any manipulation, start by preparing a suitable plaster back slab. The *length* should be equal to the distance from the olecranon to the metacarpal heads (1). The *width* in an adult should be 6″ (15 cm), and it should be about 6 layers thick. The slab should be trimmed with a tongue (2) for the first web space, a large radial curve to allow elbow flexion (3) and allowance for ulnar deviation (4).

20. *Reduction technique (3)* The essential first stage in the reduction of a Colles fracture is to disimpact the distal radial fragment. The elbow is flexed to a right angle and the arm held by the interlocked fingers of an assistant (1). Traction is applied in the line of the forearm (2).

21. *Reduction technique (4)* Traction need only be applied for a few seconds, and disimpaction may be confirmed by holding the distal fragment between the thumb and index. It should be easy to move anteriorly and posteriorly.

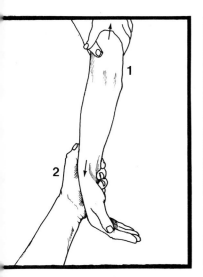

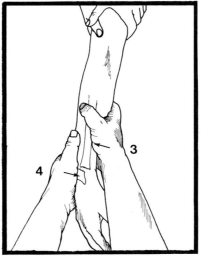

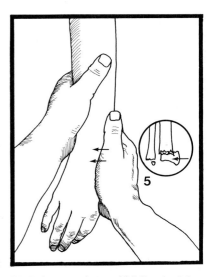

22. *Reduction technique (5)* The elbow is now extended (1). The heel of one hand should be placed over the dorsal surface of the distal radial fragment, and the fingers curled round the patient's wrist and palm (2). This grip allows traction to be re-applied to the disimpacted fracture.

23. *Reduction technique (6)* Now, by using the heel of the other hand as a fulcrum (3) firm pressure directed anteriorly (4) will correct all the remaining deformities normally visible in lateral radiographs of the wrist (posterior displacement, anterior angulation).

24. *Reduction technique (7)* Still maintaining traction, alter the position of the grip so that the heel (here of the right hand) is able to push the distal fragment ulnarwards and correct the radial displacement (5). Ulnar angulation, the other deformity seen in the A.P. radiograph, is corrected by placing the hand in full ulnar deviation at the wrist.

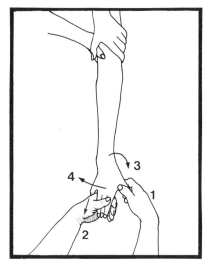

25. *Reduction technique (8)* Change the grip to allow free application of the plaster. Note that one hand holds the thumb fully extended (1). The other holds three fingers (to avoid 'cupping' of the hand) maintaining slight traction (2). The limb should be in full pronation (3), *full* ulnar deviation at the wrist (4) and *slight* palmar flexion.

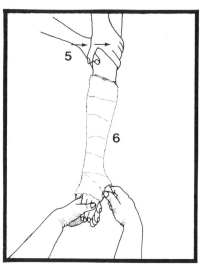

26. *Reduction technique (9)* Note that the elbow must be *extended* (either by an assistant (5), or by resting the upper arm against the edge of the table) to maintain this position. The skin may be protected with wool roll (6). If stockingette is preferred, it must be applied prior to reduction.

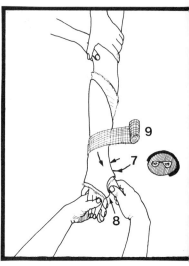

27. *Reduction technique (10)* The wetted slab should now be positioned so that it covers the anterior, lateral and posterior aspects of the radius (7). The tongue should be carefully turned into the palm (8). The slab should be held in position with two wetted 4″ (10 cm) open weave bandages (cotton, gauze or 'Kling' bandages) (9). The end can be secured with a wetted scrap of plaster bandage.

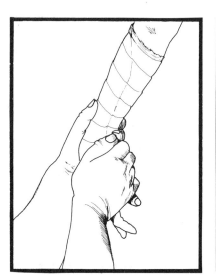

28. *Reduction technique (11)* Before the plaster sets, many surgeons like to apply further pressure over the postero-lateral aspect of the distal fragment, and maintain this until setting occurs ('final moulding'). This precaution ensures maintenance of the reduction, but care should be taken not to dent the plaster.

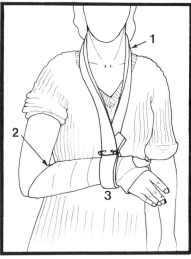

29. *Reduction technique (12)* A collar and cuff sling should be applied (1). Make sure that there is no constriction at the elbow (2) or at the wrist (3), and try to flex the elbow beyond a right angle so that the forearm is not dependent.

30. *Alternative techniques:* It is not unexpected that in this common fracture methods of reduction are legion. As it is generally an easy fracture to reduce, it follows that success can rightly be claimed for many techniques. The method given is logical in so far as it correlates with the pathology as seen on the radiographs.

Note, however, (A) a direct, simple and extremely effective procedure is to disimpac the fracture (20), apply a plaster slab (27), and correct the deformity before the plaster sets by applying pressure on the postero-lateral aspect of the distal fragment (as in 28). (B) In the elderly patient, unfit for general anaesthesia (but preferably after intravenous diazepam) a *marked* dorsal displacement may be corrected by quick application of pressure (without previous disimpaction) over a dorsal slab.

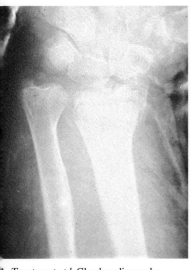

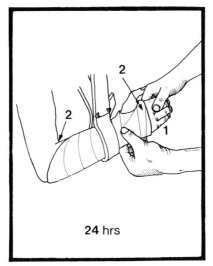

24 hrs

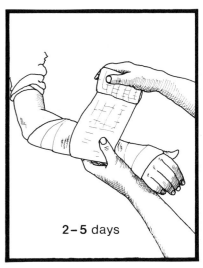

2–5 days

1. *Treatment ctd.* Check radiographs ould be studied. Severe persisting formity, *especially in the A.P. projection* l.) should not be accepted, and re-anipulation should be undertaken. If fficulty is anticipated, radiographs may be tained before discontinuing the aesthetic. If the position is acceptable, the tient is shown finger exercises and advised garding normal plaster care.

32. *After care (1)* The patient is seen the next day and the fingers examined for adequacy of the circulation and the degree of swelling (1). The palm, fingers, thumb and elbow are checked for constriction caused by bandaging or elbow flexion, and any adjustments made (2). Thereafter the patient should be seen within the next 2–5 days with a view to completion of the plaster.

33. *After care (2)* At the next review (usually a fracture clinic) finger swelling is checked: if slight, the plaster is completed (if marked, completion is delayed). *Superficial* layers of cotton bandage are removed, the slab retained, and encircling plaster bandages applied. The patient is instructed in elbow and shoulder exercises, and unless there is still a fair amount of swelling, the sling may be discarded.

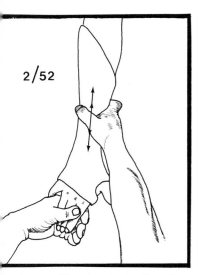

2/52

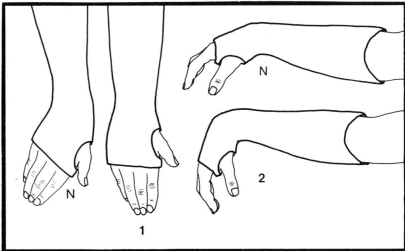

4. *After care (3)* At 2 weeks the plaster is ecked for slackness (treated, if marked, by e careful application of a new plaster) for ftening (reinforce) and for technical faults ee 35). Freedom of movement in the ngers, elbow and shoulder are noted. In me centres check radiographs are taken at is stage. Slight fracture slipping is evitable: gross slipping (rare) may be an dication for re-manipulation.

35. *After care (4) Positional errors:* (1) The commonest fault is lack of ulnar deviation. This should be sadly accepted if discovered at 2 weeks, (but re-plastered in the correct position if discovered earlier). Lack of ulnar deviation increases the risks of late problems arising from disruption of the inferior radio-ulnar joint; non-union of the ulnar styloid is common, with frequently some restriction of pronation and supination and local pain. (2) Excessive wrist flexion is liable to lead to difficulty in recovering dorsiflexion and a useful grip, and if present, the plaster should be re-applied with the wrist in a more extended position. (Full wrist flexion was once advocated in the treatment of Colles fracture—the Cotton-Loder position—but has been abandoned for the reasons given.)

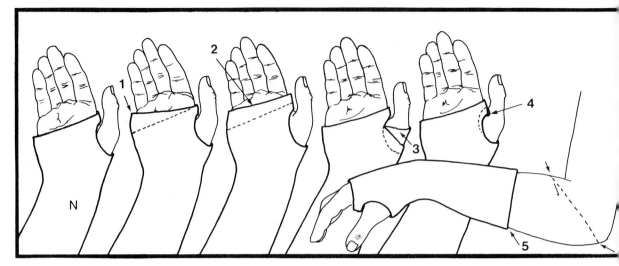

36. *After care (5) Plaster faults:* Errors in plastering technique should not occur, but nevertheless are often discovered at this stage. The following faults are common. (1) The distal edge of the plaster does not follow the normal oblique line of the M.P. joints, and movements of the little and sometimes the ring finger are restricted. The plaster should be trimmed to the dotted line. (2) All the M.P. joints are restricted by the plaster which has been continued beyond the palmar crease. Trim to the dotted line. (3) The thumb is restricted by a few turns of plaster bandage. Again the plaster should be trimmed to permit free movement. (4) The plaster is digging into the skin of the first web and should be trimmed back to the dotted line. (5) The plaster is too short. Support of the fracture is greatly impaired; the plaster should be extended to the olecranon behind, and as far in front as will still permit elbow flexion.

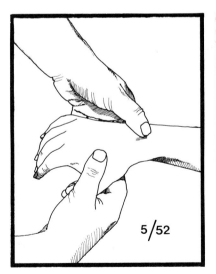

37. *After care (6)* The plaster should be removed at 5 weeks (or 6 weeks in badly displaced fractures in the elderly) and the fracture assessed for union. (Radiographs are of limited value.) *If there is marked persisting tenderness*, a fresh plaster should be applied and union re-assessed in a further 2 weeks.

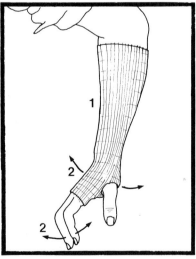

38. *After care (7)* If tenderness is minimal or absent, (1) a circular woven support (e.g. Tubigrip) or a crepe bandage may be applied (to limit oedema and to some extent increase the patient's confidence). (2) The patient is instructed in wrist and finger exercises and encouraged to practise these frequently and with vigour. (3) Arrangements are made to review the patient in a further 2 weeks.

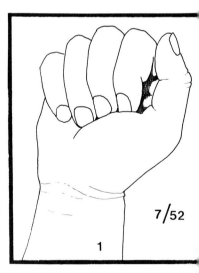

39. *Need for rehabilitation (1)* Now, about weeks post injury, you must decide whether to discharge the patient or refer her for rehabilitation. Base your decision on (a) finger movements (b) grip strength (c) wrist movements (d) the patient's occupation.

For example, (a) if finger 'tuck-in', i.e. the last few degrees of flexion cannot be carried out (loss illustrated) physiotherapy should be considered.

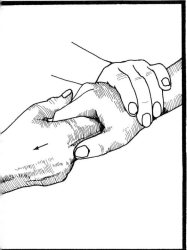

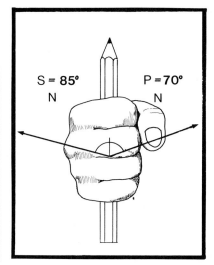

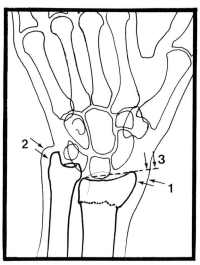

. *Need for rehabilitation (2)* (b) Assess the patient's grip strength by first asking her to squeeze two of your fingers as tightly as possible while you try to withdraw them. Compare one hand with the other. Repeat with a single finger. Marked weakness is an indication for physiotherapy.

41. *Need for rehabilitation (3)* (c) Assess wrist movements. Initially, material restriction of *palmar flexion* is normal and by itself is of little importance. If, however, the total range of *pronation and supination* is less than half normal, physiotherapy is advisable. (d) Where there is only slight restriction of movements and power, rehabilitation may still be indicated through the special requirements of the patient's work.

42. *Complications (1) Persistent deformity or mal-union (a)* Radial drift of the distal fragment results in prominence of the distal radius (1). Radial tilting and bony absorption at the fracture site lead to relative prominence of the distal ulna (2) and tilting of the plane of the wrist as seen in the A.P. radiographs (3). These deformities may be symptom free, and surgery on purely cosmetic grounds is seldom indicated.

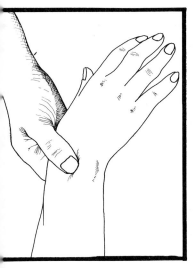

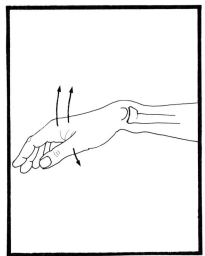

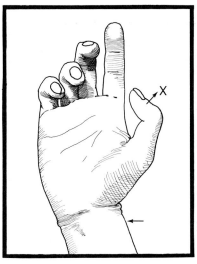

. *Mal-union (b)* In some cases there is quite marked pain in the region of the distal radio-ulnar joint, due to its severe disorganisation. There is generally quite marked *local tenderness* and supination in particular is reduced. Physiotherapy in the form of grip strengthening and pronation/supination exercises is indicated. If symptoms remain severe, excision of the distal end of the ulna may be considered.

44. *Mal-union (c)* Uncomplicated persistence of dinner-fork deformity (i.e. persistent deformity in the lateral, but not in the A.P. radiographs) is accompanied by some loss of palmar flexion, but significant functional disturbance is unusual. This type of residual deformity is generally accepted.

45. *Complications (2) Delayed rupture of extensor pollicis longus* may follow Colles fracture, and be due to attrition of the tendon by roughness at the fracture site, or by sloughing from interference with its blood supply. Disability is often slight, and spontaneous recovery may occur. There is no urgency regarding treatment, and in the elderly this complaint may be accepted or treated expectantly. In the young, extensor indicis proprius tendon transfer is advocated.

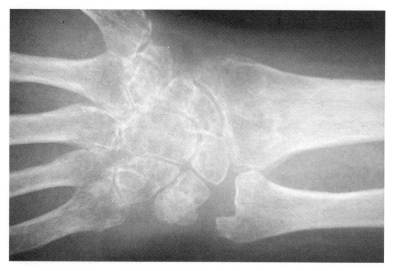

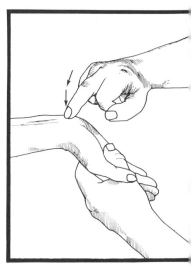

46. *Complications (3) Sudeck's atrophy:* This is often detected about the time the patient comes out of plaster. The fingers are swollen and finger flexion is restricted. The hand and wrist are warm, tender and painful. Radiographs show diffuse osteoporosis (ill.).
Treatment: (1) The mainstay of treatment is intensive and prolonged physiotherapy and occupational therapy, but (2) if pain is very severe, a further 2–3 weeks rest of the *wrist* in plaster may give sufficient relief to allow commencement of effective finger movements. (3) If the M.P. joints are stiff in extension and making no headway, manipulation under general anaesthesia followed by fixation in plaster (M.P. joints flexed, I.P. joints extended) for 3 weeks only may be effective in initiating recovery.

47. *Complications (4) Carpal tunnel (median nerve compression) syndrome:* Paraesthesiae in the median distribution is the main presenting symptom, and the diagnosis may be confirmed by other symptoms and signs (e.g. tapping (ill.), nerve stretching, tourniquet and plaster fixation tests). Surgical decompression is advocated at an early stage, as the symptoms in this situation tend to be persistent and progressive.

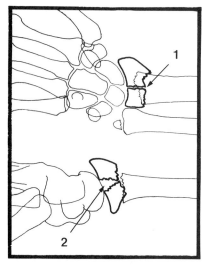

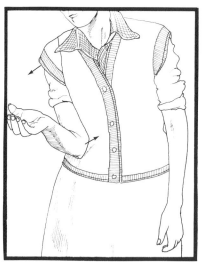

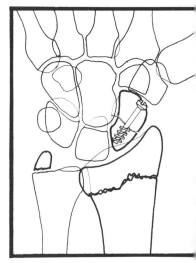

48. *Complications (5) Comminution of the radial fragment:* Sometimes there may be a small vertical crack through the radial fragment, showing in the A.P. radiograph (1). In other cases the fracture may run horizontally, and the scaphoid or lunate may separate the fragments (2). In both types, physiotherapy is necessary after union, and in the latter, marked permanent restriction of movements is the rule.

49. *Complications (6) Persisting stiffness:* Restriction of movements, even after prolonged physiotherapy, is not uncommon, but is seldom severe enough to impair limb function to a material extent. This is due to compensatory (trick) movements developed by the elbow, shoulder and trunk. (For example, in case of loss of supination.)

50. *Complications (7) Associated scaphoid fracture:* This may be treated by manipulation of the Colles fracture and application of a scaphoid plaster. After the Colles fracture has united, further immobilisation may be required for the scaphoid. Alternatively, the scaphoid fracture may be fixed with a screw (ill.), the Colles fracture manipulated, and fixation discontinued as soon as the latter has united

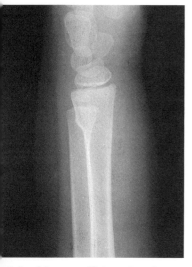

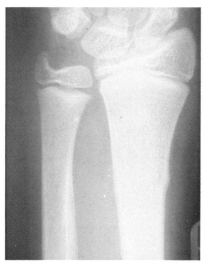

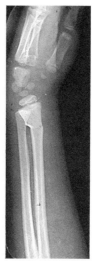

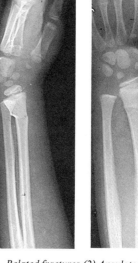

Related fractures (1) A number of ...ctures involving the distal end of the ...lius, produced by falls on the outstretched ...nd, have certain similarities to the ...ssical Colles fracture. The commonest of ...se is the *undisplaced greenstick fracture* ...he radius. In its most minor form it may ...overlooked; the only sign may be slight ...al buckling.

52. *Undisplaced greenstick fracture of the radius ctd.:* The level of the fracture is rather variable, and it may be situated fairly proximally. These fractures may be treated like undisplaced Colles fractures by the application of a plaster slab. This may usually be completed after 1–2 days. Fixation for about 3 weeks only is usually all that is necessary.

53. *Related fractures (2) Angulated greenstick fracture of the radius:* In this type of injury there is both clinical and radiological deformity. Manipulation is required as for a Colles fracture, and the after care is similar; the period of plaster fixation may be reduced to 3 or 4 weeks, depending on the age of the child.

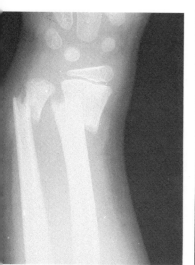

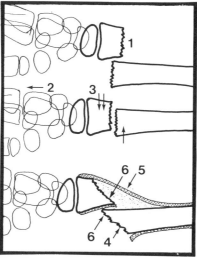

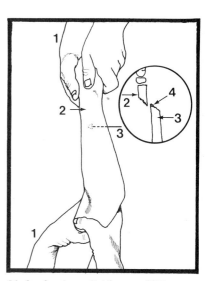

Related fractures (3) Overlapping radial ...cture (1) In children the radius often ...ctures close to the wrist, with off-ending ...he fragments. On the ulnar side there ...y be (1) detachment of the triangular ...o-cartilage (2) separation of the ulnar ...physis (3) fracture and angulation of the ...al ulna (4) fracture and displacement of ...distal ulna (ill.), in effect a fracture of ...h bones of the forearm (5) dislocation of ...ulna (Galeazzi fracture dislocation).

55. *Overlapping radial fracture (2)* If the fracture line is transverse (1) reduction is straightforward by traction (2) and local pressure (3). When, however, there is an oblique fracture running distally from front to back (4) reduction by traction is often impossible, due to the integrity of the periosteum on the dorsal surface (5) and the overlapping bony spikes (6).

56. *Overlapping radial fracture (3)* Two closed techniques may be tried. For the first, *2* assistants are essential to apply *maximal* traction to the limb (1). While this is being strongly maintained, the surgeon should press forcibly with the heel of one hand on the distal fragment (2) and use the other to apply counter-pressure (3). Reduction is achieved by shearing off one of the bone spikes (4).

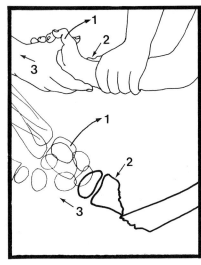

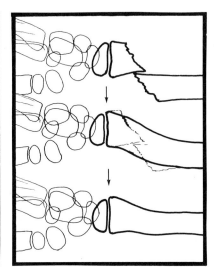

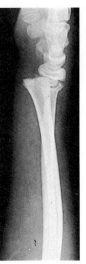

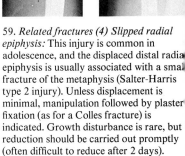

57. Overlapping radial fracture (4)
Alternatively, by *increasing* the deformity (1) and applying pressure directly over the distal radial fragment (2) whilst maintaining traction (3) reduction may be achieved. After the fragments have interlocked the angulation is corrected. Thereafter plaster fixation is carried out as in other fractures in this region.

58. Overlapping radial fracture (5) If shortening is marked, and closed methods fail, open reduction may be considered. (Performed through a small dorsal incision under a tourniquet: internal fixation is not required.) Nevertheless, if persisting overlap is reluctantly accepted, a good result from remodelling is the usual outcome (ill.) *provided* any angulation is corrected.

59. Related fractures (4) Slipped radial epiphysis: This injury is common in adolescence, and the displaced distal radial epiphysis is usually associated with a small fracture of the metaphysis (Salter-Harris type 2 injury). Unless displacement is minimal, manipulation followed by plaster fixation (as for a Colles fracture) is indicated. Growth disturbance is rare, but reduction should be carried out promptly (often difficult to reduce after 2 days).

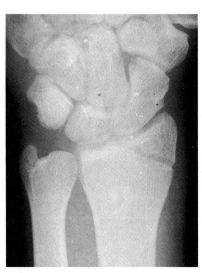

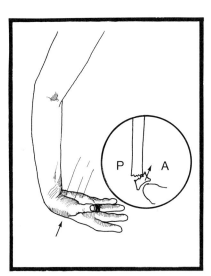

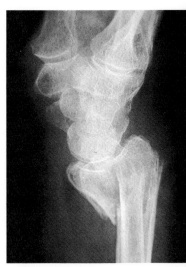

60. Related fractures (5) Fracture of the radial styloid: This fracture is sometimes caused by an engine starting-handle kickback as well as by a fall on the outstretched hand. Displacement is usually slight, and manipulation unlikely to be of value. Plaster fixation as for a Colles fracture is indicated, and physiotherapy is often required. Many of these fractures are complicated by Subeck's atrophy.

61. Related fractures (6) Smith's fracture (1) This injury frequently results from a fall on the back of the hand, although a clear history is not always obtainable. The distal radial fragment is tilted anteriorly (posterior angulation) and may be displaced anteriorly. The fracture is usually impacted.

62. Smith's fracture (2) This fracture is frequently referred to as a reversed Colles fracture because the deformities when viewed from the side clinically and radiologically are in the opposite direction those seen in a Colles fracture. (Note, however, that the two fractures may be identical in A.P. radiographs.) Comminuted Smith's fractures may involve the articular surface of the radius (ill.). Greenstick fractures are common. (See also 65.)

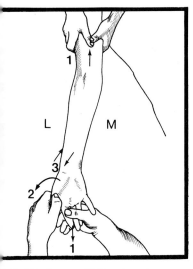

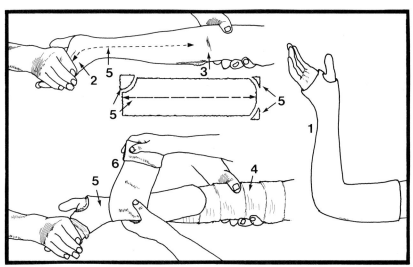

. *Smith's fracture (3)* To reduce these
ctures, traction is applied to the arm (1) in
pination (2) until disimpaction is achieved.
his may be confirmed as in a Colles
acture.) Pressure may be applied with the
els of the hands to force the distal
igment dorsally (3).

64. *Smith's fracture (4)* The reduction is difficult to hold, and a long arm plaster is required
(1). This may be more conveniently applied in two stages, and best as a complete plaster. The
arm is held in full supination and dorsiflexion (2). This is easily maintained with the elbow
extended (3). Wool roll is applied to the arm (4) and an anterior slab, trimmed as shown, may
be used (5) before completion (6). The fracture may be moulded while setting. It is then
extended above the elbow (1). *After care:* (1) Split if necessary. (2) Radiographs should be
taken at weekly intervals for the first 3 weeks to detect any significant slipping (treated by re-
manipulation or moulding). (3) A slack plaster should be changed with care. (4) 6 weeks'
fixation is usually required, with physiotherapy after removal of the plaster.

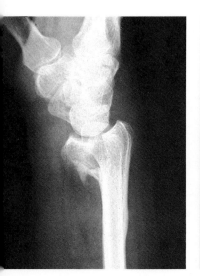

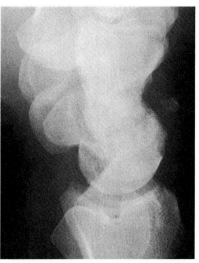

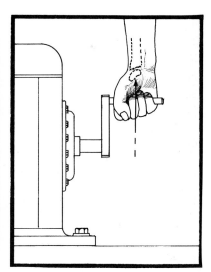

. *Related fractures (7) Barton's fracture:*
is is a form of Smith's fracture in which
anterior portion only of the radius is
olved. Closed reduction may be
empted along the lines indicated for
ith's fracture. If this fails, with the carpus
dging the fragments apart, open reduction
d internal fixation is indicated in the
unger patient (e.g. by cancellous screw or
Ellis buttress plate).

66. *Related fractures (8)* Forcible palmar
flexion may result in a *minor avulsion
fracture of the carpus* at a ligament insertion
(ill.). (9) If the wrist is forcibly palmar flexed
or dorsiflexed, the carpus impinging on the
distal end of the radius may produce a
marginal chip fracture of the radius.
Symptomatic treatment only is required for
any of these injuries (e.g. 2–3 weeks in a
plaster back slab).

67. *Fractures of the scaphoid: Mechanisms
of injury:* Scaphoid fractures often result
from 'kick-back' when using starting handles
on internal combustion generators, pumps,
compressors and inboard marine engines.
(The motorist's avoidance of this fracture is
his only dividend from the unfortunate
abolition of car starting handles.) Otherwise
the fracture may be acquired by falls on the
outstretched hand.

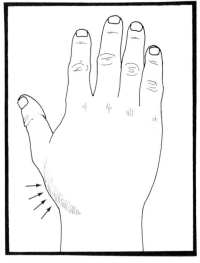

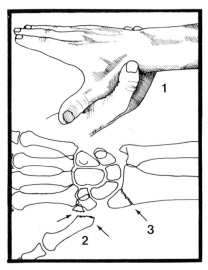

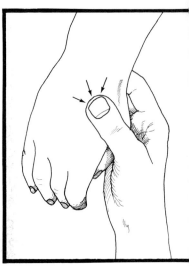

68. *Fractures of the scaphoid: Diagnosis (1)* Fracture of the scaphoid may be suspected when there is complaint of pain on the lateral aspect of the wrist following any injury. In those cases which follow starting handle accidents there may be marked and rapid swelling of the hand and wrist.

69. *Diagnosis (2)* Tenderness in the anatomical snuff box (1) is suggestive of this injury, but by no means diagnostic. Many wrist sprains without fracture give rise to tenderness in this site. Beware too of tenderness which may be the result of a Bennett's fracture of the thumb metacarpal (2) or of a fracture of the radial styloid (3).

70. *Diagnosis (3)* In a true scaphoid fracture, tenderness will also be elicited on the application of pressure over the *dorsal aspect of the scaphoid*, and also on pressure over the palmar aspect. Tenderness in these additional sites very seldom occurs in other injuries in this area, no matter how severe.

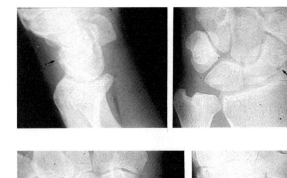

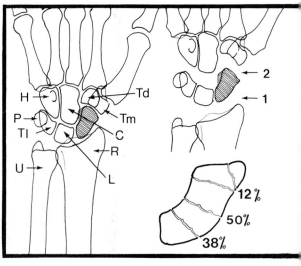

71. *Diagnosis (4) Radiographs:* Radiography is required in all suspect cases. Note the following important points: (1) Request cards should be clearly marked 'scaphoid' and not 'wrist', to ensure that (2) at least 3 views of the scaphoid are obtained (A.P., lateral and 1 or 2 oblique projections). The fracture is often hair-line and hard to see, so that (3) in all suspected but unconfirmed cases, the radiographs should be repeated 10–14 days after injury (when decalcification at the fracture site should render any fracture visible). Illustrated: fracture of distal waist, 4 views.

72. *Anatomical features (1)* The scaphoid plays a key role in wrist and carpal function, taking part in the radio-carpal joint (1) and in the joint between the proximal and distal rows of the carpus (2). It articulates with the radius (R), trapezium (Tm), trapezoid (Td), capitate (C) and lunate (L). The commonest site for fracture is the waist (50%). 38% of fractures occur in the proximal half, and 12% in the distal half. (U = ulna, H = hamate, P = pisiform, Tl = triquetral.)

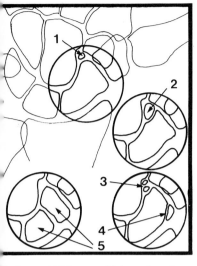

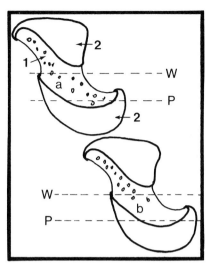

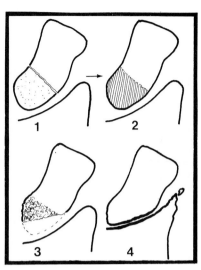

3. *Anatomical features (2)* A number of abnormalities in ossification may be confused with fractures. The *os centrale* may be small (1) large (2) or double (3). The *os radiale externum* (4) lies in the region of the tubercle and in some cases may represent an old, un-united fracture; certainly the so called 'bi-partite scaphoid' (5) is now generally regarded as being due to this. (Rounded edges differentiate these from fracture.)

74. *Anatomical features (3)* The blood supply of the scaphoid is through small vessels which enter the ligamentous ridge (1) lying between the two main articular surfaces (2). When these vessels are well scattered as at (a), ischaemia following fracture is uncommon. If all the vessels enter the distal part of the ridge (b), fractures of the waist (W) and proximal poles (P) may be followed by avascular necrosis.

75. *Anatomical features (4)* Avascular necrosis is of immediate onset, but 1–2 months may elapse before increased density betrays its presence on the radiographs (2). There is usually slow but progressive bony collapse (3) and radio-carpal osteo-arthritis (4). This leads to worsening pain and stiffness in the wrist. This complication occurs in about 30% of fractures of the proximal pole of the scaphoid.

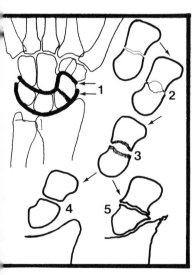

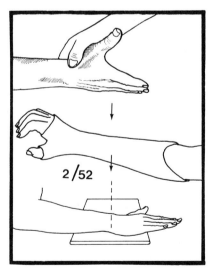

78. *Suspected fracture (2)* (a) If after two weeks repeat films confirm a fracture, a fresh plaster is applied and the patient treated as for a frank scaphoid fracture. (b) If the radiographs are negative, the patient is presumed to have suffered a sprain, and is treated accordingly, either being left free or given a crepe bandage or similar support. If after a further 2 weeks' freedom symptoms recur, further careful radiographic examination is essential. (See 102.)

6. *Anatomical features (5)* Because of its role in two major joints (1) movement of the fragments is difficult to control, and non-union may occur in waist fractures. Cystic changes at the fracture site (2) are followed by marginal sclerosis (3). The edges may round off and become symptomless (4) or osteo-arthritis may supervene (5). Note that non-union can occur without avascular necrosis, and that most fractures with avascular necrosis are united.

77. *Treatment: Suspected fractures (1)* When there is localised scaphoid tenderness, but no radiological confirmation of fracture, a scaphoid plaster is applied (usually with a sling for a few days, especially if swelling is marked). The plaster is removed after two weeks and fresh radiographs taken. Absorption of bone at the level of a fracture generally reveals any hair-line crack.

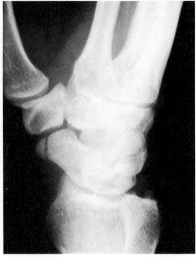

79. *Fractures of the tuberosity of the scaphoid:* Avascular necrosis never occurs in fractures of this type, and non-union here does not give rise to significant symptoms. Symptomatic treatment only is needed (e.g. crepe bandage or plaster, depending on pain). Some extend this to include all distal pole fractures, but generally plaster fixation is the mainstay of treatment of all fractures through the body of the scaphoid (but see 90).

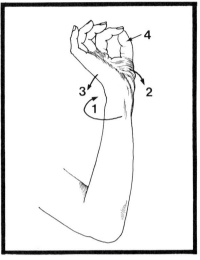

80. *Treatment of undisplaced fractures of the body of the scaphoid: The scaphoid plaster (1)* The position of the hand is of some importance and this should be made quite clear to the patient prior to the application of the plaster. The wrist should be fully pronated (1) radially deviated (2) moderately dorsiflexed (3). In addition, the thumb should be in mid abduction (4).

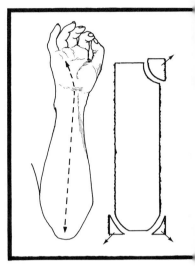

81. *The scaphoid plaster (2)* An anterior plaster slab, although by no means essential is frequently used. This may be made from 6–8 layers of 4″ (10 cm) plaster bandage, or from a slab dispenser. The proximal corners should be trimmed and a cut-out made to accommodate the swell of the thenar muscles.

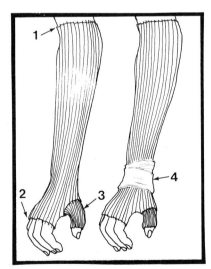

82. *The scaphoid plaster (3)* Stockingette is applied from just above the elbow (1) to the proximal phalanges (2) allowing for subsequent turn-down. A smaller gauge may be used for the thumb (or wool roll) (3). A turn of wool is used to protect the bony prominences of the wrist (4). If there is a lot of early swelling suggesting more to come, more generous wool padding is applied round the wrist and hand.

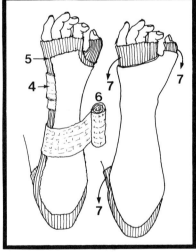

83. *The scaphoid plaster (4)* The plaster slab may then be wetted and applied to the forearm, taking care not to extend it beyond the proximal palmar crease (5). Encircling plaster bandages are then applied, using 6″ (15 cm) bandages for the forearm, 4″ (10 cm) for the wrist and 3″ (7.5 cm) for the thumb (6). The edges of the stockingette are turned down before completion (7).

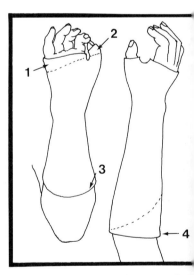

84. *The scaphoid plaster (5) Common faults* Plaster including M.P. joints of fingers, restricting flexion (1). Terminal phalanx of thumb included, preventing inter-phalangeal joint flexion (2). Plaster too short (3). Plaster restricting flexion of the elbow (4).

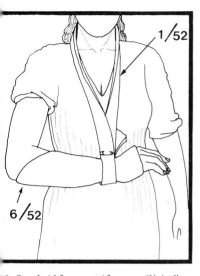

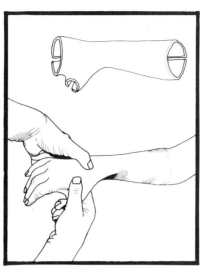

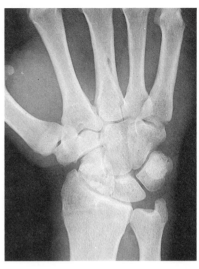

5. *Scaphoid fracture: After care (1)* A sling should be worn for the first few days until swelling subsides. Analgesics are usually required initially. The patient is reviewed at weeks (assuming the initial plaster check as been satisfactory). If on this visit the plaster is unduly slack, it should be changed. Any softening in the palm should be reinforced.

86. *After care (2)* At 6 weeks the plaster should be removed and the scaphoid assessed clinically and with radiographs. There are several possibilities: (a) if there is no tenderness over the dorsal surface and in the snuff-box, and the fracture appears united on the radiographs, the wrist should be left free and reviewed in 2 weeks (usually for discharge, or further radiographs if pain recurs).

87. *After care (3)* (b) The fracture line may still show clearly on the radiographs. (c) The radiographs may suggest union, but there is marked local tenderness. (d) There is some uncertainty on either score. These possibilities are all suggestive of delayed union, and a further 6 weeks of plaster fixation is desirable.

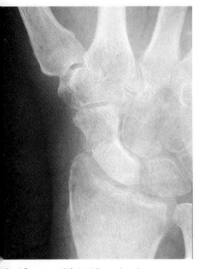

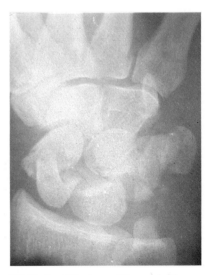

89. *After care (5)* At 12 weeks (ctd.) there may be: (d) no evidence of union radiologically, but no sclerosis of the bone ends. Union may nevertheless still occur. If there is no significant tenderness, the wrist should be left free, and re-assessed in a further two weeks. (See below also.)
(e) evidence of delayed union, with marked local tenderness and severe pain on movement. In such a case the patient should be given the option of a further period of plaster fixation, or of internal fixation of the fracture with a cancellous bone screw. The same advice should be offered in situation (d) above where pain recurs on leaving the wrist free.

8. *After care (4)* At 12 weeks, there may be: (a) evidence of *avascular necrosis* (note density of proximal half in radiograph) (b) clear evidence, clinically and radiologically, of *union* (c) *established non-union*, with sclerosis of the bone ends
   In all these circumstances, there is no need and no advantage in continuing with plaster fixation.

90. *Displaced fractures of the scaphoid:* Where there is marked displacement of a fractured scaphoid, careful analysis of the radiographs should be made to exclude a carpal dislocation. There is much to be said for primary internal fixation of this type of fracture, and this is certainly indicated if conservative treatment is attempted, and check radiographs through plaster show persistent displacement.

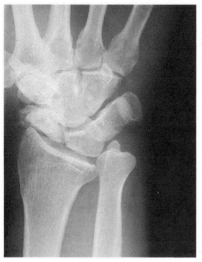

91. *Complications:* (1) *Sudeck's atrophy*—treat as in 46. (2) *Avascular necrosis:* Surgery should be carried out before secondary changes occur in the wrist. Illustrated: the scaphoid is collapsing, and although there is as yet little evidence of osteo-arthritis, further delay would be unwise. The scaphoid should be excised, with or without the insertion of a silastic spacer.

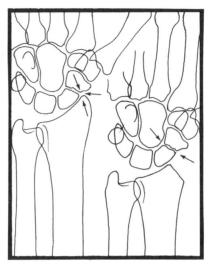

92. *Complications:* (3) *Non-union:* (a) This may remain symptom free, and active treatment is then inadvisable. (b) If symptoms are marked, and it is seen early, internal screw fixation and bone grafting may be considered. (c) If an early impingement osteo-arthritis threatens, satisfactory results may be obtained from excision of the radial styloid even although the mid-carpal joint is unaffected by this (ill.).

93. *Complications:* (4) *Advanced osteo-arthritis:* This generally occurs as a sequel to avascular necrosis or non-union. The following treatments may be considered: (a) *Wrist joint (radio-carpal) fusion:* Pronation and supination movements are retained, but all other wrist movements are lost. This is the most reliable procedure and is the only one which should be considered in the patient who undertakes heavy manual labour. (b) Where the retention of some wrist movement is essential, excision of the proximal row of the carpus may be considered. The results are a little unpredictable in terms of final range of movements, strength, and freedom from pain. (c) Where surgery is thought inadvisable, good results in terms of relief from pain, with reasonable function may be obtained by the use of a block-leather support, or similar orthotic device.

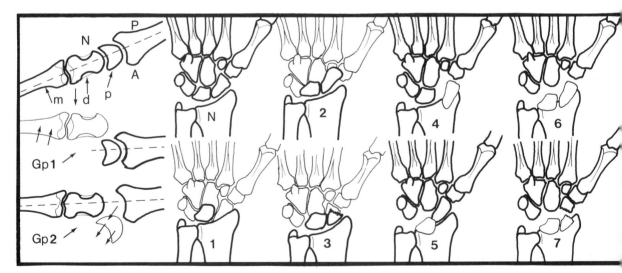

94. *Dislocations of the carpus:* These may result from a fall on the outstretched hand, and are comparatively uncommon. There are two main groups. In the first, the metacarpals (m), the distal row of the carpus (d) and part of the proximal row (p) dislocate backwards. In classifying injuries within this group, the prefix 'peri' is used to describe undisplaced structures in the proximal row. Occasionally one of the carpal bones fractures, part remaining in alignment, and part displacing with the distal row of the carpus. Note in the illustrations that structures drawn in feint lines are *displaced*. N = normal appearance from the side or *volar* aspect.
(1) Peri-lunar dislocation of the carpus;
(2) peri-scapho-lunar dislocation of the carpus; (3) trans-scapho peri-lunar dislocation of the carpus. (Not illustrated are the rare trans-capitate, trans-triquetral peri-lunar dislocations and others.) In the second main group of injuries, the distal row re-aligns with the radius and part of the proximal row is extruded: hence
(4) dislocation of the scaphoid;
(5) dislocation of the lunate; (6) dislocation of the lunate and scaphoid; (7) dislocation of the lunate and part of the scaphoid. (Note correspondence between 1 and 5, 2 and 6, 3 and 7.)

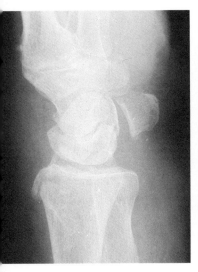

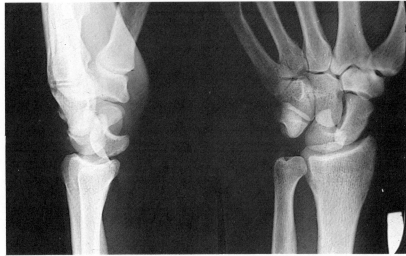

5. *Dislocation of the lunate:* This is the commonest of all the carpal dislocations, and generally results from a fall on the outstretched hand. It is frequently overlooked, and this is nearly always due to failure in interpretation of the radiographs. Note in the *normal* radiographs of the carpus (ill.) that the pisiform bone stands out to a varying degree from the rest of the volar surface.

96. *Dislocation of the lunate:* The *shape* of the dislocated lunate is quite different from the ovoid/quadrilateral mass of the pisiform. The *concave surface* in which the capitate usually sits is *rotated* anteriorly, and the crescent moon shape of the bone (and hence its name) is rendered obvious. The articular surfaces of the scaphoid and triquetral remain aligned with the radius while the lunate is *displaced* anteriorly. In the A.P. projection, the lunate is sector shaped (resembling a foil-wrapped cheese segment). *Diagnosis:* This is established on the basis of a history of injury, local tenderness, and the radiographs. Evidence of median nerve involvement is very suggestive (may result from direct pressure of the displaced bone on the nerve).

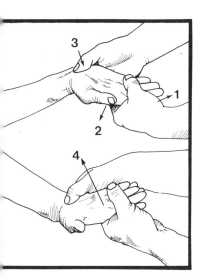

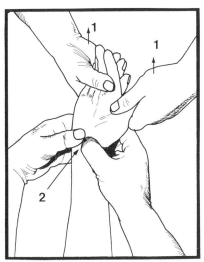

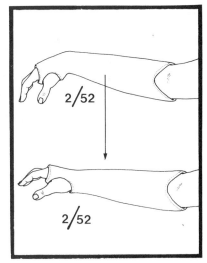

97. *Treatment (1)* Reduction can generally be achieved by closed methods under general anaesthesia. (1) Apply traction to the supinated wrist. (2) Extend the wrist, maintaining traction. (3) Apply pressure with the thumb over the lunate. (4) Flex the wrist as soon as you feel the lunate slip into position.

98. *Treatment (2)* Alternatively, if an assistant is available, he should apply traction in supination and extension as before (1) while you use both thumbs to push the lunate posteriorly and distally (2). When it is felt to reduce, the wrist is once again flexed. The reduction should be checked with radiographs before the anaesthetic is discontinued. (Failure is an indication for open reduction.)

99. *Treatment (3)* (a) The wrist is encased in plaster in a position of moderate flexion for 1–2 weeks (1). (b) The plaster is then changed for one with the wrist in the neutral position for a further 2 weeks (2).
(c) Physiotherapy may then be required, depending on the degree of residual stiffness. Swelling may be a problem initially, and the usual precautions should be taken (e.g. generous padding, elevation, sling, etc.).

100. *Complications:* (1) *Late diagnosis:* If there is delay in making the diagnosis, manipulative reduction becomes increasingly difficult, and after a week may not be possible. Open reduction is then necessary, and carries with it the greatly increased risk of avascular necrosis. Surgery should be performed through an anterior incision, and every effort made to reduce the bone without disturbing any of its ligamentous attachments, (evidence suggests the major blood supply enters anteriorly) or further damaging the median nerve.
(2) *Median nerve palsy:* Prompt reduction of the dislocation is usually followed by early complete recovery. After late reduction recovery may be incomplete, but seldom requires separate treatment. (3) *Sudeck's atrophy:* This is a common complication and is treated along previously described lines (46).

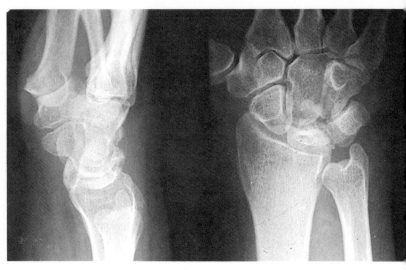

101. *Complications:* (4) *Avascular necrosis:* This leads to collapse of the lunate and secondary osteo-arthritis which advances with great rapidity. *All cases of dislocated lunate should have monthly radiographs for 6 months* to allow early detection of this complication. If detected early, excision, with or without prosthetic replacement, may prevent progressive osteo-arthritis. In many cases, and certainly at the later stages, arthrodesis of the wrist is preferable.

Note that repeated trauma to the wrist without frank dislocation of the lunate may lead to similar radiographic appearances (Kienbock's disease); this condition is found particularly in manual workers such as carpenters, cobblers and pneumatic drill operators, etc.

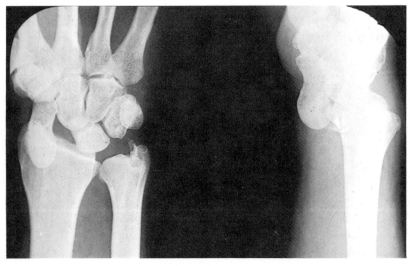

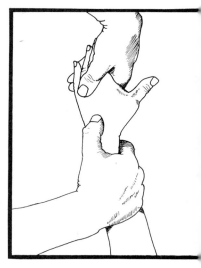

102. *Dislocations and subluxation of the scaphoid:* These uncommon injuries are diagnosed radiologically and if suspected, A.P. projections in both radial and ulnar deviation may be helpful. The most striking feature is the widening of the space between the scaphoid and lunate. *Treatment:* (a) If the displacement is anterior and complete as shown, manipulate as for dislocation of the lunate. (b) In many cases, dislocation is incomplete, with the proximal pole being tilted posteriorly, and the distal pole anteriorly. Such injuries have often a toggle-like instability within the dorsiflexion/palmar flexion range (and the stable position within this phase must be found by trial and error during reduction).

103. *(b) ctd.:* Reduction may be achieved by pressure over the dorsal pole. The wrist should be kept in plaster in the stable position with added radial deviation for 6 weeks. Check films are mandatory. Note (1) Slight residual displacements should be accepted—the late results are usually excellent. (2) Gross displacements should be reduced through a *posterior* incision, with reefing of the posterior (scapho-lunate) capsule.

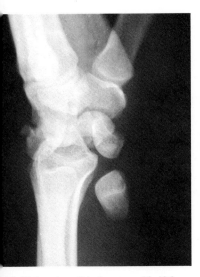

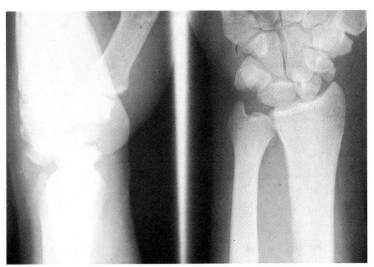

04. *Dislocation of the lunate and half the scaphoid:* This may be treated initially by closed reduction in the same way as an uncomplicated dislocation of the lunate. Thereafter, however, the scaphoid fracture dominates the picture, and the treatment should follow the lines described for that injury. If after reduction there is gross carpal instability, internal fixation of the scaphoid should be considered.

105. *Trans-scapho peri-lunar dislocation of the carpus:* This injury corresponds to dislocation of the lunate and half the scaphoid just described. It is the commonest of the first group of carpal dislocations. In some cases there may be associated fractures of the styloid processes of the radius and the ulna. *Treatment:* Reduction by traction is usually easy. Thereafter the management is that of fracture of the scaphoid. If, however, the scaphoid reduction is poor or if the wrist is very unstable, internal fixation of the scaphoid must be considered.

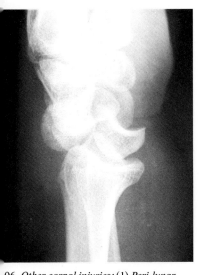

107. *Other carpal injuries ctd.:* (2) *Dislocation of both the lunate and scaphoid:* This should be treated as for dislocation of the lunate (95). (3) *Peri-scapho-lunar dislocation of the carpus:* This should be treated in the same way as peri-lunar dislocation of the carpus (105). (4) *Dislocation of the trapezium, trapezoid or hamate* are rare. Closed reduction should always be attempted, but open reduction is frequently required. In the face of instability, transfixion by Kirschner wires may be helpful. (5) *Fractures through the bodies of any of the carpal bones other than the scaphoid* are rare, and should be treated symptomatically by 6 weeks' fixation in a Colles or scaphoid plaster (depending on the injury). Fractures of the hamate and pisiform may be complicated by ulnar nerve palsy which should be treated expectantly. (6) *Small chip fractures of the carpus* are common and generally result from hyper-flexion or hyper-extension injuries of the wrist. Direct violence is sometimes responsible. The bone of origin is often in doubt. Rest of the wrist in plaster for 3 weeks is all that is required, and full recovery of function is the rule.

06. *Other carpal injuries:* (1) *Peri-lunar dislocation of the carpus:* This corresponds to isolated dislocation of the lunate. *Treatment:* (a) Reduce by traction. (b) Apply plaster with the wrist in flexion and retain for 1–2 weeks before (c) changing the plaster to one with the wrist in the neutral position. This should be retained for a further two weeks. (d) Thereafter physiotherapy may be required to mobilise the wrist.

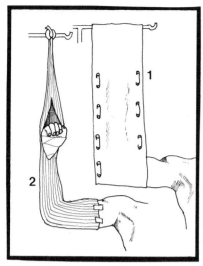

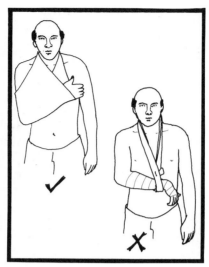

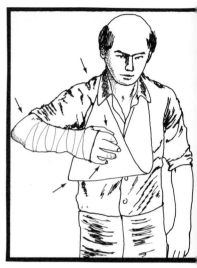

108. *Injuries to metacarpals and phalanges: General principles: Post traumatic swelling (1)* It is essential that every effort is made to limit swelling which may lead to chronic oedema and irrecoverable fibrosis. *Admission for elevation* (e.g. by roller towel (1) or stockingette (2) supported by an i.v. drip stand) is advisable if (a) there is extensive soft tissue involvement (trauma or surgery) (b) there are multiple fractures.

109. *Post traumatic swelling (2)* If the injury is less severe (e.g. a single fracture with no significant soft tissue injury) and it is thought it can be treated reasonably on an out-patient basis, elevation of the arm in a sling may be helpful, *provided the sling is applied in such a way that the hand is not dependent.* Any pressure dressing should be carefully applied to avoid local constriction.

110. *Principles of splintage:* (1) If a fracture or joint is unstable, some form of stabilising support will be required, but (2) as *few joints as possible* should be immobilised for as *short a time as possible.* The arm should be removed from any sling 2–3 times per day and the elbow and shoulder put through a full range of movements: free fingers should be vigorously exercised.

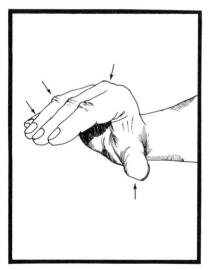

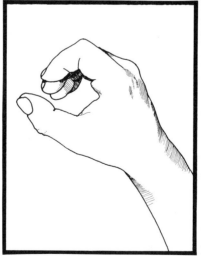

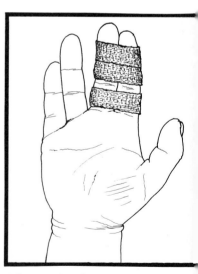

111. *Principles of splintage ctd.:* (3) The M.P. joints of the fingers should *never* be splinted in extension. When recovery of movements is hoped for, and fixation is required, the M.P. joints should be flexed to 90°, the I.P. joints extended, and the thumb abducted. In practice, it is often difficult to splint in this position, but M.P. joint extension must be studiously avoided.

112. *Principles of splintage ctd.:* (4) The previously described position, where return of function is expected, reduces the effects of fibrosis in the collateral ligaments and places the finger joints in a favourable position for mobilisation. It must be carefully differentiated from the position of *fixation* where no return of function is anticipated (e.g. the position a joint is placed in for fusion). In the latter case, the M.P. and I.P. joints are put in mid-flexion.

113. *Principles of splintage ctd.:* (5) Where a finger injury requires stabilisation in the A.P. plane (e.g. an I.P. collateral ligament avulsion fracture) or where minimal fixation is required (e.g. an undisplaced fracture of a phalanx) 'garter' strapping to an adjacent finger often provides the ideal combination of stability while retaining movement.

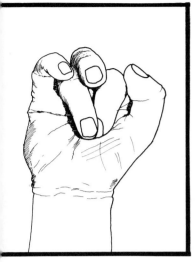

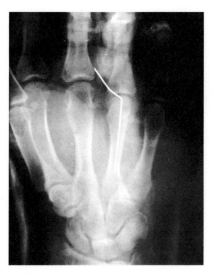

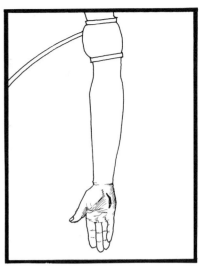

114. *Principles of splintage ctd.:*
(6) Rotational (torsional) deformity of a metacarpal or phalanx may not be noticeable in extension, but cause obvious deformity and functional impairment in flexion. Note that when the fingers are flexed individually they all touch the palm close to the scaphoid. By checking the striking point of the injured finger by flexing it prior to fixation, rotational deformity can usually be avoided.

115. *Principles of splintage ctd.:* (7) In the presence of gross instability, especially where fractures are multiple, internal fixation may be helpful. In its simplest form, percutaneous Kirschner wires are often very useful; after 3 weeks there is usually sufficient stability to allow their removal. Alternatively, the experienced surgeon may use screws (e.g. A.O. small screws) and other devices.

116. *Soft tissue management:* (1) Where there is necrotic or foreign material, a thorough debridement should be performed under a tourniquet to minimise the risks of infection. There is little tissue to spare in the hand, and wide excision of wounds is to be avoided. (2) The tourniquet should be released prior to closure to secure bleeding points and reduce wound haematoma.

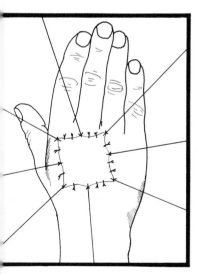

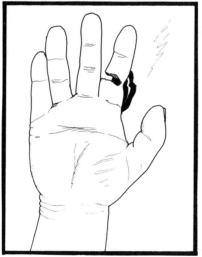

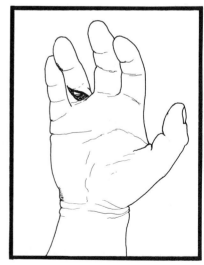

117. *Soft tissue management ctd.:* (3) Where there is skin loss, every attempt should be made to ensure that healing will be achieved as quickly as possible to permit early mobilisation. The exposure of fractures, joints and bones should be avoided, and if the situation permits, a primary skin grafting procedure or plastic repair should be carried out.

118. *Soft tissue management ctd.:* (4) If there is division of both neurovascular bundles to a finger, amputation should be advised unless facilities for micro-surgery are available and the particular circumstances (e.g. employment, hobbies, etc.) make an attempt at preservation particularly desirable. In all cases, the maximum length of thumb must be preserved.

119. *Soft tissue management ctd.:* (5) If there is appreciable risk of infection (e.g. ragged wound, dirty causal instrument) primary suture of nerves and also of tendons in the 'no man's area' of the tendon sheaths should not be undertaken. Where, however, the circumstances are ideal, the experienced surgeon may achieve the best results by primary repair.

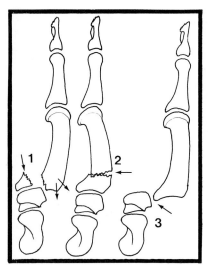

120. *Injuries to the thumb: The base:* The commonest injuries involving the base of the thumb are (1) Bennett's fracture (or Bennett's fracture dislocation as it may be more aptly called) (2) fractures of the base of the thumb metacarpal (3) carpo-metacarpal dislocation of the thumb.

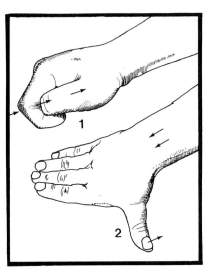

121. *Diagnosis:* Injuries of the base usually result from force being applied along the long axis of the thumb—e.g. from a fall or blow on the clenched fist (1)—or from forced abduction of the thumb (2). Any of these may be mistaken for scaphoid fracture, but tenderness is maximal distal to the snuff box (and deformity may be obvious).

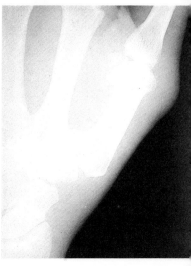

122. *Bennett's fracture:* Note the distinctive features of this fracture: (1) A small medial fragment of bone which may tilt, but maintains its relationship with the trapezium. (2) The (vertical) fracture line involves the joint between the thumb metacarpal and the trapezium (trapezo-metacarpal joint). (3) Most important, the proximal and lateral subluxation of the thumb metacarpal.

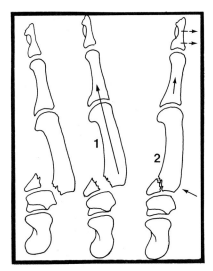

123. *Treatment (1)* The principle of reduction is straightforward: traction is applied to the thumb (1) and reduction completed by abducting it and applying pressure to the lateral aspect of the base (2). A general anaesthetic or Bier block is usually necessary. Maintaining reduction can be troublesome, and careful attention must be paid to the details of plaster fixation.

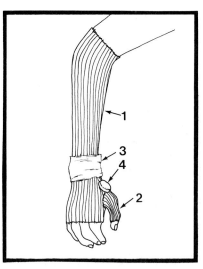

124. *Treatment (2)* (a) Begin by applying stockingette to the arm (1) and the thumb (2). Bony prominences should be protected as required with wool roll (3). (b) A small felt pad is placed over the base of the thumb metacarpal (4). (Note: adhesive felt should not be applied directly to the skin in this situation if a pustular rash is to be avoided.)

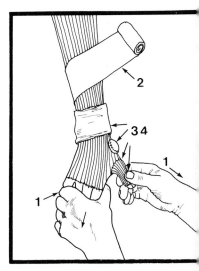

125. *Treatment (3)* (c) An assistant applies traction to the thumb and steadies the lateral three fingers (1). (d) Two to three 6″ (15 cm) P.O.P. bandages (with or without an anterior slab) are applied to the *forearm* (2). (e) Two 4″ (10 cm) P.O.P. bandages are the quickly applied to the wrist and up to the I.P. joint of the thumb.

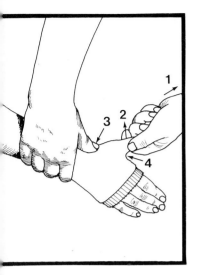

127. *After care:* (a) Check radiographs are taken to confirm that reduction has been achieved. (b) The arm may require elevating with a sling for the first few days. (c) The patient should be seen at weekly intervals for the first 2 to 3 weeks. If the plaster appears slack at any stage it must be changed. If there is evidence of slipping of the fracture, a new plaster should also be applied (no anaesthetic is generally required). During the setting of the plaster, light traction should be applied to the thumb while the plaster is well moulded round the base (in the position described for the initial reduction).
(d) Plaster fixation should be maintained for 6 weeks.

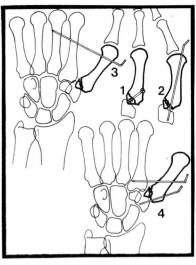

6. *Treatment (4)* The surgeon now takes ₂ thumb (the plaster being set on the ₋earm while the distal part remains soft). ₋ must apply traction (1), abduct the ₋umb (2), maintain pressure over the base the first metacarpal (3), and mould the ₋aster well into the M.P. joint on its flexor ₋pect (4).

128. *Alternative methods of treatment:* A good result is the rule following reduction and plaster fixation, but alternative methods of holding this fracture are practised. These include (1) screw fixation (e.g. A.O. small fragment set) (2) intramedullary Kirschner wire (3) Kirschner wire fixation of thumb to index and middle metacarpals (4) use of two Kirschner wires to stabilise the thumb metacarpal.

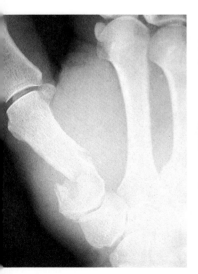

9. *Fracture of the base of the thumb ₋etacarpal:* Note that the joint surface is ₋t involved and that there is no ₋bluxation. Greenstick fractures of this ₋pe are common in children. Angulation is ₋ually slight or moderate and should be ₋cepted; gross angulations should be ₋anipulated, using the technique described ₋r Bennett's fracture. Plaster fixation for ₋out 5 weeks is desirable.

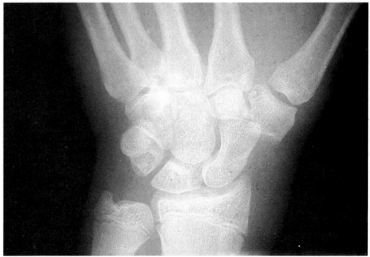

130. *Carpo-metacarpal dislocation of the thumb:* The thumb may dislocate at the joint between the metacarpal base and the trapezium; or the whole of the first ray may be involved, the trapezium remaining with the thumb metacarpal, with the dislocation taking place between the trapezium and the scaphoid (ill.). Both these injuries result from forcible abduction of the thumb. *Treatment:* Reduce by applying traction to thumb and local pressure over the base. Thereafter apply a well padded plaster of scaphoid type for 3 weeks. Elevation of the limb for the first few days is desirable. Physiotherapy is seldom required.

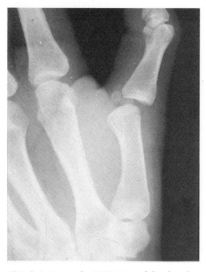

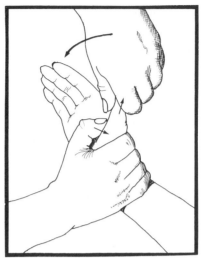

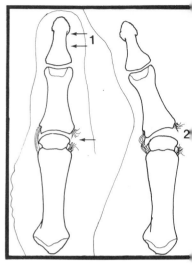

131. *Injuries at the M.P. joint of the thumb: Posterior dislocation (1)* This injury generally results from forcible hyperextension of the thumb. It is common in children. In a number of cases there is 'button-holing' of the capsule by the metacarpal head and closed methods of reduction will fail. Nevertheless, manipulation should be tried first in all cases.

132. *Posterior dislocation (2)* Manipulative reduction may often be attempted without anaesthesia (by the quick confident application of traction to the thumb with simultaneous pressure over the metacarpal head). When open reduction is required this should be performed through a lateral incision under a tourniquet. In all cases a light plaster splint should be worn for 2–3 weeks after reduction.

133. *Rupture of the ulnar collateral ligament (Gamekeeper's thumb) (1)* This injury is caused by forcible abduction (1). If unrecognised and untreated, there may be progressive M.P. subluxation (2) with interference with grasp, causing significant permanent disability. (a) *Suspect* this injury when there is complaint of pain in this region. (b) *Look for tenderness* on the medial side of the M.P. joint.

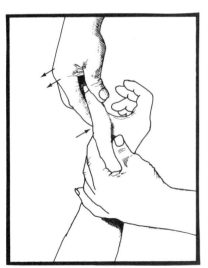

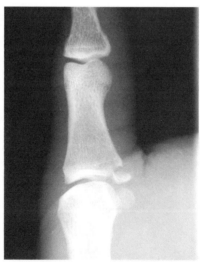

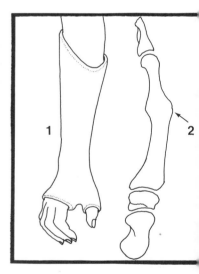

134. *Ulnar collateral ligament (2)* (c) Extend the M.P. joint fully and apply stress to the ulnar collateral ligament by abducting the proximal phalanx. Note the presence of any 'give'. Carefully compare one side with the other. If in doubt, stress radiographs should be taken.

135. *Ulnar collateral ligament (3)* (d) Study radiographs of the joint: (i) Subluxation may or may not be apparent in the unstressed films. (ii) An avulsion fracture (ill.) may betray this type of injury. If a fracture is present, note its position. (Marked displacement, or rotation so that its articular surface is pointing distally, are indications for surgery.)

136. *Ulnar collateral ligament (4) Treatment:* (a) Slight laxity (incomplete tear or minimally displaced avulsion fracture: fixation in a scaphoid-type plaster for 6 weeks (1). (b) Gross laxity (complete tear) or rotated fracture: surgical repair. (Exposure of the lesion under a tourniquet; repair of torn ligament or replacement of fracture; plaster for 6 weeks.) (c) Longstanding lesions with marked symptoms: M.P. joint fusion (2).

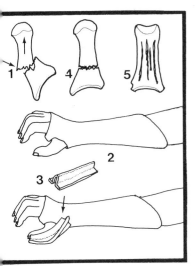

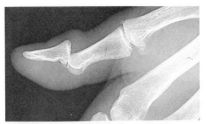

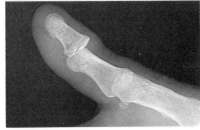

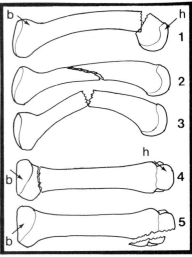

137. *Fracture of the proximal phalanx:* The severely angled fracture (1) should be reduced by traction and local pressure. Hold with a dorsal (or volar) slab (2) to which is added a girdered extension (3), held on with bandages. The minimally angled fracture (4) and the splinter fracture (5) may be protected by a local slab (similar to 3) bandaged in position. Elevation may be required.

138. *I.P. joint dislocation of the thumb:* Reduce by traction as described for M.P. joint dislocations (132). Only occasionally is anaesthesia required (ring or Bier block). Thereafter splint for 2–3 weeks with a local plaster slab. *Fractures of the terminal phalanx:* Crushing injuries are the usual cause, and any soft tissue damage takes priority in management. A light local splint (e.g. of plaster) will prevent pain from stubbing.

139. *Injuries to the fifth metacarpal:* The commonest fractures involving the metacarpal of the little finger are (1) fractures of the neck (2) spiral fractures of the shaft, usually undisplaced (3) transverse fractures of the shaft, often angulated (4) fractures of the base (5) fractures of the head. (b = base, h = head.)

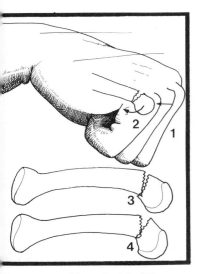

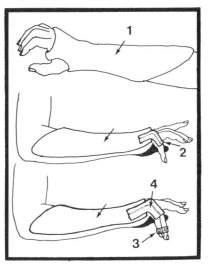

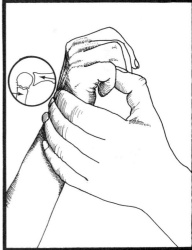

140. *Fractures of the neck of the fifth metacarpal (1)* These are nearly always caused by the clenched fist meeting resistance—for example, as a result of a fight (1). Angulation and impaction are common (2). When angulation is slight (3) or moderate (4) it should be accepted, and the fracture supported for 3–4 weeks until local pain settles.

141. *Neck of fifth metacarpal (2)* A simple dorsal slab (1) completed after a few days, may be quite satisfactory. Better fixation is achieved by the addition of a finger extension (2) to the basic slab. Still more support is provided by the use of garter strapping (3) and the inclusion of the ring and little fingers in the extension (4) (securing bandages omitted for clarity).

142. *Neck of fifth metacarpal (3)* If angulation is gross, an attempt may be made to correct it. The M.P. joint is flexed; pressure is then applied to the head via the proximal phalanx, using the thumb to do so. The fingers apply counter pressure to the shaft. Reduction is generally easy, but must be maintained during setting of the plaster.

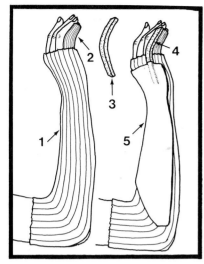

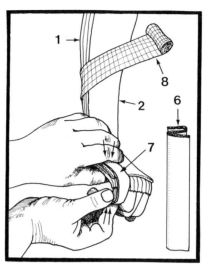

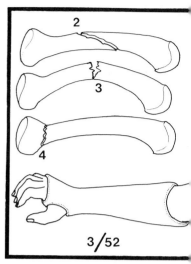

143. *Neck of fifth metacarpal (4)* The following technique may be employed. Stockingette is applied to the arm (1) and to the little finger (2). A thin strip of felt (3) is placed over the finger (4). A substantial dorsal slab is applied (5). The finger should be flexed into the palm and the striking point checked (114).

144. *Neck of fifth metacarpal (5)* A finger slab, made from a thrice folded slab formed from 3 layers or so of 4″ (10 cm) plaster bandage (6) is applied from wrist to finger tip (7). Pressure is maintained while the slab is setting (or with one hand as in 142). Meanwhile an assistant can be securing the slabs with a wet gauze bandage (8). Complete in 2–3 days and retain for 4–5 weeks only.

145. *Injuries of the fifth metacarpal ctd.:* Spiral fractures of the shaft (2), transverse fractures of the shaft with slight or moderate angulation or displacement (3) and fracture of the base (4) may be treated quite adequately by the application of a Colles plaster for 3–4 weeks.

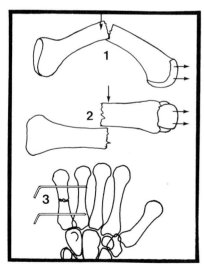

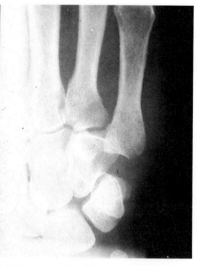

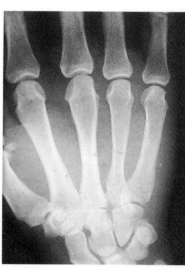

146. *Injuries of the fifth metacarpal ctd.:* Marked angulation of a shaft fracture should be treated by traction and local pressure prior to plaster fixation (1). Displaced fractures may be similarly reduced (2) but soft tissue between the bone ends may render reduction possible only by open methods. If that is required, reduction may be maintained by percutaneous (3) or intramedullary Kirschner wiring.

147. *Injuries of the fifth metacarpal ctd.:* (5) Fractures of the *head* of the fifth metacarpal (see 139, 5) may be treated by garter strapping and early mobilisation; if symptoms are marked a dorsal slab may also be used for the first 1–2 weeks. (6) Dislocation of the base of the metacarpal (ill.) is usually easily reduced with traction, but may need Kirschner wire stabilisation.

148. *Injuries to the index, middle and ring metacarpals:* The commonest fracture is a spiral fracture of the shaft (especially of the ring metacarpal), but fractures involving the base and neck are frequent, as are transverse fractures of the shaft (ill.). Undisplaced fractures may be supported by a Colles type slab, but be on guard for swelling which can be severe, especially in multiple fractures.

49. *Injuries to the index, middle and ring etacarpals ctd.:* Severely displaced actures of the index metacarpal should be nanaged along the lines described for actures of the fifth metacarpal. In articular, badly displaced fractures should e reduced, and if necessary secured by ttramedullary or transfixion Kirschner ires (146). These wires may be retained for weeks; plaster fixation may be needed for further 2 weeks.

When the A.P. radiographs show the resence of an isolated off-ended fracture of e middle or ring metacarpals, or moderate ngulation or shortening, the position can enerally be accepted. The striking point of e finger should be checked, a dorsal slab pplied, and the limb elevated to counteract velling. If off-ending or angulation is nspicuous in the *lateral projection,* eduction by manipulation should be ttempted.

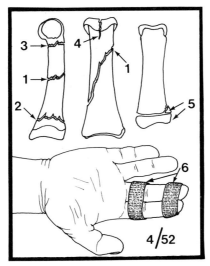

150. *Fractures of the proximal and middle phalanges (1)* Undisplaced, simple fractures—e.g. of the shaft (1), base (2), neck (3), intercondylar region (4), or epiphyseal injuries (5)—seldom present any problem. Garter strapping (6) for 3–4 weeks may give adequate support, but if symptoms are marked, this may be supplemented by the use of a volar or dorsal slab, with finger extension.

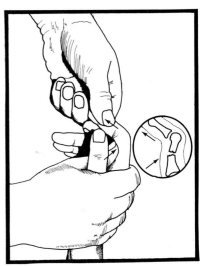

151. *Proximal and middle phalanges (2)* There is a tendency for angulation to occur due to intrinsic muscle pull; if more than 15° this should be corrected under general anaesthesia by gentle traction, using the thumb as a fulcrum. Generally these fractures are stable in flexion, and the affected finger may require to be fixed initially in this position.

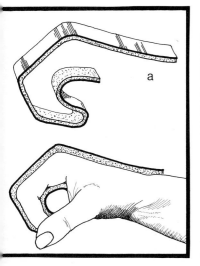

52. *Proximal and middle phalanges (3)* here are various methods of fixation: these clude (a) foam-plastic covered malleable luminium splinting. Although this may hold e finger well, there may be difficulty in rapping it securely to the hand, and corporation in a dorsal slab may be elpful. Great care must be taken to check e strike point and avoid undue local ressure which may lead to skin sloughing.

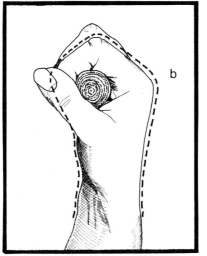

153. *Proximal and middle phalanges (4)* (b) If a rolled bandage can be held in the palm, this may be used as a fulcrum, the injured finger being flexed over it and secured with adhesive tape. Additional encircling bandaging is required for security, but even so dislodging may occur. Some surgeons use a (wetted) P.O.P. bandage in the palm.

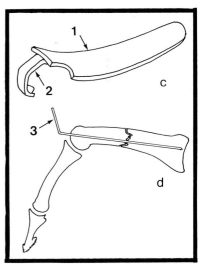

154. *Proximal and middle phalanges (5)* (c) A volar P.O.P. slab (1) with a substantial finger extension (2) may be used, moulding the fracture while this is setting; thereafter, the plaster is secured with wet open-weave bandages. If this arrangement appears too flimsy, it may be reinforced with a dorsal slab and dorsal finger extension.
(d) Intramedullary wires may be used (3) especially in the case of open and multiple fractures.

155. *After care:* In all cases (a) uninjured fingers should be left free and exercised, (b) rigid fixation should be discarded as soon as possible. In many situations garter strapping may be substituted after 2 weeks, and often all support after 4. *In no instance should the M.P. joints be fixed in extension.* *Complications:* (a) *Finger stiffness* is the commonest and most disabling complication, and is due to joint adhesions, fibrosis in the adjacent flexor tendon sheaths, and collateral ligament shortening. Infection in open fractures may be a major contributory factor. Stiffness may be minimised by the procedures described (e.g. elevation, correct splinting, early mobilisation) and by intensive physiotherapy and occupational therapy. Physiotherapy

and occupational therapy should be continued with vigour until the range of movements and finger power become static. This implies careful recording, at frequent intervals, of these parameters. Early return to work should be encouraged to foster re-adaption. Inability to work and a static response to physiotherapy requires most careful assessment of the following: (a) Possibility of redeployment (b) Possiblity of improvement from further surgery (e.g. tenolysis) (c) Amputation.

Amputation as primary treatment must be raised in compound phalangeal fractures when they are associated with flexor tendon division. Division of one or both neurovascular bundles, skin loss or severe crushing are additional factors weighing in

favour of this procedure (in contrast to attempted repair where treatment is likely to be prolonged and the final result uncertain). With these factors must be considered the patient's age, sex and occupation. (b) *Malunion:* Problems may arise from (i) recurrence of deformity (ii) failure to correct initial deformity (iii) torsional deformity. In some cases (iv) epiphyseal displacement may have escaped attention. In the latter case, re-modelling may lead to correction, and in the others, trick movements and postural adaptations may remove the patient's initial strong desire for corrective surgery. It is wise not to offer surgical correction until at least 6 months have passed since the injury.

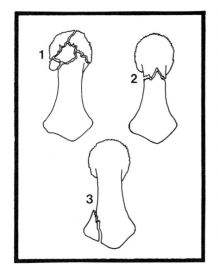

156. *Fractures of the terminal phalanx:* Fractures of the terminal tuft (often comminuted) (1), of the neck (2), and the base (3) are painful but relatively unimportant injuries. Treatment of any associated soft tissue injury takes precedence (e.g. debridement and suture of pulp lacerations).

Nevertheless, strapping the finger to a spatula or use of a plastic finger splint may relieve pain and prevent any painful stubbing incidents.

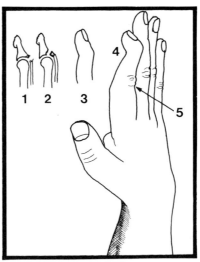

157. *Mallet finger (1)* This is caused by forcible flexion of the finger from the extended position. The distal slip of the long extensor tendon tears from its attachment to the phalanx (1), or avulses a fragment of bone (2). The patient is unable to extend the distal I.P. joint fully; drooping of the distal phalanx may be slight (3) or severe (4). In late cases there may be hyperextension of the proximal I.P. joint (5).

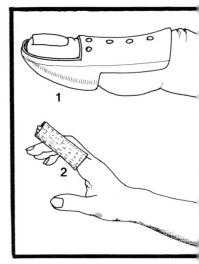

158. *Mallet finger (2) Treatment:* Splint in extension for six weeks, using if available an ABUNA plastic extension splint (1). Alternatively, the finger may be held in extension by a padded spatula, trimmed to include the distal joint only, and strapped to the volar surface. Plaster may also be used: begin by forming a tube of 4 thicknesses of 4″ (10 cm) dry plaster bandage round the finger (2).

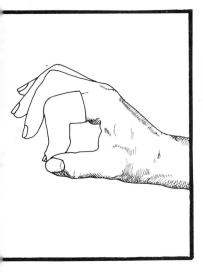

59. *Mallet finger (3)* The patient's hand is then dipped momentarily in water: he is asked to flex the proximal I.P. joint and extend the distal joint against the thumb while the plaster is smoothed off. If the deformity recurs on removal of the splint, immediate operation is not advised, as (1) disability may be slight (2) spontaneous (fibrotic) healing may occur after 6 months (3) the results of tendon suture are uncertain. I.P. fusion gives the best overall results.)

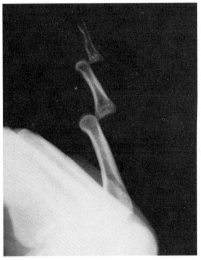

160. *M.P. and interphalangeal joint dislocations:* These may be simple or multiple (ill.) and as they result from hyperextension are almost always posterior dislocations. Reduce as described for the thumb (132). Thereafter garter strapping should be applied for 2 weeks unless there is any evidence of instability—when plaster of Paris splintage may be required for a slightly longer period.

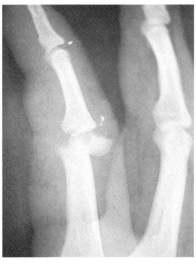

161. *Fracture dislocations:* It is essential that the joint surface is correctly re-located, and important that mobilisation is commenced as soon as possible. Open reduction is usually required, and fixation may be achieved with an intramedullary Kirschner wire. This should be removed after 2–3 weeks and mobilisation commenced using garter strapping for the first week or so until the fracture becomes more stable.

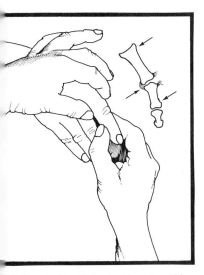

62. *'Sprains' and lateral subluxations (1)* These are usually caused by falls in which the side of a finger strikes some resistant object. There is avulsion or tearing of a collateral ligament. Spontaneous reduction is the rule. *Diagnosis:* The injury should be suspected on the basis of the history and the presence of local tenderness. Confirmation is obtained by noting instability on stressing the collateral ligament.

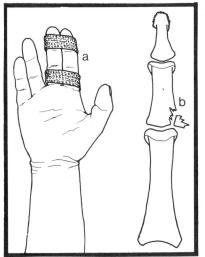

163. *Sprains and lateral subluxations (2)* Radiographs may show a tell-tale avulsion fracture. If doubt remains, stress films may be taken. *Treatment:* (a) Garter strapping for 5 weeks should be adequate. (b) If an avulsion fracture is present and has rotated, it should be replaced. *Complications:* Fusiform swelling of the finger may persist for many months even in the treated injury.

Self test
164. Radiograph of a patient complaining of pain in the hand after being involved in a fight. What pathology is shown?

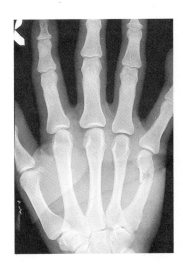

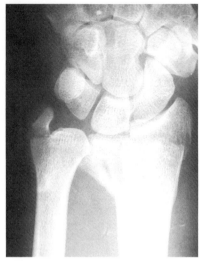

165. Describe this A.P. radiograph of the wrist; the history is of pain and marked swelling following a fall on the outstretched hand.

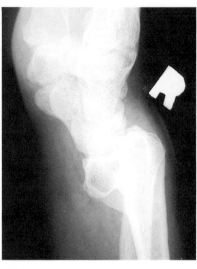

166. History of deformity of the wrist persisting after an injury some years previously: diagnosis?

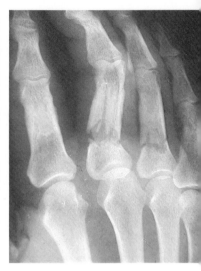

167. History of a crushing injury of the hand and fingers. Describe the radiograph.

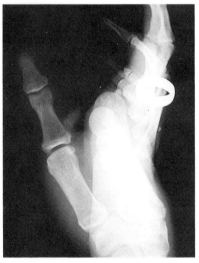

168. The complaint is of pain and deformity of the hand following an injury in which the fingers were forced backwards. What does the radiograph show?

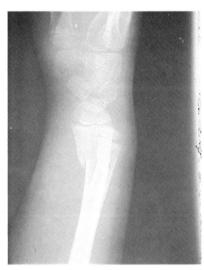

169. Describe this injury sustained by a child in a fall.

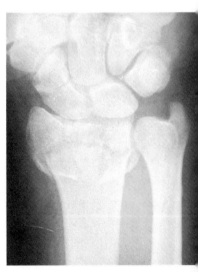

170. Describe the radiographic appearances. The history is of a fall on the outstretched hand.

64. Fracture of the neck of the fifth metacarpal.

65. Fracture of the distal radius; comminution of the distal fragment, with the fracture line involving the radio-carpal joint; fracture of the ulnar styloid.

66. Mal-union of a Smith's fracture.

67. (1) There is a transverse fracture of the base of the proximal phalanx of the ring finger; the single film suggests that there is no significant angulation or displacement. (2) There is a fracture of the base of the proximal phalanx of the middle finger, with vertical splinter fractures running into the proximal I.P. joint. There is angulation of the fracture. The single oblique view suggests that this is mainly anterior angulation.

168. Posterior dislocation of all the fingers at the M.P. joints. The thumb is not affected.

169. Greenstick fractures of the radius and ulna just proximal to the epiphyseal lines. There is slight subluxation of the distal ulna whose angulation is less than that of the radius. The deformity corresponds to that found in a Smith's fracture, and the combination of fracture of the radius with ulnar subluxation has some of the features of the Galeazzi lesion.

170. (1) There is a highly comminuted fracture of the distal radius with the radial displacement, ulnar angulation and impaction usually associated with a comminuted Colles fracture with involvement of the radio-carpal joint. A lateral projection would be required to differentiate it with certainty from a Smith's fracture. (2) There is a fracture through the waist of the scaphoid.

10. The spine

General principles: (1) *The main concern in any spinal injury is not with the spine itself,* but with the closely related neurological elements (the spinal cord, issuing nerve roots and cauda equina). (2) *If there is no neurological complication* risks of later neurological involvement must be assessed; if there is some risk of this, *precautions must be taken to see that this is avoided at all stages.* (3) *If there is an incomplete paraplegia* complicating the injury *great care must be taken to see that no deterioration is allowed to occur.* (4) *If paraplegia is present and complete*, the prognosis regarding potential recovery must be firmly established as early as possible. Only if this is pronounced *total and permanent* can vigilance in the handling of the spinal injury be relaxed.

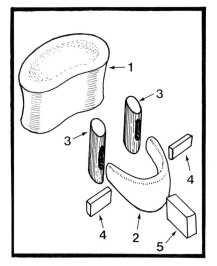

2. *Anatomical features (after Kapandji) (1)* The components of a typical vertebra have a complex relationship, and can be illustrated with an exploded diagram. The elements comprise the vertebral body (1) composed of cancellous bone covered with an outer shell of cortical bone, the horse-shoe shaped neural arch (2), two articular masses or processes which take part in the facet (interarticular) joints (3) and the transverse (4) and spinous (5) processes.

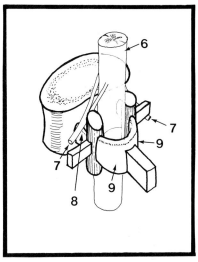

3. *Anatomical features (2)* When these components are brought together they form a protective bony covering for the cord (6) and the issuing nerve roots (7). The neural arch (2) is divided by the articular processes (3) into pedicles (8) and laminae (9).

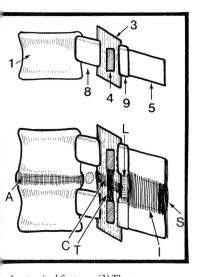

4. *Anatomical features (3)* The same components may be seen when the model is viewed from the side (numerical key as in 2, 3). The relationship of the vertebrae is maintained under normal circumstances by the shape and integrity of the bony structures and by the following ligaments: interspinous (I), supraspinous (S), intertransverse (T), annular (A), facet joint and capsular (C), and ligamenta flava (L).

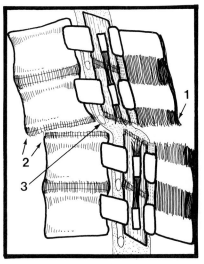

5. *Anatomical features (4)* The interspinous and supraspinous ligaments are of paramount importance, and form the so-called 'posterior ligament complex'. If this is torn (1) the other ligaments offer little resistance and the spine may sublux or dislocate (2). Subluxation may also occur if the neural arch or articular facets are fractured, and in either circumstance *the spine is said to be unstable.* The neurological structures (3) may be damaged (complicated fracture of the spine); if they escape initially, they nevertheless remain at risk, and it is vital to ensure that *delayed neurological involvement* does not occur.

If the neural arch, articular facets and posterior ligament complex remain intact, the injury is described as a *stable* one, neurological damage is uncommon, and the prognosis is generally excellent. (Exceptions include burst fractures of the spine, some lateral wedge fractures, and extension injuries of the cervical spine.)

Summary:

Stable injuries: Posterior ligament complex and neural arch intact. Generally uncomplicated.

Unstable injuries: Posterior ligament complex ruptured ± fracture of the neural arch or facet joints. May be complicated; if not, there is potential for neurological involvement.

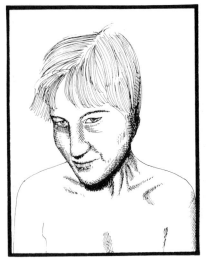

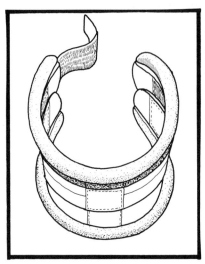

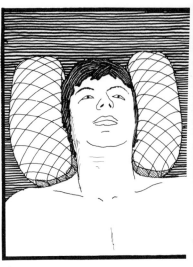

6. *Diagnosis:* Suspect involvement of the cervical spine where the patient
(a) complains of neck, occipital or shoulder pain after trauma, (b) has a torticollis (ill.), complains of restriction of neck movements, or supports the head with the hands, or (c) is found unconscious after a head injury, especially in road traffic accidents. In all cases, further investigation by radiographs is essential.

7. *Initial management: (1)* If you suspect that the cervical spine has been injured, your first move should be to safeguard the cord by controlling neck movements. The simplest and best way of doing this is by applying a cervical collar. (Ill: commercially available collar adjustable in depth and girth.) At the roadside, an adequate collar may be fashioned from rolled newspapers pushed into a nylon stocking and wrapped round the neck.

8. *Initial management: (2)* Alternatively, if the patient is on a trolley, the head may be supported by sandbags. *Do not allow the head to flex forwards, and do not hyperextend.* Keep the head in a neutral position wherever possible, and in the conscious patient quickly check that there is active movement in all limbs.

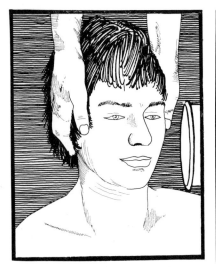

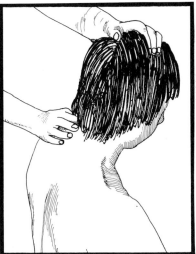

9. *Initial management: (3)* Especially if there is some evidence of neurological involvement, *do not* check the range of movements in the cervical spine. Accompany the patient to the X-ray department, supporting the head during the positioning of the tube and making sure that the spine is not forced in to flexion. For initial screening an A.P., lateral, and a through-the-mouth projection of C1 and C2 should be taken.

10. *Initial management: (4)* If these films appear normal, you may proceed in reasonable safety to (i) further examination of the neck for localising tenderness, restriction of active movements, and protective spasm, and (ii) a more thorough neurological examination. If these show no departure from normal, the patient may be treated with a cervical collar, with a follow-up review in one week.

11. *Initial management: (5)* If there is, however, persistent material limitation of movements or evidence of neurological disturbance further investigation is necessary. The following additional radiographs should be taken: (a) two more lateral projections, one in flexion and one in extension. These again should be supervised. (b) right and left oblique projections of the cervical spine. The commonest difficulty is the technical one of visualising the lower cervical vertebrae in the stocky patient. The upper border of T1 *must* be seen. *Accept that* detail may be poor. *Do not accept* that the spine cannot be shown in sufficient detail to exclude dislocation of one vertebra over another. If necessary, assist the radiographer by arranging for traction to be applied to the arms—one in adduction and the other in abduction; slight angulation of the tube and increase in exposure may be helpful.

In some cases screening of the cervical spine movements may be useful.

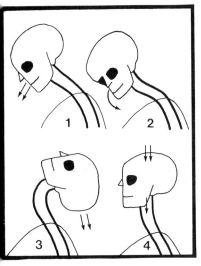

12. *Classification of cervical spine injuries:* Injuries of the cervical spine may be grouped according to the mechanism of injury: (A) Flexion injuries, 1. (B) Flexion and rotation injuries, 2. (C) Extension injuries, 3. (D) Compression injuries, 4.

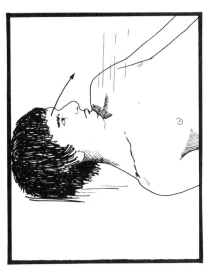

13. *Causes of flexion and flexion/rotation injuries:* These may result from (a) falls on the back of the head leading to flexion of the neck—for example, in motor cycle spills, diving in shallow water, pole vaulting, and rugby football (b) blows on the back of the head from falling objects (e.g. in the building and mining industries) (c) rapid deceleration in head-on car accidents.

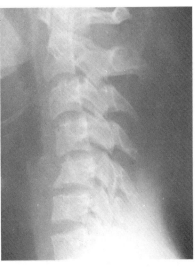

14. *(A) Flexion injuries: Stable anterior wedge fracture (1)* The vertebral body is wedged anteriorly, while the posterior part is generally intact. Before the injury can be declared stable, there must be (1) no evidence of injury to the posterior ligament complex—no separation or avulsion of the vertebral spines, or clinical evidence of ligament tear (see 91)—(2) no damage to the neural arches or facets. (3) In addition, flexion and extension laterals must be taken, and must show no vertebral instability.

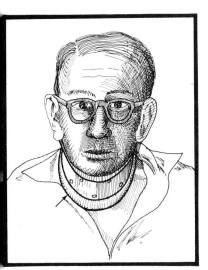

15. *Stable anterior wedge fracture (2)* Assuming these criteria are satisfied, neurological disturbance is rare and the prognosis excellent. Treat with a cervical collar for six weeks. Rarely when there is a degree of lateral wedging there may be troublesome nerve root involvement usually with (mainly) sensory disturbance in the corresponding dermatome. *If instability is at all suspected, treat as a cervical dislocation* (see 38).

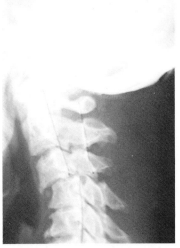

16. *(B) Flexion/rotation injuries:* (a) *Unilateral dislocation with a locked facet joint* (1) One facet joint dislocates, so that in the lateral projection of the cervical spine one vertebral body is seen to overlap the one below by about a third. The A.P. view may not be helpful, or it may show mal-alignment of spinous processes. There is often little difference between laterals taken in flexion and extension.

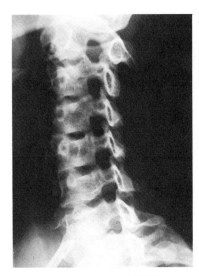

17. *Unilateral dislocation* (2) Oblique projections will, however, confirm the diagnosis. On one side the columnar arrangement of bodies, foramina and facet joints will be regular (ill.), while on the other it will be broken. Damage to the posterior ligament complex is variable, and *after reduction* these injuries may be quite stable: *BUT NOTE:* if there is an associated fracture involving a facet joint, the injury is MOST CERTAINLY UNSTABLE, and fusion will be required after reduction.

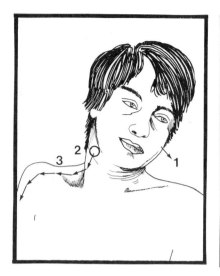

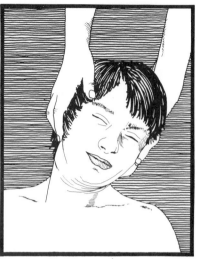

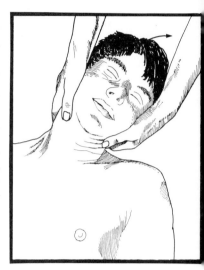

18. *Unilateral dislocation* (3) On clinical examination of the patient with a unilateral dislocation, the head is slightly rotated and inclined to the side (1) away from the locked facet (2). There is often great pain with radiation (3), due to pressure on the nerve root at the level of the affected joint, and there may be cord involvement.

19. *Treatment* (1) The initial aim in treatment is to reduce the dislocation, and the secrèt of this is well controlled traction. (A) The patient is given a general anaesthetic; the head must be well supported during induction, the administration of any muscle relaxant, and intubation (which must be carried out without undue extension of the neck). (B) X-ray facilities should be available. (Preferably an image intensifier.)

20. *Treatment* (2) (C) The surgeon must have freedom to manipulate the head, and may do this with the patient fully on the table, or pulled up till the head is supported in the lap of the surgeon seated at the top end of the table. Place the thumbs under the jaw, clasp the fingers behind the occiput, and apply firm traction in *lateral flexion* away from the side of the locked facet, i.e. in the direction the head is usually inclined.

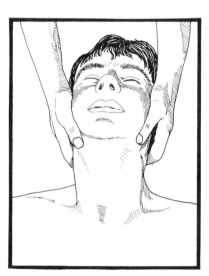

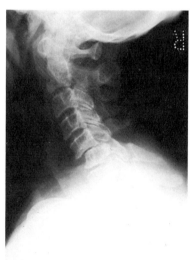

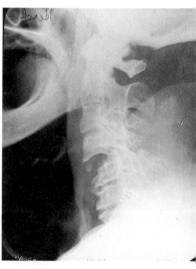

21. *Treatment* (3) (D) Maintaining traction, bring the head into the mid-line position, correcting the rotation element *before* lateral flexion. Release the traction, support the head (e.g. with foam plastic blocks) while check radiographs are taken. If reduction has not been achieved, repeat the manoeuvre with greater anaesthetic relaxation. Screening may be used. (If reduction fails (rare), or if preferred, use skull traction as at 32 et seq.)

22. *Treatment* (4) (E) Once reduction has been achieved, a cervical collar should be applied, and worn cominuously for 6 weeks. (F) Fortnightly radiographs of the neck should be taken, and flexion and extension laterals at the end of the 6 weeks' fixation. *If there is any evidence of late subluxation* (ill.) the patient should be admitted for local cervical fusion.

23. *(B) Flexion/rotation injuries:*
(b) *Unstable injuries:* The commonest injury of this type is one where there is a pure cervical dislocation without fracture. Displacement may be severe, and there is frequently locking of both facets (ill.). Damage to the posterior ligament complex is always present, and is generally obvious from the degree of vertebral displacement.

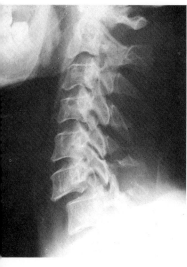

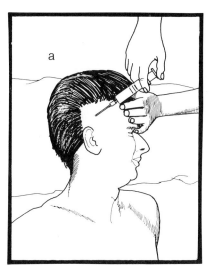

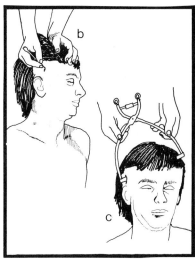

. Unstable injuries (2) There may be other idence of instability associated with sruption of the posterior ligament complex, g. (1) avulsion fracture(s) of a spinous ocess, (2) widening of the gap between two inous processes or (3) *evidence of forward p on the flexion lateral of the spine mpared with the extension lateral.*

25. *Unstable injuries* (3) *Treatment* (1) Unstable injuries without fracture require fusion; skull traction will be required to achieve and maintain reduction and should be applied without delay. Several types of calliper are available, and the following description applies to those of Cone's pattern (but see 29). (a) Shave the skin round the proposed insertion points (approximately 6–7 cm above the external meati) and infiltrate the areas deeply with local anaesthetic.

26. *Treatment* (2) (b) Make a small incision (about 1 cm in length) on each side down to bone. Bleeding is usually brisk, but generally controllable by firm local pressure applied for a few moments; if not, secure and tie off any remaining bleeding points. (c) Now insinuate one point holder through the temporalis muscle fibres until it is in contact with the skull.

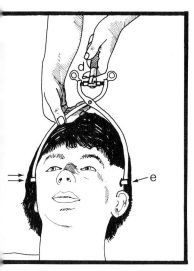

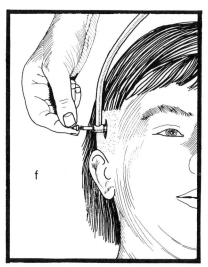

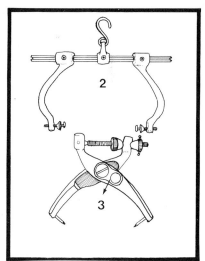

. Treatment (3) (d) Keep the point holder essed firmly against the skull: straighten t the calliper, and close it with the ¬nbuckle spanner. (e) Guide the second ¬int holder through the skin wound; ¬cillate the calliper slightly to allow its ¬ered end to part the temporalis fibres on ¬ second side. Close the calliper until both ¬int holders are in firm but not hard ¬ntact with the skull.

28. *Treatment* (4) (f) Now screw the points in (you should check that their protrusion is limited to about 3 mm) to penetrate the outer cortex only; tighten them with a key. If the points fail to enter, either they are blunt or the bone unduly hard. In these circumstances, a small awl may be used as a starter, taking great care to avoid penetration of the inner cortex. (g) Now seal the wound with strips of gauze soaked in Nobecutane or a similar preparation.

29. *Other traction devices:* (2) *Blackburn callipers* are designed to hook into the diplöe of the skull, and a trephine is used to remove a tiny lid of outer cortex. Occasionally no diplöe is present, and the points must hook under the full thickness of the skull, and come in contact with the dura.
(3) *Crutchfield traction tongs* are inserted nearer the vertex than the other two devices.

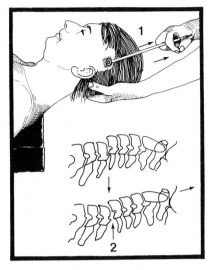

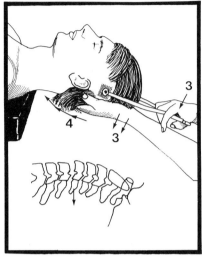

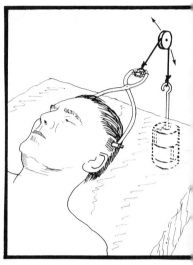

30. *Reduction* (1) If reduction is required, many surgeons prefer to do this manually under general anaesthesia with good relaxation. X-ray facilities are essential, and great care must be taken during induction and throughout the procedure to avoid uncontrolled movements of the head. When all is ready, the head is supported and the end of the table dropped; firm traction is applied in the neutral position or slight flexion (1) to unlock the facets (2).

31. *Reduction* (2) Maintaining firm traction the neck is slowly extended (3). The hand supporting the occiput may be moved in anticipation down the neck to act as a fulcrum (4). The traction is then slowly reduced, the table end raised, and whilst maintaining a little controlling traction, the position is checked with radiographs.

32. *Reduction* (3) *Alternative techniques:* Continuous (weight) traction may be used t overcome muscle tension and unlock over-riding facets. The *direction* of traction may be controlled by altering the position of the traction pulley, or by the use of pads under the head or shoulders. The *amount* of traction can be adjusted by the weights. Th duration of maximal traction is monitored by radiographs.

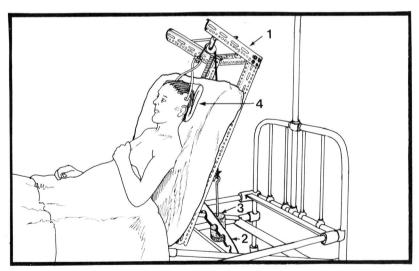

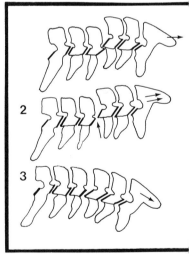

33. *Reduction* (4) A better arrangement is for traction to be applied with the patient in a sitting-up position. Traction is more efficient, being countered by the body weight: the patient can see what is going on, and if paraplegic, breathing is easier as the diaphragm is unobstructed. A framework of slotted angle (e.g. Dexion) (1) may be attached to the mattress frame if the hospital bed has not this facility; and the frame may be racked up and down (2) while pressure points are being attended to. The weight required (3) will be found to vary from about 15 lb (7 kg) for a light adult woman to 30 lb (14 kg) + for a heavy man. The line of traction should start in the neutral position or *slight* flexion (4). The patient should be sedated, *and in the recently injured patient radiographs to check progress should be taken every 15 minutes.*

34. *Reduction* (5) As soon as the neck has been stretched sufficiently to allow the locked facets just to clear one another (2), the neck should be extended to complete th reduction (3). If the injury is longstanding (say 1–3 weeks) progress will be much slower, and in extreme cases can extend to days.

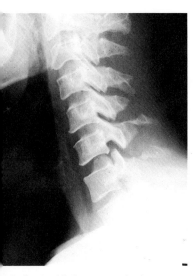

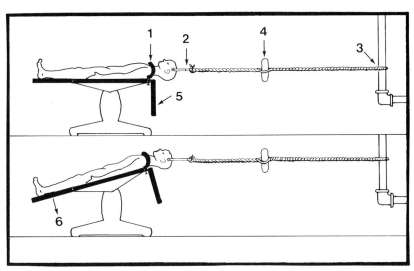

. *Reduction* (6) As soon as check
diographs confirm the reduction (ill:
duction of case shown in 24) the traction
ould be reduced to about 6 lb (2.5 kg). *On*
account should the neck be allowed to
er distract.

36. *Reduction* (7) *Alternative techniques: Sillar's method:* The patient is anaesthetised and
placed on the theatre table with the break at shoulder level. Shoulder rests are fitted (1) and
traction cord stretched between the skull callipers (2) and some theatre fixture (3). The cord is
tightened with a windlass (4) and when sufficient tension is present the end of the table can be
dropped (5). Thereafter the spine should be visualised with image intensifier screening or
serial radiographs. The windlass is tightened until the facets unlock. Thereafter the cervical
spine may be extended by tilting the table (6), and the traction slackened off. The advantage
of this method is that reduction is rapid and that there is fine *linear* control of the spine (as
opposed to the trial and error method of weight adjustment over an indefinite time).

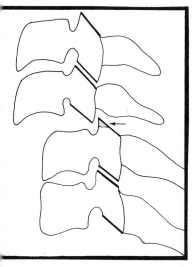

38. *After care:* In the common situation where there is dislocation of the cervical spine
without fracture, the posterior ligament complex never regains its former strength irrespective
of the method of reduction or duration of subsequent traction. Spontaneous recurrence of the
displacement is inevitable unless posterior fusion is carried out. The decision about surgery
depends on your assessment of the neurological picture, and may be deferred until this is
reasonably clear. In the interval traction should be maintained. The following situations are
common: (a) If there is no neurological disturbance, spinal fusion should be carried out; it is
reasonable to do this as a carefully planned procedure after a few days. (b) If there is an
incomplete paraplegia, there may be a reasonable delay of 1–2 weeks. (c) If paraplegia is
complete, fusion is not required. Traction may be discontinued and a collar substituted after
4–6 weeks. (d) Where the injury is accompanied by fracture, and union in this fracture may
result in stability (e.g. fracture of the *base* of a spinous process) traction may be continued
until union occurs (say after 8 weeks). The final stability of the spine should nevertheless
always be checked by flexion and extension laterals.

. *Reduction failure:* Failure to obtain
duction is unusual in recent injuries, but
ere may be difficulty after 3–4 weeks.
ssuming that there is not complete
raplegia, open reduction should be
tempted by local trimming of those parts
the facets which are blocking reduction
cetectomy). Note that in very
ngstanding dislocations, spinal stability is
ore important than accurate reduction,
d the spine may be fused in the dislocated
sition if reduction cannot be obtained.

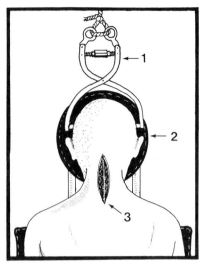

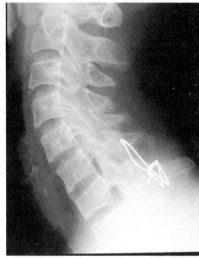

41. *(C) Extension injuries: Mechanisms:* Commonly (a) as a result of a fall downstairs, striking the forehead against the ground (b) in front impact car accidents where the forehead strikes the car roof, fascia or bonnet (3rd, 4th and 5th phases of injury) (c) in rear impact car accidents in which the neck extends due to the inertia of the head.

Pathology: These injuries are particularly common in the middle-aged and elderly who suffer from cervical spondylosis. Osteo-arthritic rigidity in the spine may lead to excessive concentration of violence at any area of the spine retaining mobility. A similar pre-disposition is found in those suffering from ankylosing spondylitis, sever rheumatoid arthritis, or congenital deformit of the spine with localised areas of fusion (e.g. Klippel-Feil syndrome).

39. *Cervical fusion* (1) Under the circumstances of a posterior ligament complex rupture, anterior cervical fusion is unreliable, and a posterior fusion is advocated. Note (a) Traction is maintained during the procedure (1). (b) After carefully controlled intubation, the patient is turned to the prone position, with the head supported in a head ring (2). (c) The cervical spines are exposed through a mid-line incision (3).

40. *Cervical fusion* (2) (d) The ruptured posterior ligament is identified and the adjacent spinous processes, laminae and facet joints rawed. (e) The spines are wired together (ill.). (f) Two iliac bone grafts are placed (and sometimes wired together) on either side of the spines, bridging them. (g) Cancellous bone chips are packed into the area before closure. (h) Traction is continued for 6–8 weeks and a collar substituted when there is evidence of graft incorporation.

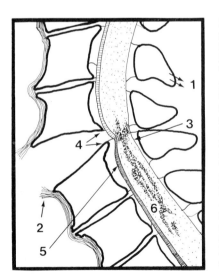

42. *Pathology ctd:* The neck hyperextends (1) leading to tearing or avulsion of the anterior longitudinal ligament (2). During the period of extension the cord may be stretched at the level of the vertebral lesion (3). At the same time, or when the vertebrae snap together again, the cord may be nipped

by backward projecting osteophytes (4) (in the patient with advanced spondylosis). Stretching and kinking of spinal vessels may lead to extensive spreading thrombosis (5). The cord damage is often diffuse and may not correspond exactly with the level of injury (6). Spread of thrombosis may lead to a deteriorating neurological picture. As far as the cord is concerned sole involvement of the central area is rare, but when it occurs the effect is (a) Motor loss, if present, tends to be greater in the legs than in the arms. (b) Temperature and pain conduction are more likely to be affected than proprioception and light touch, which are frequently spared.

Diagnosis: (1) The history of injury, pain in the neck, and complaint of weakness in the arms are suggestive. (2) Where the causal force is anterior (41, a, b,) bruising or laceration of the forehead is an invaluable sign.

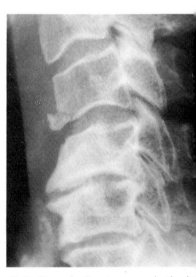

43. *Radiographs:* Spontaneous reduction is the rule, so that the radiographs *may be quite normal.* Nevertheless, evidence of injury may be present. (1) The anterior longitudinal ligament may avulse its attachment to the vertebral body (ill.) or an osteophyte. (2) Haemorrhage may lead to anterior displacement of the pharyngeal shadow. Rarely there may be (3) fractures c the laminae or spinous processes or (4) tearing open of a vertebral body.

4. *Treatment:* Extension injuries of the ⹁ine are stable. *Local treatment* consists of ⹁e judicious use of a collar till local pain ⹁d cervical muscle spasm settle. *The ⹁neral treatment* is that of the ⹁ccompanying neurological problem which ⹁ay be minor or profound.

⹁) Compression fractures of the cervical ⹁ine: Mechanisms: These injuries may be ⹁used by (a) heavy objects falling on the ⹁ad (b) the vertex striking the ground as in ⹁lls, diving and other athletic accidents (c) ⹁e head striking the roof in head-on car ⹁cidents (phase 2).

⹁agnosis: (a) The history of injury may be ⹁ggestive. (b) There may be tell-tale ⹁cerations on the crown of the head. ⹁) Complaint of pain in the neck should lead ⹁ the taking of the radiographs which will ⹁arify the diagnosis.

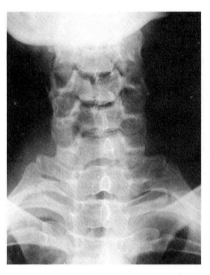

45. *Radiographs* (1) The appearances are dependent on the degree of causal violence. When the forces are moderate, a fissure fracture of the vertebral body may be produced, most obvious in the A.P. projection (ill: vertical fracture through the body of C5, with a similar but less marked fracture of C6).

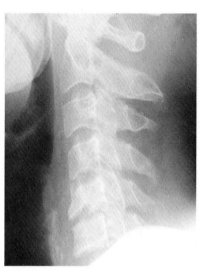

46. *Radiographs* (2) In more severe injuries the vertebral body may be comminuted and flattened. Fragments of the vertebral body may be extruded in any direction; when this occurs the cord may be endangered. (Ill: compression fracture of C5: note the encroachment on the neural canal by the posterior part of the body.)

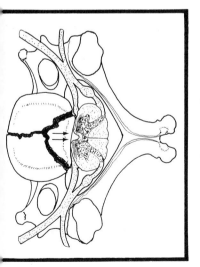

⹁7. Neurological involvement: The most ⹁lnerable part of the cord lies anteriorly, ⹁fecting firstly the motor supply of the ⹁pper limbs *before* the motor pathways to ⹁e lower limbs: hence paralysis tends to be ⹁aximal in the upper limbs. Next to be ⹁volved are the spino-thalamic tracts ⹁rrying pain and temperature, and lastly, ⹁e posterior columns. (Proprioception and ⹁ht touch.)

48. Neurological assessment: On admission, a complete neurological examination should be carried out: this should involve testing (1) all the main muscle groups in the upper and lower limbs, (2) the skin and tendon reflexes, (3) sensation to pin prick and light touch, (4) proprioception. If the paralysis is bilateral, symmetrical and complete, testing should be repeated meticulously at 6 hours, 12 hours, and 24 hours post injury. No recovery after 24 hours in injuries at cervical level almost certainly indicates a hopeless prognosis. *Be careful to note, however, that a profound neurological loss cannot be declared complete unless proprioception and light touch have been most carefully assessed.* Many apparent recoveries in lesions first described as complete may well have been due to failure in carrying out a careful examination of these modalities of sensation.

Treatment: (1) The posterior ligament complex is intact, and once these fractures have healed there is no tendency to subsequent displacement. They are generally best treated by cervical traction for 6 weeks until cancellous union has occurred. Traction also minimises the chances of backward displacement of bone fragments. (2) Laminectomy is sometimes carried out to allow removal of backward projecting bone fragments causing cord compression. This is fully justifiable in the face of the following criteria: (i) an incomplete cord lesion, (ii) a deteriorating neurological picture, (iii) a local block on myelography. Laminectomy is considered by many to be a dubious procedure in the presence of a complete neurological lesion.

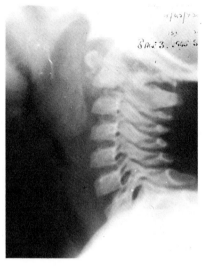

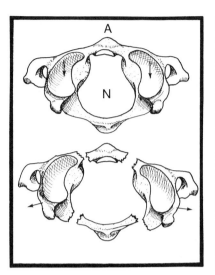

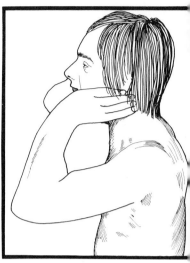

49. *The upper two cervical vertebrae:* (A) *Atlanto-occipital subluxations and dislocations:* Traumatic lesions at this level are usually fatal, but a few survive. Subluxations from rheumatoid arthritis and spinal infections (ill: cervical tuberculosis: atlanto-occipital subluxation and retro-pharnygeal abscess) are seen more frequently. Cervical fusion (occiput to C1 and C2) with a period of halo traction (see 60) is generally advocated.

50. *(B) Fractures of the atlas* (1) The usual pattern of fracture is *quadripartite*, and is produced as a result of severe downward pressure of the occipital condyles on the atlas. Such force may result from (a) a weight falling on the head (e.g. in the construction industry) (b) the head striking the roof of a car in a road traffic accident (c) from a fall from a height on to the heels.

51. *Fracture of the atlas* (2) Clinically, if the patient is conscious he may resent sitting up and may support the head with the hands. There may be complaint of severe occipital pain due to local pressure on the great occipital nerve. About 50% of patients survive this injury without significant neurological involvement.

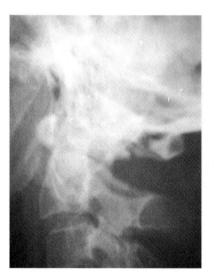

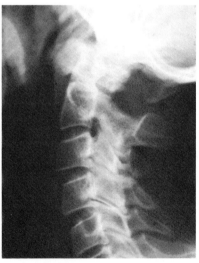

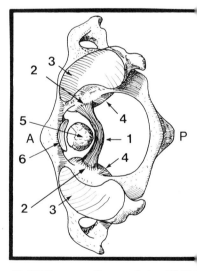

52. *Radiographs* (1) The *lateral* radiograph may show the fracture of the posterior arch. The plain A.P. view is generally unhelpful. A through-the-mouth projection is generally most valuable and should reveal the lateral displacement of the lateral masses. Nevertheless pain and resistance to all movement may lead to failure; if this is the case, an oblique lateral centred on C3 and A.P. and lateral tomography may be useful.

53. *Radiographs* (2) Congenital absence of part of the posterior arch may cause confusion, but in itself is of no significance, being a stable condition. *Treatment of arch fractures:* These cannot be reduced; with *slight* displacement a well fitting collar for 6 weeks with observation in hospital for 2–3 weeks *at least* is desirable. With more severe displacements, 6 weeks skull traction is advisable.

54. *(C) Transverse ligament lesions* (1) The transverse ligament (1) runs between two bony tubercles (2) which lie between the joint surfaces (3) which articulate with the occiput and those which articulate below with the axis (4). The odontoid process (5) articulates with the anterior arch (6) and the transverse ligament restrains its backward travel.

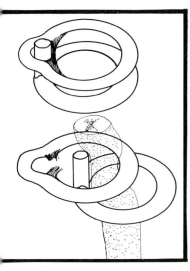

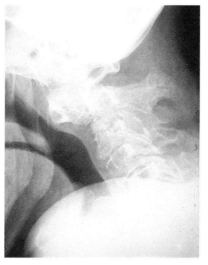

are pathological. (Illustrated: gross shift in an arthritic spine) (ii) There is generally a degree of rotatory deformity, and a through-the-mouth view may show an asymmetrical location of the odontoid peg relative to the lateral masses of the atlas. (iii) If there is remaining doubt, flexion and extension laterals should be taken under close supervision. An abnormal excursion of the odontoid peg in relation to the anterior arch of the atlas is diagnostic.

. *Transverse ligament* (2) The ligament ay be torn in sudden flexion injuries; it ay become attenuated or rupture in eumatoid arthritis (or in soft tissue ections of the neck in children). In either se the risk to the cord is great as it comes pinched between the posterior arch the atlas and the odontoid peg (as shown re diagramatically).

56. *Transverse ligament* (3) *Diagnosis:* The condition may be suspected from the history, by pain in the neck *and the head*, and by the presence of marked cervical spasm. *Radiographs:* The diagnosis is established by radiographs. (i) Plain lateral films should be examined and the gap between the posterior face of the anterior arch and the odontoid carefully measured. In the adult, the upper limit of normal is 4 mm, and measurements in excess of this

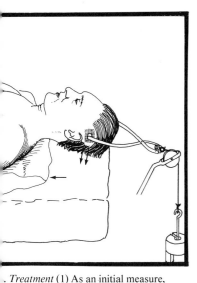

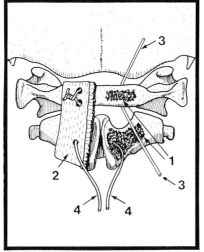

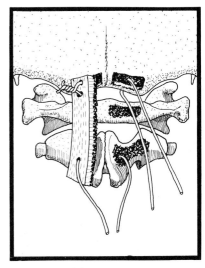

. *Treatment* (1) As an initial measure, ull traction of about 6–7 lb (3 kg) in tension should be set up. In children, a riod of six weeks traction alone may ffice to restore stability to the spine. This especially so where the pathology has en due primarily to local infection and this s been in addition adequately dealt with.

58. *Treatment* (2) Where the pathology is secondary to rheumatoid arthritis, local cervical fusion is generally advised to prevent subluxation of C1 on C2. The posterior arches of C1 and C2 are rawed (1). Two stout grafts (from tibia or iliac crest) are wired in position (one side only shown) (2). The upper wires (3) pass round the arch while the lower (4) is passed through a hole drilled in the spine of C2. The area is packed with bone chips.

59. *Treatment* (3) If the posterior arch of C1 is very frail, it may be necessary to include the occiput in the grafted region: great care must be taken in passing the fixing wires through holes drilled in the edge of the foramen magnum.

After surgery, traction is maintained for 6 weeks, and a collar is generally worn for a further 2–3 months.

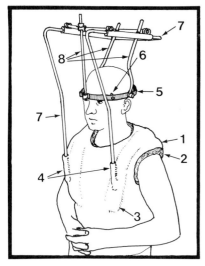

head is shaved; the skull callipers are removed and replaced with the halo (5). This metal ring is attached to the skull with four diametrically opposed metal points (6) screwed into position in a similar manner to the points in Cone's callipers. Once this is securely in position the cantilever frame (7) shaped like a bent 'U' is attached to the sockets in the plaster. The halo is connected to the cantilever frame by three bars (8) which have adjustable couplings at both ends.

When the device is finally removed, stability must be assessed with flexion and extension laterals; if there is evidence of persisting instability, fusion will be needed.

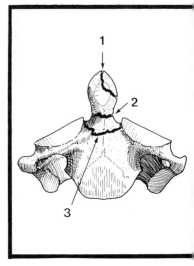

60. *Treatment:* If the dislocation is due to recent trauma, conservative treatment by the use of halo traction over a period of 8 weeks may be successful. The apparatus is cumbersome and the patient must be well motivated. A plaster jacket (1) is applied over stockingette and generous wool and felt padding (2) to cushion the weight of the plaster and the apparatus. A rigid metal frame (3) is buried in the plaster. It incorporates tubular sockets (4) to take the main frame. When the plaster has dried, the

61. *Odontoid fractures* (1) The odontoid process (dens) may fracture at any one of three levels: (1) Fractures at the tip are generally quite stable injuries, requiring on symptomatic treatment with a collar. (2) T commonest fracture is one occurring at the junction of the process with the body. (3) Fractures involving the body have a good prognosis with respect to union.

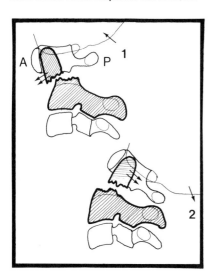

62. *Odontoid fractures* (2) Fracture may result from sudden severe flexion (1) or extension (2) of the neck (flexion and extension fractures). *Diagnosis:* This injury may be suspected from the history and the site of pain and protective muscle spasm. Occasionally the original injury may be ignored, and only discovered on investigation of an advancing ataxia or other neurological disturbance.

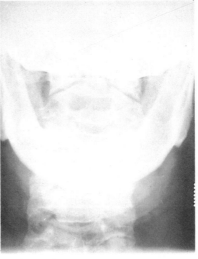

63. *Odontoid fractures* (3) The diagnosis may be readily confirmed by routine radiography; the fracture may show clearly in the through-the-mouth A.P. projection (ill: fracture of the base) and/or in the standard lateral view. Only if there is doubt need carefully supervised flexion and extension laterals be taken, or tomography carried out. Confusion can sometimes arise, however, from certain congenital abnormalities.

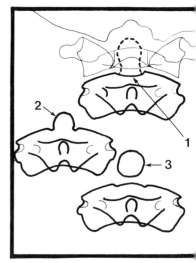

64. *Congenital abnormalities* of the odontoid include (1) complete absence (pr disposing to dislocation): (2) hypoplasia: (3) non-fusion of the odontoid process (persistent os odontoideum). (The ossification centre for the apex normally appears at 2 years with fusion occurring b 12.) Rounded edges and a separate articulation with the atlas may help to distinguish it from a fracture (even though may behave as such).

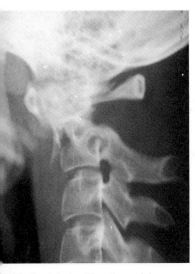

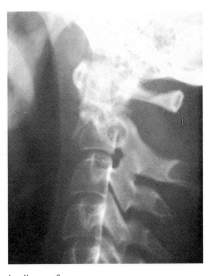

both instances, external support should be continued without interruption for 8 weeks. (3) Stability should then be assessed with flexion and extension laterals. Surgical treatment (fusion of C1 and C2) is indicated (a) if conservative treatment fails (b) if the case presents late (c) if a good reduction cannot be obtained (d) where the delays and complications of conservative management are thought to present a greater hazard than the risks of primary surgery.

5. *Flexion injuries:* The atlas and dens displace anteriorly in relation to C2. (Ill: a flexion injury made obvious by flexion and extension laterals.) There may be an associated rotational injury. If the fracture is junctional (61, 2) the incidence of non-union is about 60%, with risk of progressive subluxation and neurological involvement. *Treatment:* In spite of the risks of complications these injuries are frequently treated conservatively, especially in children and where the fracture presents a large

healing surface.
Method: (1) Reduce by applying traction in extension, using skull callipers (as in ruptures of transverse ligament, 57).
(2) After 1–2 weeks in traction, it may be possible to mobilise the patient: this is, of course, especially desirable in the elderly patient who will not tolerate prolonged traction and confinement to bed. A stout well-fitting cervical collar may be used. In the young patient, however, better support will be afforded with halo-pelvic traction. In

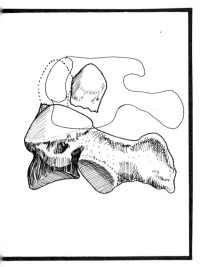

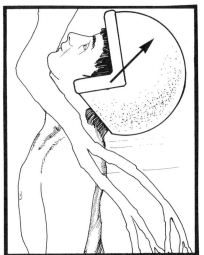

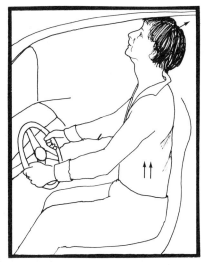

6. *Extension injuries:* Fracture with backward displacement is commoner in the elderly, and is a relatively stable lesion. *Treatment:* (1) If the shift is slight, a collar for 8 weeks should suffice. (2) If marked, apply traction in slight flexion with callipers, but slacken off the weight as soon as reduction has been achieved to avoid distraction. After 2–4 weeks a collar may be substituted.

67. *Fractures of the pedicles of C2*
(1) Fractures of the pedicles of the axis may occur in two distinct ways: (a) Fracture may follow simultaneous extension and distraction of the neck. This is the mechanism of death by hanging. Similar, and not always fatal injuries occur in cyclists who are caught under the chin by a tree branch or a rope; nevertheless, neurological disturbance is usually profound.

68. *Fractures of the pedicles of C2*
(2) (b) Radiologically identical fractures may be produced by forcible extension of the neck accompanied by compression; this may occur in road traffic accidents if the head strikes the vehicle roof and ricochets into extension. Neurological involvement here is rare. These two types of injury may be distinguished by the history, site of bruising (neck or forehead) and neurological disturbance.

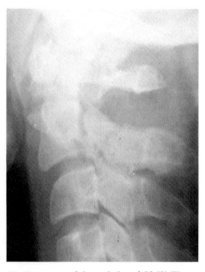

suggest distraction, or if neurological signs are advancing, traction must be abandoned. There would then be an indication for local fusion.
(b) *Extension injuries with compression:*
(i) If the injury appears stable and there is no neurological disturbance, a well fitting collar should be worn for 6 weeks. (ii) If there is neurological involvement, a 6-week period of cervical (skull) traction should be advised. Thereafter (iii) if there is any evidence of instability, fusion is indicated.

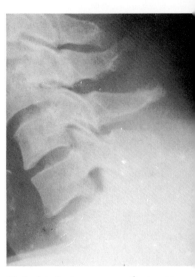

69. *Fractures of the pedicles of C2* (3) The fracture normally shows clearly in lateral radiographs of the cervical spine. Occasionally there is spondylolisthesis of C2 on C3.
Treatment: (a) *Extension injuries with distraction:* Skull traction for a period of 4–6 weeks is advocated to maintain position only. There is always the risk in this type of injury of further distraction, and it is therefore important to limit traction to a maximum of 5 lb (2 kg). If radiographs

70. *Isolated spinous process fractures:* Fracture of the spinous process of C7 or T1 (clay shoveller's fracture) may result from sudden muscular contraction (avulsion fracture). This is a stable injury, and symptomatic treatment only is required (e.g. a cervical collar for 2–3 weeks). It must be carefully distinguished from a cervical dislocation with associated fracture. (If in doubt, flexion and extension laterals should be taken.)

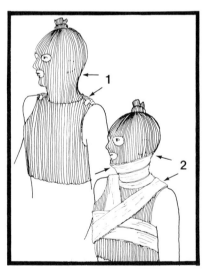

71. *Plaster fixation in cervical spine injuries* (1) Plaster fixation is occasionally indicated as a substitute for a well-fitting collar. It may afford a little more support and be helpful in treating the poorly motivated patient who may be tempted to remove the support. Stockingette is applied to the head and trunk (1), and wool padding to pressure areas (2). Felt pads to the chin and occiput are advisable.

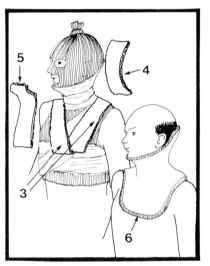

72. *Plaster fixation* (2) Four plaster slabs are prepared from 6″ (15 cm) plaster bandages: two are applied over the shoulders (3), one from mid scapular region to the occiput (4), and one over the point of the chin on to the chest (5). The slabs are joined with circular bandages; the stockingette and wool are turned down and trimmed (6). This plaster is best applied with the patient seated on a stool.

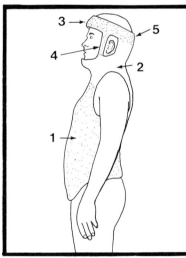

73. *The Minerva plaster:* This extensive plaster, although not giving as much support as halo-pelvic fixation, is sometimes used as an alternative, for the same indications (especially in children).
Method: A plaster jacket is applied first (1) this is extended with slabs to form a collar (as in 71, 72) (2); additional support is provided with a head band (3) and side struts (4). If to be worn for any length of time, the head should be cropped or shaved (5).

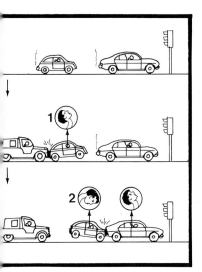

Diagnosis: The commonest symptoms are of pain and stiffness in the neck. In addition there may be radiation of pain and numbness into the arm and shoulder (often indicating a poorer prognosis) or to the intrascapular region or occiput. *Clinically* neck movements are restricted, and widespread cervical tenderness is usual; but objective neurological signs are rare. *Radiographs:* (1) There may be loss of the usual cervical curvature or localised kinking (of greater significance). (2) Occasionally there may be evidence of hyperextension (anterior osteophytic avulsion) or hyperflexion (flake fracture of the spinous processes). (3) There is some evidence that joint space narrowing and other spondylotic changes may appear 1–2 years after the incident and be related to it.

Treatment: Treatment is primarily conservative: only in the most severe and persistent case is local cervical fusion ever considered. (a) A cervical collar and analgesics are prescribed initially. (b) If after 6–8 weeks symptoms are not controlled, local heat with or without cervical traction is advised.

Note: Symptoms are usually *prolonged* (18 months—3 years is common) but the majority of cases eventually resolve completely. Poor prognostic signs include arm radiation and delay in settling any litigation.

4. *Soft tissue injuries of the neck (Whiplash Injuries):* Whiplash injuries of the cervical spine occur almost exclusively in road accidents. In the classical incident the spine is hyperextended following a rear impact collision (1) and then rapidly flexed as the vehicle in which the patient is travelling hits an object in front—usually another car (2). The term is now used loosely to cover virtually every neck injury without fracture sustained in a road accident.

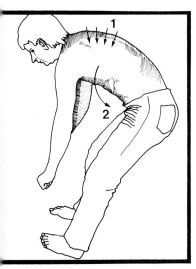

5. *Fractures of the thoracic and lumbar spine: Mechanism:* Fractures of the thoracic and lumbar spine occur most frequently as a result of forces which tend to produce flexion of the spine (1). A rotational element is frequently present (2).

Causes: The many possible causes of this type of injury include (a) falls from a height on to the heels, where the normal curvature of the spine results in further flexion (b) blows across the back and shoulders which cause the spine to jack-knife at the thoraco-lumbar junction—for example, injuries in the mining and construction industries (c) flexion and rotational forces transmitted to the spine from road or vehicle impact in car and motor cycle accidents (d) heavy lifting, especially in the middle aged and elderly, where there is often the pathological element of osteoporosis or osteomalacia. Less commonly malignancy (especially metastatic deposits) may be a factor, when the causal force may be slight or not even remembered.

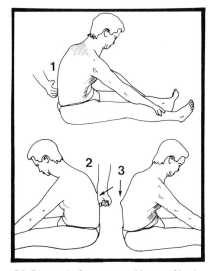

76. *Diagnosis:* Suspect on a history of back pain after trauma, especially if there is local spinal tenderness (1), pain on spinal percussion (2), or especially if there is an angular kyphosis (3). Thoracic or abdominal radicular pain may wrongly divert attention to the chest or abdomen, and in the elderly there may be no convincing history of injury; any suspicion merits radiography.

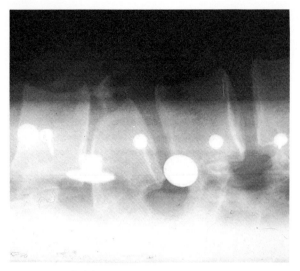

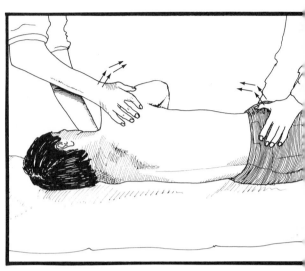

77. *Radiographs* (1) A.P. and lateral radiographs only should be taken in the first instance. In the obviously seriously injured patient there may be difficulty in obtaining a lateral because of severe pain, or through fear of causing cord damage. In these circumstances, a shoot-through lateral may be taken using a fixed grid or chest bucky. (Ill: shoot-through lateral: note tacks securing canvas to stretcher poles: but detail sufficient to show a wedge fracture of L3, with anterior subluxation and obvious instability.)

78. *Radiographs* (2) If these measures are unsatisfactory you should *personally* supervise the turning of the patient on his side in order to obtain a lateral projection; in essence you should see that the patient is turned gently and smoothly in such a way that the upper part of the spine with the shoulders is rotated in pace with the pelvis, and that the patient remains well supported (e.g. by pillows) when he is on his side.

79. *Note:* (1) The most important decision to make in any spinal injury is whether it is stable. This profoundly influences treatment. (2) *Most stable fractures* are uncomplicated by damage to the cord or cauda equina, although bursting, compression fractures are an occasional exception. (3) *Unstable fractures* of the spine may be accompanied by neurological involvement. If this is incomplete, there is always hope of recovery. There is the risk that further displacement at the fracture site may jeopardise this, or convert an uncomplicated injury to a complicated one. Treatment is, therefore, vitally important. (4) The commonest spinal injury *by far* is the wedge compression fracture. (5) In practice, the most frequent problem is to recognise a wedge fracture and decide whether it is stable. (6) Other types of injury are most often unstable.

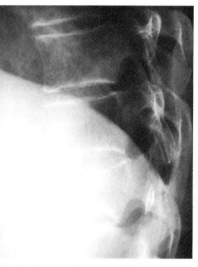

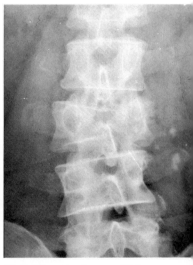

80. *Stable wedge fractures* (1) Wedge fractures are most commonly observed in the lateral radiographs (anterior wedge fractures) and are caused by pure flexion forces. (Illustrated: wedge fracture of D11; note the difference in height between the anterior and posterior margins of the vertebral body.)

81. *Stable wedge fractures* (2) Less commonly, when there is a rotational element added to forward flexion, vertebral wedging may be apparent in the A.P. projection (lateral wedging). (Ill: lateral wedging of L3.) This form of wedging is often associated with root compression on the narrowed side, and these injuries have a poorer prognosis regarding ultimate functional recovery and freedom from pain.

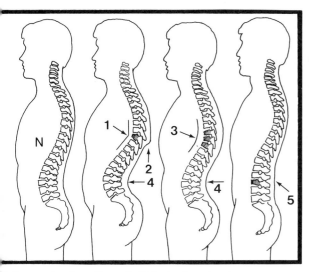

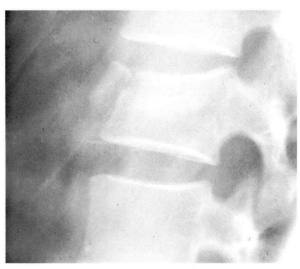

2. *Interpreting the radiographs* (1) In the thoracic spine, an anterior wedge fracture of a single vertebra will lead to localised kinking (1) with or without an overlying gibbus (2). Multiple fractures in the thoracic spine, especially when wedging is slight in each of the affected vertebrae, will lead to a more regular kyphosis (3). In either of these circumstances, the increased thoracic curvature will tend to produce an increased lumbar lordosis (4) and/or hyperextension in the hip joints. In the case of the lumbar spine, anterior wedge fractures lead to obliteration or reversal of the normal lumbar lordosis (5). (Compare with the normal profile, N.)

83. *Interpreting the radiographs* (2) In anterior wedge fractures, the anterior border of the vertebra will measure less than the posterior border. The crushing of the anterior portion may be quite regular, or may result in a marginal shearing fracture (generally the anterior superior corner) (ill.). If the posterior margin is decreased in height relative to the vertebrae above and below it is evidence of increased violence, and the possibility of bony fragments encroaching on the vertebral canal must be borne in mind.

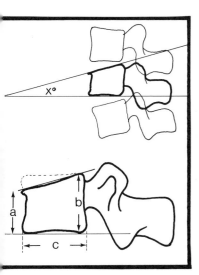

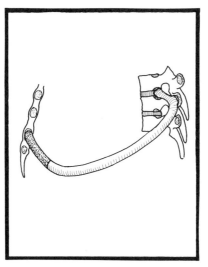

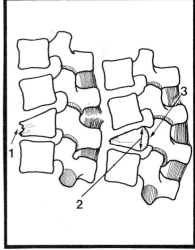

4. *Interpreting the radiographs* (3) Assess the amount of wedging: the fracture is likely to be stable if the height of the anterior margin still amounts to two-thirds or more of the posterior margin, or putting this another way if the degree of wedging is 15° or less, or if the width of the body divided by the difference in the heights is greater than 3.75

i.e., $x < 15°$, or $\dfrac{c}{b-a} > 3.75$).

85. *Interpreting the radiographs* (4) In the case of the upper 8 thoracic vertebrae, note any associated fractures of the sternum. Each of the upper thoracic vertebrae is linked by ribs to the sternum, and *appreciable* wedging cannot take place without involvement of these structures.

86. *Unstable fractures* (1) Marked wedging (20° or more, or collapse of the anterior margin to less than half the posterior) (1) is likely to denote instability (as it is associated with posterior ligament complex rupture). If the posterior margin is reduced in height (2) a greater degree of wedging is possible without rupture of the posterior ligament complex. Posterior *lumbar* bulging (3) is less serious than in the dorsal spine where the canal is narrow.

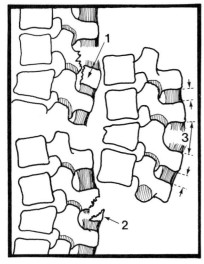

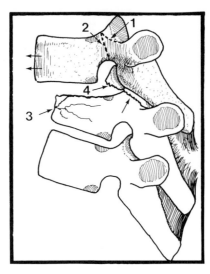

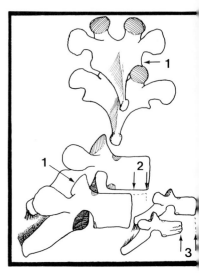

87. *Unstable fractures* (2) Look for other evidence of damage to the posterior ligament complex and associated structures, fundamental to spinal stability. Note especially avulsion fracture of a spinous process (1), avulsion fracture of the tip of a spinous process (2), wide separation of the vertebral spines at the level of injury (3).

88. *Unstable fractures* (3) Examine the radiographs carefully for evidence of fractures at the level of the facet joints (1) or pedicles (2). A comminuted fracture of a vertebral body (3) with involvement of these structures (ill: facet joint fracture, 4) is generally unstable: bilateral pedicle fractures are invariably unstable.

89. *Unstable fractures* (4) Look for shift of one vertebra relative to another. This is an invariable sign of instability. Vertebral displacement patterns include the following: (a) Ruptured posterior ligament with unilateral facet joint displacement (1). In the lateral projection, the degree of forward shift is about a third or less (2); (b) Bilateral dislocated facet joints, often with body fracture and a greater degree of displacement (3).

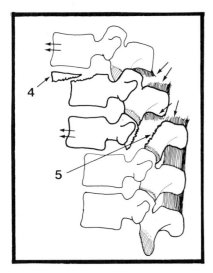

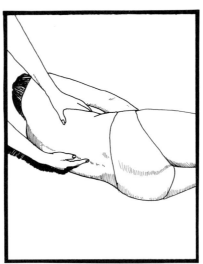

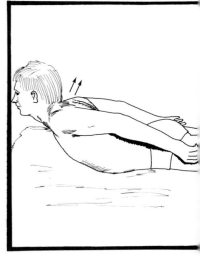

90. *Unstable fractures* (5) (c) Shearing fracture of a vertebral body (4); (d) Bilateral neural arch fractures and traumatic spondylo-listhesis (5). *Note in all these injuries there is damage to the posterior ligament complex.* If there is any remaining doubt the following additional radiographs should be taken: (1) oblique projections (2) a further lateral, *supervised*, in slight flexion.

91. *Unstable fractures* (6) The spinal radiographs may give unequivocal evidence of instability. In other cases where there is the *slightest* suspicion of the posterior ligament complex being involved, that structure must be carefully examined clinically. Press firmly between successive spines, preferably in slight flexion. If the interspinous ligaments are torn, the examining finger will encounter a boggy softness instead of the normal resistance to pressure.

92. *Treatment: Stable fractures:* (1) Admit for complete bed rest in recumbency with one pillow. (2) Analgesics as required. (3) When acute symptoms have settled (say after one week) extension exercises should be commenced and vigorously practised (ill.). (4) The patient can be allowed up and home at 6 weeks. This programme may be compressed if wedging is minimal.

93. *Treatment of unstable fractures, either with no neurological lesion or an incomplete neurological lesion* (1) The aims of treatment are (a) To reduce any displacement that is present. (b) To prevent any recurrence of displacement (with risks of neurological disasters) until stability is regained.

Stability may be achieved in the following ways: (a) By the occurrence of spontaneous anterior fusion (b) By healing of the torn posterior ligament complex (very uncertain in its occurrence and something that cannot be relied upon, especially in cases uncomplicated by fracture) (c) By surgical fusion.

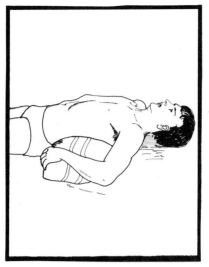

94. *Treatment* (2) Reduction can generally be achieved by gently extending the spine with a pillow or a sandbag at the level of injury. If this is unsuccessful, or if there are locked facets, open reduction will be required. After reduction, further care is dependent on the nature of the injury and the availability of equipment.

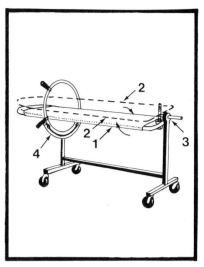

95. *Treatment* (3) (a) The patient may be nursed in a Stryker frame. This special bed allows the patient to be rotated from the supine to the prone position with minimal nursing effort. During the manoeuvre, the patient is sandwiched between two mattresses (1, 2) which are locked together, and turned round a pivot at one end (3) and a quadrant (4) at the other. The frame is then locked and the uppermost mattress removed.

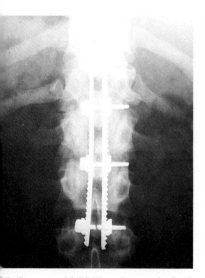

96. *Treatment* (4) (b) The spine may be fixed internally. This is especially applicable if open reduction is required. Paired Meurig-Williams plates are secured with set screws (bolts as they are usually wrongly called) passed through spinous processes above and below the level of the fracture. The nuts are keyed in to the plates. This form of fixation almost invariably cuts out, and can only be relied on for about 4 weeks.

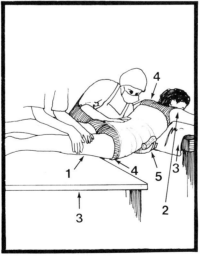

97. *Treatment* (5) (c) A plaster jacket may be applied with the spine in extension. The sedated but conscious patient supports himself by the thighs (1) and shoulders (2) between two tables (3) while the plaster is applied. Stockingette (4) with felt and wool pads to protect the bony prominences is applied prior to encircling plaster bandages (5) and slabs. The patient is lifted on to pillows and the plaster trimmed when dry.

98. *Treatment* (6) Methods (a) (b) (c) may be used as definitive treatment or to give time to make arrangements for fusion and give the patient a chance to recover from his injuries. Surgery is indicated (1) If there is any evidence of recurrence of displacement after conservative treatment or (2) If rupture of the posterior ligament complex is the principal element of the injury. A posterior fusion is generally employed, using bone grafts from the ilium wired to spinous processes above and below the injury. The spinous processes and laminae have their surfaces rawed and bone chips are also packed into the area. After a fusion the patient may be nursed in a Stryker frame (or a plaster bed with anterior and posterior turning shells) for approximately 6–8 weeks. As a plaster bed takes 1–2 weeks to manufacture, preliminary internal fixation may be required if this line of treatment is going to be employed. (But note: a plaster bed is contra-indicated in the presence of paraplegia.)

Treatment of unstable fractures with a complete, irrecoverable cord lesion: (a) If the spine is grossly unstable internal fixation may be indicated (i) to facilitate nursing (ii) to reduce chronic back pain from local root involvement (iii) to prevent mal-union and a degree of spinal deformity which would make sitting and rehabilitation difficult.

(b) If the spine is not wildly unstable, and first class nursing is available, there is less need for internal fixation, and the treatment is then of the accompanying paraplegia.

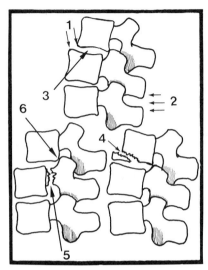

99. *Other spinal injuries* (1) *Retrospondylolisthesis* (1) especially at the thoraco-lumbar junction may result from a blow in the sacral or lower lumbar region (2). There may be shearing through the disc (3), the vertebral body (4) or the pedicles (5) so the articular processes impinge on the vertebral body (6). Neurological involvement if present is seldom complete. The posterior ligament complex is damaged: treat as unstable unless strong contrary evidence.

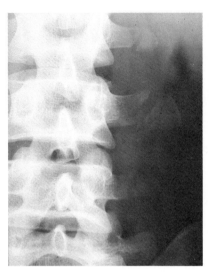

100. *(2) Fractured transverse processes:* Lumbar transverse processes may be fractured by (1) avulsion (quadratus lumborum), (2) direct trauma, (3) rotational injuries of the spine. Symptomatic treatment with analgesics and bed rest is all that is usually needed, but if multiple fractures are present, there may be substantial retro-peritoneal haemorrhage leading to shock and paralytic ileus. These are treated along routine lines.

101. Neurological assessment

(1) Where there is evidence of a deficit, a thorough neurological examination is required on admission. This must include as a minimum:

(a) Testing for evidence of muscle activity and its power in all muscle groups below the level of injury.

(b) Testing sensation to pin prick and light touch over the entire area affected.

(c) Testing proprioception.

(d) Testing the reflexes—the tendon reflexes; the plantar responses; the anal reflex (stimulation of the perineum leading to contraction of the external anal sphincter) and the glans-bulbar reflex (compression of the glans leading to perineal muscle contraction).

(2) If the findings indicate a complete spinal lesion, the examination should be repeated after 6 hours, 12 hours and 24 hours.

The common lesions: (a) Spinal concussion causes a temporary arrest of conduction within the cord; its effects are patchy, and recovery is rapid. If, for example, there is a *complete* spinal lesion on first examination, spinal concussion is an unlikely, but possible cause. If after 12 hours the lesion remains complete, spinal concussion is *not* the cause.

(b) If there is any evidence of voluntary motor activity, skin sensation or proprioception below the level of the lesion, the cord has not been transected, (and further recovery is possible).

(c) After an injury to the cord, the reflexes generally disappear for at least some hours, and sometimes for as long as 2 weeks. Return of reflex activity with continued absence of all sensation and voluntary muscle contraction confirms a *transection of the cord*.

(d) Where the injury is at a level where there is potential damage to lumbar nerve roots or the cauda equina (e.g. injuries at the thoraco-lumbar junction persistent absence of reflexes would confirm such damage.

(e) Note that cord transection is irrecoverable, but there is potential recovery where there is involvement of nerve roots and the cauda equina.

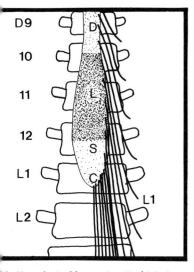

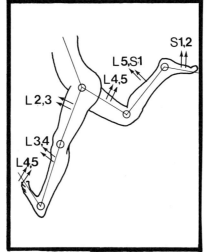

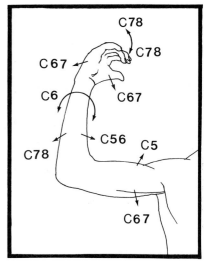

2. *Neurological lesions in spinal injuries:* ote (1) The spinal cord ends at L1; any jury distal to this can involve the cauda t not the cord. (2) All the lumbar and cral segments of the cord lie between D10 d L1 only. (3) Injuries at the thoraco-mbar junction produce a great variety of urological disturbances as (a) the cord ay or may not be transected (b) the nerve ots may be undamaged, partly divided, or mpletely divided.

103. Cord or root damage is reflected in disturbance of myotomes or dermatomes. *Myotomes* (1) As a rule, motion in each joint is logically controlled by 4 myotomes in sequence: viz. *Hip flexion*, L2, 3, extension L4, 5. *Knee extension*, L3, 4 (including knee jerk), flexion L5, S1. *Ankle dorsiflexion* L4, 5, plantar flexion S1, S2 (including ankle jerk). (In addition, inversion is controlled by L4 and eversion by L5, S1.)

104. *Myotomes* (2) In the upper limb, the arrangement is less regular: *Shoulder abduction* C5, adduction C6, 7. *Elbow flexion* C5, 6 (including biceps jerk), extension C7, 8 (including triceps jerk). *Wrist flexion and extension;* both C6, 7. *Finger flexion and extension*, C7, 8. *Pronation and supination* C6 (including supinator jerk). *Hand intrinsic muscles* T1.

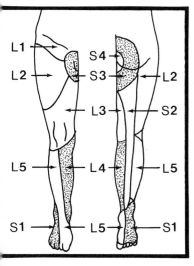

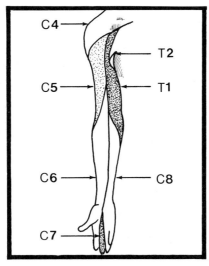

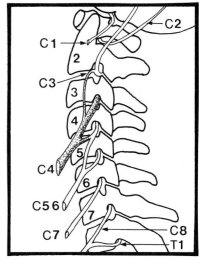

5. *Dermatomes* (1) The lumbar and sacral rmatomes have a complex arrangement hich is difficult to commit to memory. emember by the facts that (a) the outer order of the foot is supplied by S1 (b) the edial part of the foot and the lateral part of e leg by L5 (c) the 'stocking top' area is pplied by L2 and (d) the saddle area by 3.

106. *Dermatomes* (2) In the upper limb, the anterior axial line follows the lie of the second rib from the angle of Louis, and continues down the anterior aspect of the arm, splitting near the middle finger which is supplied by C7. The other dermatomes are arranged in a regular fashion on either side of the axial line.

107. *Cervical cord: special features:* Note (a) the phrenic nerve arises from C4, with minor contributions from C3 and C5. Cord section proximal to the phrenic nerve will lead to rapid death from respiratory paralysis. Those with lesions at C4–5, and more distal, are capable of respiration without external support. (b) C2 and C3 supply the vertex and occiput (accounting for pain here in upper cervical lesions). C5–T1 contribute to the brachial plexus. (Drawing diagramatic.)

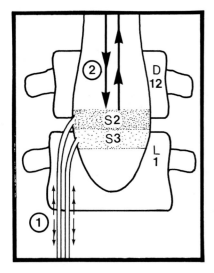

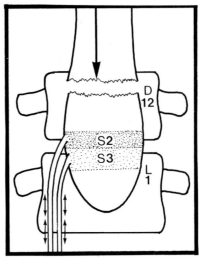

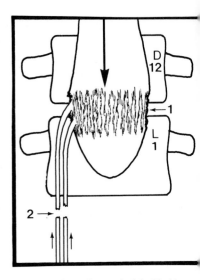

108. *Neurological control of the bladder:* Note (a) Autonomic fibres controlling the detrusor muscle of the bladder and the internal sphincter travel from cord segments S2 and 3 to the bladder via the cauda equina (1). (b) Under normal circumstances bladder sensation and voluntary emptying are mediated through pathways stretching between the brain and the sacral centres (2).

109. *Neurological control of the bladder ctd.:* (c) If the cord is transected above the S2, 3 segments (e.g. by a thoracic spine fracture) voluntary control is lost, but the potential for co-ordinated contraction of the bladder wall, relaxation of the sphincter, and complete emptying remains. (Normally 200–400 cc of urine is passed every 2–4 hours, the reflex activity being triggered by rising bladder pressure or skin stimulation.) (Automatic bladder or cord bladder.)

110. *Neurological control of the bladder ctd.:* (d) Injuries which damage the sacral centres (1) or the cauda (2) prevent co-ordinated reflex control of bladder activity. Bladder emptying is always incomplete and irregular, and occurs only as a result of distension. Its efficiency varies with the patient's state of health, the presence of urinary infection, and muscle spasms. (Autonomous or isolated atonic bladder.)

111. Treatment of spinal paralysis

1. The aim of treatment is (a) maximal physical recovery and mental readjustment, with ideally (b) complete physical independence and (c) retur to full-time employment.

2. These ideals can be most fully realised through the special resources and environment of a paraplegic unit, and no effort should be spared in having the patient transferred to such a unit at the earliest convenience.

3. Pending transfer, and assuming the injury has been dealt with in an appropriate fashion, it is vital that attention is paid to the problems of the skin and bladder.

(a) The skin: If pressure is applied to the skin it becomes ischaemic; if pressure is maintained, necrosis from tissue anoxia results. The skin of the elderly is thin, and least able to tolerate pressure. Poorly nourished skin, anaemia, and local skin damage such as abrasions (which increase oxygen demand) are also adverse factors. The most important points, both of whic are amenable to treatment, are (i) the duration of ischaemia (ii) the amount of pressure applied to the skin.

The *duration of pressure* applied to any one area is in practice regulated by regular turning of the patient. During the initial weeks of treatment it is essential that the patient does not lie for longer than two hours in one position. If the patient is being nursed on a Stryker frame, then he alternate from the prone to the supine; if he is being nursed in bed, then he alternates between lying on each side and in the supine position. It is important to note that regular turning of the patient should start from the time of injury; irreversible damage may be done on the day of admission when other problems allow this vital aspect of treatment to be overlooked for some hours.

The *amount of pressure* applied to the skin is obviously important: if the body weight is locally concentrated ischaemia will be complete. If the skin loading is reduced by being spread over a large area, then ischaemia will be less severe and more tolerable. Because of these loading factors, pressure sores tend to commence over bony prominences—the sacrum, the trochanters, the heels, the elbows, and the malleoli. Particular attention should be paid to these areas, and local padding over the ankles and elbows may help. To distribute the body weight more evenly, the patient may be nursed on pillows laid across the bed from head to foot. When the patient is lying on his back, additional pillows, laid horizontally, may be used to support the elbows and arms. Pillows may also be placed under the legs so that the heels are relieved of pressure. When the patient is lying on his side, a pillow may be placed between the legs, and the legs positioned in such a way that the malleoli and knees are free from pressure. In some centres, water beds or sand beds are used to help distribute the loads on the skin.

It is important to preserve the tone and general condition of the skin. If it becomes moist it becomes susceptible to bacterial invasion. If it is subjected to fixation through contact with rough, unyielding surfaces, local abrasions may occur. Local injury of this nature increases tissue demands and may initiate the production of pressure sores. To prevent this, (i) unstarched, soft bed linen should be used and non-porous surfaces avoided. Nursing the patient on sheepskin is sometimes advocated. (ii) the skin should be protected from incontinence. (iii) skin hygiene should be maintained by frequent, thorough cleansing with soap and water. After washing, the skin must be thoroughly dried; rubbing with alcohol may help this, and at the same time lead to temporary, local vaso-dilatation. Talcum powder is also used to help drying and reduce friction between the skin and the bedlinen.

If pressure sores occur, preventative measures should be tightened up, and any underlying anaemia corrected. Any local sloughs or sequestra should be removed. If the area involved is small, healing may be achieved with local dressings, going through the stages of granulation and contraction. If a large area is involved, rotational flaps usually afford the best means of closure. If sores persist, they are frequently followed by progressive anaemia, deterioration in general health and well being, and often amyloid disease.

(b) The bladder: The effects of spinal paralysis on the bladder are dependent on the level of injury, and have been described. The immediate problem is prevention of over-distension of the bladder while minimising the risks of infection. The methods available include (i) Intermittent supra-pubic cystostomy using plastic tubing. This method is demanding on staff and facilities, and carries the risk of pelvic infection.

(ii) Intermittent catheterisation: If properly performed with a full aseptic ritual, the risks of infection are probably lowest with this method, but it is very demanding on staff.

(iii) Indwelling catheterisation: This is probably the commonest method employed, but is almost invariably accompanied by some degree of urinary infection.

Mechanical emptying of the bladder by one of these methods is usually required for 3–4 weeks, after which, in the appropriate lesions, automatic function will be starting to take over. This should be assessed by (i) removing the catheter and (ii) giving copious fluids. (iii) When filling of the bladder is apparent, trying to achieve emptying by stroking the skin in the inner groin area or by applying manual pressure over the bladder.

If these measures fail, re-catheterisation will be necessary, and the procedure repeated after a week. Thereafter the efficiency of emptying should be assessed by measuring the residual urine every 3–6 months. Renal function should be reviewed by a yearly intravenous pyelogram, urine culture and estimation of the serum urea. Failure to establish a satisfactory emptying pattern will require skilled urological investigation and management.

4. *Physiotherapy and occupational therapy:* These measures should be commenced without delay, attention being paid to the following aspects of management.

(i) Chest: The risks and effects of respiratory infection should be minimised by deep breathing exercises, the development of the accessory muscles of respiration, assisted coughing, percussion and postural drainage.

(ii) The joints: Mobility should be preserved in the paralysed joints by passive movements. This must be done with caution if there is any spasticity; over-stretching must be avoided to minimise the risks of myositis ossificans.

(iii) The unparalysed muscles: These should be developed for compensatory use—e.g. shoulder girdle exercises to make unaided bed—wheelchair transfers possible. Troublesome muscle spasms may be controlled with diazepam.

Depending on the level of the lesion the patient may require assistance in some or all of the following areas:

(iv) Regaining balance for sitting or standing.

(v) Tuition in calliper walking (or gait improvement in partial lesions).

(vi) Overcoming problems of dressing.

(vii) Help with alterations and adjustments within the home to permit wheelchair use.

(viii) Industrial re-training or other measures to help return to employment.

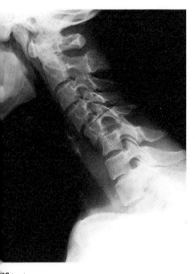

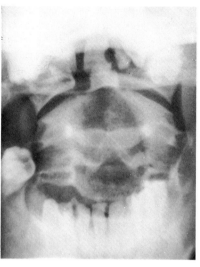

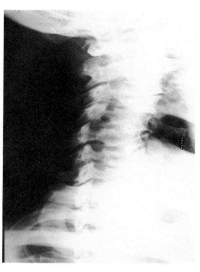

f test
2. Describe the lesion shown. Is the injury ble or unstable?

113. Describe this through-the-mouth view of the first two cervical vertebrae.

114. Is there any abnormality showing in this oblique projection of the cervical spine?

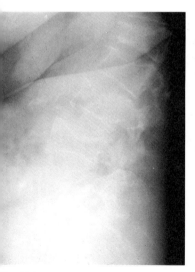

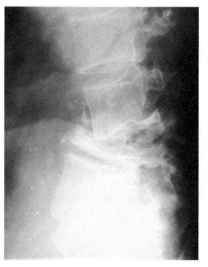

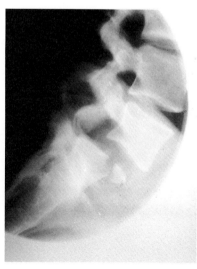

5. This lateral radiograph is of an elderly ient complaining of pain in the back after ing a heavy weight. What do the liographs show?

116. Describe this fracture: is it likely to be stable or unstable, complicated or uncomplicated?

117. Describe this injury. What treatment would be required?

112. Dislocation of C5 on C6 with bilateral locked facets. 50% forward shift is present and the injury is unstable. There is no accompanying fracture.

113. There is a congenital deformity of the odontoid process (hypoplasia). No fracture is present and there is no evidence of other injury. The shadow lying above the hypoplastic odontoid process is that of one of the incisors.

114. There is a subluxation of C4 on C5 involving the facet joint on the right side. The articular surfaces are still in contact and the subluxation has not reached the stage of a frank dislocation with locking of the facet joint.

115. Anterior wedge fractures of L1, L2, L3. Central ballooning of the disc into L4. Gross demineralisation of the spine, probably secondary to osteoporosis or osteomalacia (i.e. pathological fracture).

116. Gross wedging of L4, with comminution and posterior displacement of fragments into the spinal canal. This is an unstable fracture and there was neurological involvement (cauda equina lesion).

117. Anterior dislocation of L5 on the sacrum, with bilateral locked facets and a fracture of the anterior margin of the first piece of the sacrum. Open reduction would be required in this injury.

11. Fractures of the pelvis, hip and femoral neck

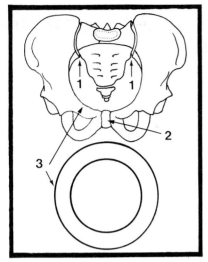

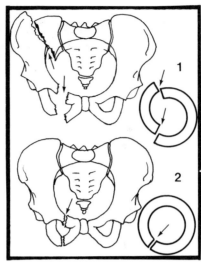

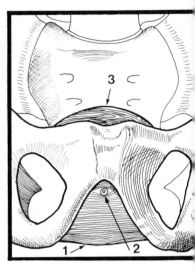

1. *General principles* (1) The two halves of the pelvis are joined to the sacrum by the immensely strong sacro-iliac ligaments (1). In front they are united by the symphysis pubis (2). This arrangement forms a cylinder of bone (the pelvic ring) (3) which protects the pelvic organs.

2. *General principles* (2) When the pelvic ring is disrupted at two levels, wide separation of the parts may occur (1). It is important to recognise this possibility. Isolated injuries on the other hand (2) do not have this tendency. *The primary classification of pelvic fractures is in to those with an intact pelvic ring and those with opening of the pelvic ring.*

3. *General principles* (3) The urogenital diaphragm (1) is pierced by the membrano urethra (2), and the bladder (3) lies behind the pubic bones. Fractures of the pelvis, especially in the region of the symphysis a pubic rami, are often associated with damage to the urethra or bladder. Rarely there may be involvement of the rectum.

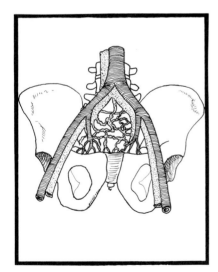

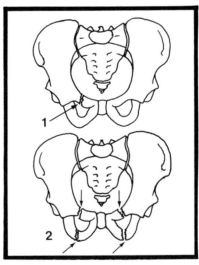

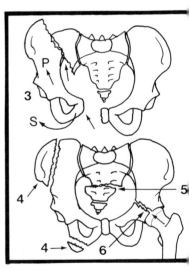

4. *General principles* (4) The pelvis is richly supplied with blood vessels which are frequently damaged by fractures. *Internal haemorrhage is often severe, leading to shock which can be rapidly fatal.* N.B. (1) Shock should be *anticipated* in pelvic fractures and the appropriate replacement steps taken. (2) Unaccountable shock following trauma is an indication for radiology of the pelvis.

5. *General classification of pelvic fractures:* (1) Isolated fracture of the pelvic ring. *There is no tendency to separation.* (2) Stable. double fracture of the pelvic ring. *Although the ring is broken in two places, the main fragments maintain their relationship.*

6. *General classification ctd.:* (3) Double fracture of the pelvic ring with separation. (Ill: disruption at symphysis pubis with fracture of the ilium.) The separation may take two forms—lateral rotation or splaying (S) or proximal shift (P). (4) Avulsion fractures. (5) Fractures of th sacrum and coccyx. (6) Central dislocatio of the hip: here the acetabular floor is involved.

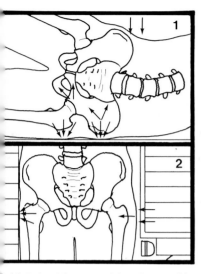

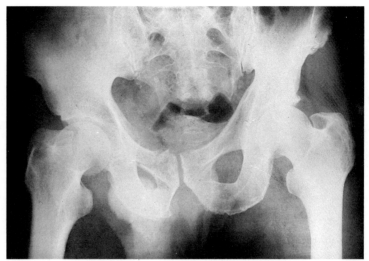

7. (1) *Isolated fractures of the pelvic ring* (1) These, like many other pelvic fractures, may result from a fall on the side (1), force being transmitted through the trochanter or iliac crest, or from crushing accidents (e.g. from reversing vehicles (2), rock falls, etc.), or through violence transmitted along the femoral shaft (e.g. road traffic accidents, falls from a height, etc.).

8. *Isolated fractures of the pelvic ring* (2) By far the commonest pelvic fracture is one involving the superior pubic ramus. This is seen frequently in the elderly patient following a fall on the side. Osteoporosis or osteomalacia are frequently contributory factors. *This injury is often missed* and should always be suspected if there is difficulty in walking after a fall, and a femoral neck fracture has been excluded. Clinically there will be tenderness over the superior pubic ramus: pain on side-to-side compression of the pelvis: movements of the hip may be relatively free. Radiographs of the hip may fail to visualise the area and full pelvic films are required.

Treatment is by bed rest for 2–3 weeks till pain settles and mobilisation can be commenced.

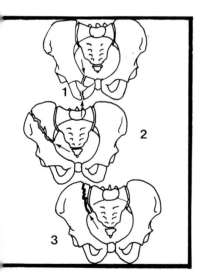

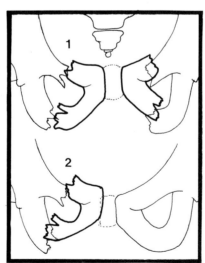

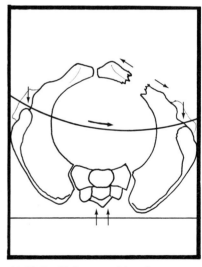

9. *Isolated fractures of the pelvic ring* (3) Other fractures of this type include (1) Fractures of two rami on one side, (2) Fracture of the ilium running into the sciatic notch, (3) Fracture of the ilium involving the sacro-iliac joint, or subluxation of the sacro-iliac joint. The treatment of these injuries, assuming they are uncomplicated, is as for isolated fracture of the superior pubic ramus.

10. (2) *Stable double fracture of the pelvic ring:* These injuries usually result from compression of the pelvis, often in the A.P. plane. The commonest is the quadrilateral or butterfly fracture (1). Less frequently there is fracture of two rami on one side with symphyseal subluxation (2). *Anticipate shock and damage to the urethra or bladder*, but otherwise treat by 6 weeks recumbency.

11. (3) *Double fracture of the pelvic ring with separation* (1) These injuries usually result from A.P. compression of the pelvis, e.g. in run-over injuries when the wheel of a vehicle forces the anterior spines backwards splaying the pelvis, or when the pelvis is compressed by falling rock or masonry, pinning the patient on his back to the ground. They may also be caused by forces transmitted up the limb.

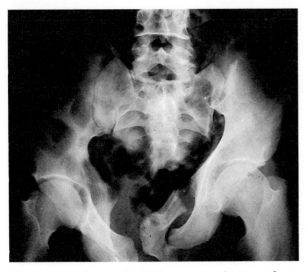

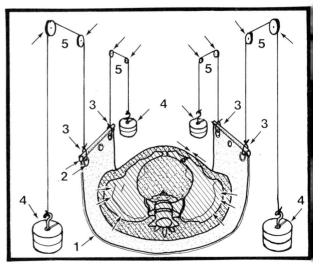

12. *Fractures with separation* (2) There are several patterns of injury within this group, e.g. (ill.) fracture of two rami on one side, dislocation of the sacro-iliac joint, some splaying of the pelvis, and proximal migration of the hemipelvis. *Treatment: N.B.* (a) Look carefully for other injuries requiring prior treatment. (b) Take blood for emergency grouping and cross matching in anticipation of a large replacement, and set up a good i.v. line. (c) Exclude damage to the urethra, bladder or viscera and (d) silent rupture of the diaphragm, a commonly associated injury (X-ray chest).

13. *Treatment:* (e) If *splaying* is the main element in the deformity, this should be corrected by side-to-side compression of the pelvis. This may be achieved by the use of a canvas sling (1) reinforced at the edges with steel rods and eyelets (2). It may be lined with wool prior to positioning under the pelvis. Traction cords are attached to the corners (3) and weights (×4) of 2–4 kg (4) applied through pulleys (5) on a Balkan beam. The sling compresses the pelvis and generally produces a satisfactory reduction.

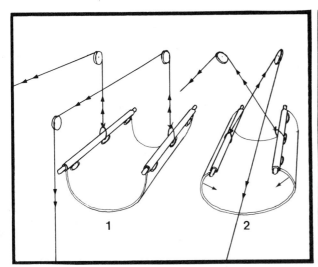

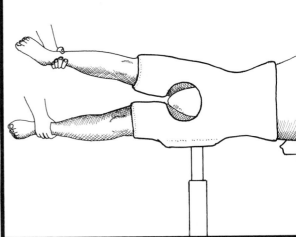

14. *Treatment ctd.:* In many cases it is possible to simplify this rather complex arrangement of weights and cordage by arranging the traction from the centre of the pelvic sling on both sides (1). Check radiographs are taken. If reduction is incomplete, the weights may be increased, or more side thrust may be gained by crossing the traction cords (2). Canvas sling support should be continued for 6 weeks, and weight bearing permitted after 8 weeks.

15. *Treatment ctd.:* Alternatively, a plaster spica ('plaster pants') may be applied: this is of particular value for patient transport. The patient is anaesthetised and laid *on his good side* on a small pelvic rest on an orthopaedic table (ill.). The hips should be slightly flexed. The weight of the limb should close the gap. This should be confirmed by radiographs prior to plastering. If the gap fails to close, the patient should be laid *on the injured side*. Adequate padding is essential. On completion, the pelvic rest should be cut free and the defect filled.

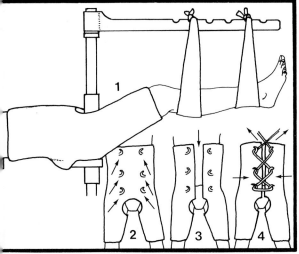

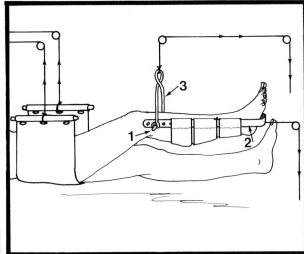

16. *Treatment ctd.:* Alternatively, a hip spica may be applied in the traditional manner on the orthopaedic table, with the hips in about 30° of flexion (1), metal hooks being incorporated anteriorly (2). When the plaster has set, a 3″ (7.5 cm) strip is cut from the front (3). The gap is then closed by cross lacing (4). If hooks are not available, the plaster may be closed with elastic bandaging.

Internal fixation with a plate and screws is often followed by a disabling osteitis of the symphysis, and should only be considered if bladder exploration is required, if prolonged immobilisation is undesirable or symphyseal instability persists.

17. *Treatment ctd.:* Where one half of the pelvis has displaced proximally, it becomes necessary to apply traction as well as side-to-side compression. This may be achieved by Steinman pin traction (1) using a metal loop (2) and stirrup (3). Treatment is maintained for 6 weeks. Slight persistent proximal subluxation is not likely to lead to material disability and may be accepted.

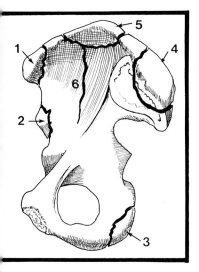

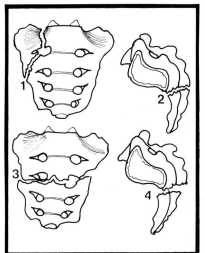

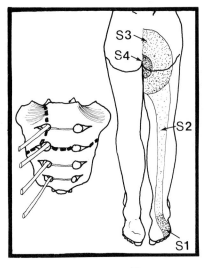

18. (4) *Avulsion fractures:* Sudden muscle contraction, especially in athletes, may avulse the anterior spine (sartorius) (1), the anterior inferior spine (rectus femoris) (2), the ischial tuberosity (hamstrings) (3), the posterior spine (erector spinae) (4), and the crest (abdominal muscles) (5). The crest and blade may also be fractured by direct violence (6). In all cases there is local tenderness, and symptomatic treatment (a few days bed rest) is all that is required.

19. (5) *Fracture of the sacrum* (1) *The ala of the sacrum* (1) may be fractured as a result of either side-to-side or antero-posterior compression of the pelvis. *Transverse fractures of the sacrum* usually result from falls from a height on to hard surfaces. These fractures may be undisplaced (2); or they may be associated with some lateral (3) or anterior displacement (4).

20. *Fractures of the sacrum* (2) In some cases there may be involvement of sacral nerve roots, leading to sensory disturbance, weakness in the leg(s), or saddle anaesthesia and incontinence. In the majority of cases neurological disturbance is due to a lesion in continuity, and is transitory; but if displacement of the fracture is gross, the changes may be permanent. Treatment of sacral fractures is symptomatic, with bed rest for 2–3 weeks.

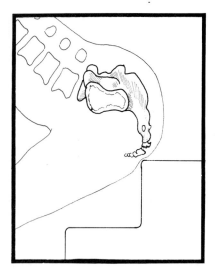

21. *Coccygeal injuries* (A) The coccyx is usually injured by a fall in a seated position against a hard surface—e.g. the edge of a step. There is local pain and tenderness, and sometimes pain on defaecation. Sitting on hard surfaces is always painful. (Note that coccygeal pain may also be caused by lumbar disc prolapse, pelvic inflammatory disease, chordoma and other tumours of the sacrum.)

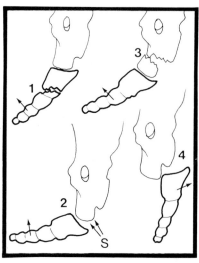

22. *Coccygeal injuries* (B) The main patterns of injury are (1) fracture of the coccyx, with a varying degree of anteversion (2) anterior subluxation of the coccyx (3) anterior displacement of the coccyx secondary to fracture of the end piece of the sacrum (4) rarely, posterior subluxation of the coccyx.

23. *Diagnosis:* (1) Clinically, there is local tenderness. (2) When there is anterior subluxation, the prominent sharp edge of t sacrum may be obvious on palpation (S). (3) The displacement may be detected on rectal examination. The diagnosis is confirmed by localised radiographs of the region, although film quality may be poor the obese patient.

Treatment: (a) Sitting on hard surfaces should be avoided, and initially the patient should use an inflatable rubber ring cushio The patient should not be allowed to beco constipated. (b) If symptoms become chronic, local short wave diathermy or ultrasound may be tried: alternatively the painful area may be injected with a long acting local anaesthetic—e.g. 10 ml of 0.5 Bupivaine Hydrochloride (Marcaine). (c) all conservative measures fail, excision of coccyx should be considered.

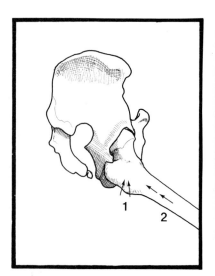

24. (6) *Central dislocation of the hip:* In this group of injuries the pelvis is fractured as a result of force transmitted through the femoral head. This may occur from a blow or fall on ths side (1) or when force is transmitted up the limb (2) via the foot, as in a fall from a height, or through the knee as in a car dashboard injury.

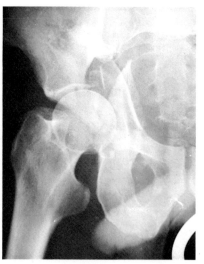

25. *Diagnosis* (1) The fracture is easily diagnosed by routine radiographs which reveal characteristic disturbance of the acetabulum. There are, however, many patterns of injury due to variations in the amount and direction of the causal force. Pending full assessment, the patient should be treated for any accompanying shock, and skin traction (*c.* 4 kilos) applied to the limb.

26. *Diagnosis* (2) When the hip joint is seriously disorganised, open reduction and internal fixation of the fragments can give good results. Nevertheless, it is clear that a very careful analysis of these fractures is necessary to select the few cases suitable fc this type of treatment. The first screening procedures should be (1) a standard A.P. projection of the *pelvis* showing both hips the one film, along with (2) a lateral projection of the hip. If there is any significant displacement of the fragments of the femoral head, further films will be required to answer the questions posed in t following frames.

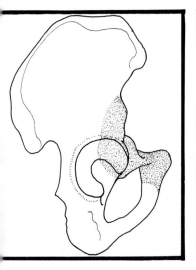

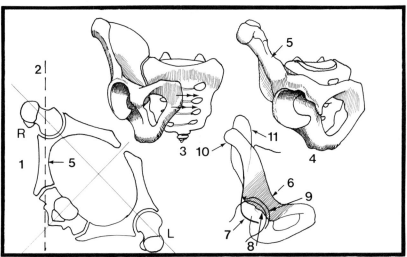

. (a) *Is the anterior column intact?* (1) The terior column is the name given to the ass of bone which stretches downwards om the anterior inferior iliac spine, and :ludes the pubis and the anterior part of e acetabular floor. To help clarify this, a ree-quarter internal oblique view of the hip ould be obtained.

28. (a) *Is the anterior column intact?* (2) Foam wedges are placed under the buttock on the *affected* side until the pelvis is tilted at 45° (1). This rotation of the pelvis from the A.P. plane (3) to the oblique position (4) places the blade of the ilium in profile (5) to the central ray (2). The radiographic appearances are complex, especially if the fracture is badly displaced: but note on the films the state of the shaded portion (6) which represents the anterior column. Note also the easily identified posterior margin of the acetabulum (7), its less obvious anterior margin (8) and its floor (9). (10 and 11 are the anterior superior iliac spine and the iliac crest.) *Isolated fractures of the anterior column are uncommon, but are important to recognise as they require an anterior surgical approach for reduction.*

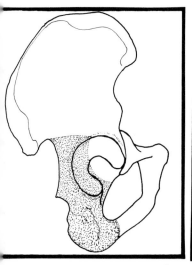

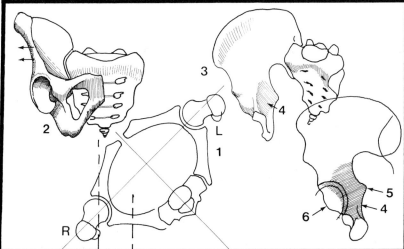

. (b) *Is the posterior column intact?* (1) e posterior column stretches upwards om the ischial tuberosity to the sciatic tch, and includes the posterior part of the tabular floor. To clarify this a second lique projection is often helpful (three-arter external oblique projection).

30. (b) *Is the posterior column intact?* (2) The pelvis is tilted 45° towards the injured side by sandbags under the good side (1). This rotation of the pelvis from the normal position (2) to the oblique (3) throws the area of the posterior column (4) away from the rest of the pelvis. Note on the radiographs the area of the posterior column (shaded), the ischial spine (5), and the anterior lip of the acetabulum (6). Careful study of the A.P., lateral and two 45° obliques may allow you to assess the state of the columns, but if there is still some doubt, the following procedures may be of value: (a) Stereo radiography. (b) Tomography. (c) Intensifier screening (rotating the pelvis into different planes under the beam and moving the femur in relation to the main fragments).

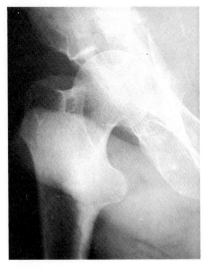

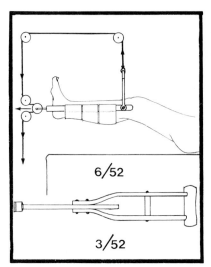

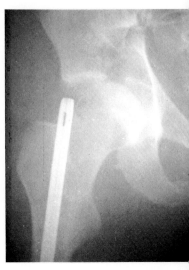

31. (c) *Is the floor of the acetabulum highly comminuted?* (1) Comminution of the acetabular floor may be obvious on the radiographs, and should be carefully assessed. If present, attempts at restoration by surgery are unlikely to be successful, *and these injuries should generally be treated conservatively.*

32. *Comminution of the acetabular floor ctd.* (2) Hamilton-Russell traction (e.g. of about 3 kg) may be used, and this should be maintained for 6 weeks; *the hip should be mobilised during this period.* Thereafter a further 3–4 weeks should elapse before full weight bearing. Some permanent restriction of hip movements is inevitable, but overall function may be good, and further treatment unnecessary unless secondary osteo-arthritis supervenes.

33. (d) *Is the weight bearing portion of the acetabulum intact, but the femoral head displaced?* Such cases should be considered for surgery, and your analysis of column involvement determines the surgical approach, viz: (i) Anterior column only—anterior approach. (ii) Posterior column only *or* both columns—posterior approach. (Illustrated: fracture of both columns, with associated nailed fracture of femur.)

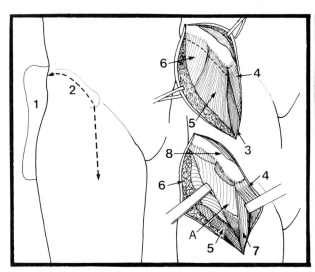

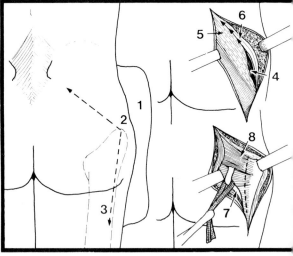

34. *Anterior (Smith Petersen) approach to the hip:* A sandbag (1) is placed under the buttock and the skin incision (2) made along the crest to the anterior spine and downwards about 4″ (10 cm) in the direction of the lateral patellar margin. The interval (3) between sartorius (4) and tensor fascia lata (5) is opened up; gluteus medius (6) and the tensor are reflected to expose the lateral lip of the acetabulum (A). The anterior lip is visualised by dissecting rectus femoris (7) medially. Dissection close to bone on the medial side of the ilium (8) will expose the pelvic side of the anterior column by reflection of iliacus.

35. *Posterior approach to the hip:* A sandbag (1) is placed under the hip. The skin incision starts well lateral to the posterior (superior) iliac spine, bisects the tip of the greater trochanter (2) and extends 3″ (7.5 cm) down the lateral aspect of the femur (3). The incision is deepened over the trochanter to expose the extensive sub-trochanteric bursa (4). The fibres of gluteus maximus (5) are easily ripped from their attachment to the ilio-tibial tract (6). The sciatic nerve (7) is identified, taped, and gently retracted medially. It may require gentle teasing away from the fracture. The short rotators (8) are divided close to the femur to expose the acetabulum from the sciatic notch to the ischium.

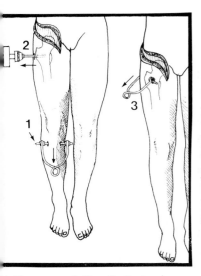

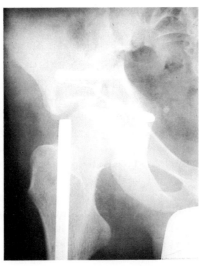

6. *Treatment ctd.:* Once the fracture has been exposed by the most appropriate approach, reduction may be facilitated by traction. Longitudinal traction may be carried out with a Steinman pin through the tibial tubercle (1). Lateral traction is generally more useful: a threaded pin, inserted percutaneously into the trochanter may be employed (2) or even a Steinman pin carefully inserted in the sagittal plane (3).

37. *Treatment ctd.:* If the fracture can be reduced, it may be held by a small plate or cross screwing. If the fracture cannot be closed, heavy gauge wire can be drawn round two large cancellous screws with wire tighteners, pulling the fragments together (ill: compare with 33). Complete reduction may prove impossible; nevertheless, any improvement may be of value if further surgery becomes necessary.

38. *Treatment ctd.:* After surgery, traction is advisable for 2–3 weeks, with mobilisation of the hip as soon as pain will allow. Weight bearing may be permitted at about 10 weeks, although the patient can often be allowed up non-weight-bearing with crutches at 6 weeks.

Note again that surgery is not advocated for minimally displaced fractures, fractures in which the acetabulum is highly comminuted, or fractures in which the head of the femur remains in alignment with the main weight-bearing portion of the acetabulum. (Treat as 32.)

39. Complications of pelvic fractures

1. Haemorrhage

(1) Substantial internal haemorrhage is common, particularly where there is disruption of the pelvic ring. Shock must be anticipated in all but the most minor of fractures by (a) routine blood grouping and cross matching (b) setting up a good intra-venous line (c) monitoring the pulse rate, blood pressure, and where applicable, the urinary output. Replacement requirements are frequently substantial (transfusion in excess of 5 litres of whole blood not being uncommon) and additional measures for monitoring response (such as measuring central venous pressure) may be required. The effects of massive transfusion must be kept in mind and appropriate precautions taken (e.g. blood warming, addition of calcium, etc.).

(2) Bruising appearing in the scrotum or buttock, or spreading diffusely along the line of the inguinal ligament are indicative of a major internal haemorrhage. In the abdomen a large retro-peritoneal haemorrhage may be felt as a discrete mass on palpation. If the peritoneum on the posterior abdominal wall has been broached, blood may escape into the abdominal cavity. Intra-peritoneal haemorrhage may also result (rarely) from the tearing of mesenteric vessels. This is a serious complication and may be suspected by loss of bowel sounds, abdominal guarding, a progressive increase in abdominal girth, and a blood-stained peritoneal tap; it is an indication for abdominal exploration. Where haemorrhage is extra-peritoneal, exploration is generally unprofitable and likely to aggravate blood loss; treatment should be by replacement only in the first instance.

(3) Ischaemia in one leg is a grave sign and may be due to rupture or intimal damage to an iliac artery. If the patient's condition will permit, exploration of this vessel is indicated.

(4) In the uncommon case of a severe retro-peritoneal haemorrhage, where in spite of a massive transfusion programme, losses continue to gain over replacement, exploration may be reconsidered. It is seldom that a single bleeding source can be found, bleeding generally arising from massive disruption of the pelvic venous plexus. Occasionally successful results have been claimed in these circumstances from ligation of one or both internal iliac arteries.

2. Damage to the urethra and bladder

Incidence: Out of every hundred fractures of the pelvis, roughly 5 are likely to have a urinary tract complication; more than two-thirds involve the urethra. Butterfly fractures are the main cause of urethral damage, whilst displaced fractures of the hemi-pelvis are generally responsible for the sharp edge of a superior pubic ramus rupturing the bladder.

Types of injury: (a) *Rupture of the membranous urethra:* the majority of cases are partial ruptures, with an intact portion of the urethral wall still connected to the bladder. Less commonly there is complete rupture with the bladder losing all continuity with the urethra; the bladder often displaces upwards.

(b) *Extra-peritoneal rupture of the bladder:* This is usually caused by a

COMPLICATIONS OF PELVIC FRACTURES 207

sharp spike of bone penetrating the anterior wall.

(c) *Intra-peritoneal rupture of the bladder:* This may result from the same mechanism, but only occurs if the bladder is full at the time of injury.

(d) *Rupture of the penile urethra:* Injuries of this type generally follow a fall astride a bar or similar object.

Diagnosis: (1) Suspicion should be particularly aroused if the radiographs show either of the fractures described.

(2) Highly suggestive is the presence of perineal bruising.

(3) Diagnostic is the presence of blood at the tip of the penis.

(4) If there is no penile blood, and damage to the bladder or urethra thought possible but not probable, the patient should be asked to attempt to pass urine. (The dangers of urinary extravasation have been exaggerated in the past and are no longer considered to be of import.) If clear urine is passed, no further investigation or treatment is required. A positive chemical test for blood in the presence of macroscopically clear urine should in these circumstances be ignored. If after several tries the patient fails to pass urine, the patient should be re-assessed. The palpability of the bladder should be determined and catheterisation considered.

(5) Catheterisation carries the risk of converting a partial urethral tear into a complete one, and of introducing infection. A diagnostic catheterisation should be approached with caution: a full aseptic regime should be followed, and a fine catheter employed. The procedure should be quickly abandoned if the catheter cannot be introduced with ease. If the tap is dry, this suggests intraperitoneal rupture of the bladder; if blood-stained urine is obtained, this suggests an extra-peritoneal tear of the bladder or a partial tear of the urethra; if blood only is obtained, this suggests a major tear of the posterior urethra.

(6) If there are strong grounds for suggesting significant damage to the bladder or urethra (e.g. penile blood) a urethrogram should be performed in preference to catheterisation. The end of a syringe containing 20 ml of 45% Hypaque is introduced into the urethra and injected: the penis is closed off with the fingers and radiographs taken. The volume injected may be doubled if required. The following are common findings. (a) The bladder shadow is clearly outlined without spillage: *no significant abnormality is likely to be present.* (b) The bladder is partly filled and there is extravasation of the radio-opaque dye to the side: this suggests *extra-peritoneal rupture of the bladder.* (c) The bladder fails to fill, and there is extravasation of the dye into the pelvic floor: there is *rupture of the membranous urethra.* (d) The bladder fails to fill, and there is extravasation of dye beneath the pelvic floor: there is *rupture of the penile urethra.*

Treatment of injuries to the urethra and bladder. *(1) Intra-peritoneal rupture of the bladder:* The bladder is explored and the tear located and sutured. The bladder is drained subsequently with a Foley catheter.

(2) Extra-peritoneal rupture of the bladder: The bladder is explored and the diagnosis confirmed. The rupture is repaired and drained by by-pass (suprapubic) catheterisation.

(3) Incomplete tear of the urethra: If there is evidence of tearing of the membranous urethra, but the bladder is undisplaced, it is likely that some urethral tissue remains in continuity; a suprapubic drain is inserted and the

urethrogram repeated after 10 days. If the circumstances are favourable, a Foley catheter may be introduced at this stage and the suprapubic catheter withdrawn. Later serial bouginage may be required.

(4) Complete rupture of the urethra: If the bladder is floating free it must be drawn down to position. This may be achieved by opening the bladder and rail-roading a Foley catheter downwards. After the balloon has been inflated, the catheter may be used for applying gentle traction. The bladder is drained by a suprapubic catheter which is kept in position for several days. The retro-pubic space may require separate drainage.

(5) Rupture of the penile urethra: An incision is made over the tip of a catheter passed to the level of the obstruction. The catheter is then passed into the bladder through the other end of the urethra. If this cannot be located, the bladder will require opening and the distal end of the urethra identified by instrumentation from above. The urethra is then repaired, usin the catheter as a stent.

3. Injury to the bowel

The rectum may be torn in compound fractures with perineal involvement, and rarely in closed injuries of the central dislocation of the hip type. Injury to the small bowel (mesenteric tears or shearing injuries of the wall leading to infarction or perforation) may be produced by crushing injuries of the pelvis. Bowel involvement may be suspected in the closed injury by abdominal rigidity, loss of bowel sounds, loss of liver dullness and distension. Exploration and a de-functioning colostomy is essential.

4. Rupture of the diaphragm

Routine radiography of the chest should be performed in all major fracture of the pelvis and the standard A.P. projection should eliminate this often-missed complication. If a rupture is confirmed, a thoraco-abdominal repair through the bed of the eighth rib should be undertaken as soon as the patient's general condition will permit.

5. Paralytic ileus

This complication may result from disturbance of the autonomic outflow to the bowel due to the accumulation of a retro-peritoneal haematoma. Treatment by naso-gastric suction and intravenous fluids usually brings rapid resolution within 2–3 days.

6. Limb shortening

Shortening of one leg may result from persistent displacement of the hemi-pelvis. Clinical measurement of the amount of shortening is difficult: leg length as measured from the anterior superior spine to the medial malleolus is unaffected, heel-blocking techniques are rather unsatisfactory, and the measurement of the distance from the umbilicus or xiphisternum to the medial malleolus somewhat inaccurate. The amount of shortening may be judged with greatest accuracy from the radiographs by noting any discrepancy between the level of the iliac crests on the A.P. film (after making a little allowance for film magnification effects). A correction (raise) should be made to the footwear if there is shortening of over $\frac{1}{2}''$ (1.25 cm).

7. Neurological damage

Neurological damage may involve (a) the lumbo-sacral trunk at the triangle of Marcille where there are fractures involving displacement of the hemipelvis, (b) isolated sacral nerves in fractures of the sacrum.

Lesions in continuity predominate, and exploration is seldom indicated. Impotence occurs in about a sixth of major pelvic fractures, and in about half of those cases in which there is rupture of the urethra. It is frequently permanent.

8. Obstetrical difficulties

Even in the case of quite marked post-fracture pelvic distortion, natural childbirth is rarely affected to a degree requiring caesarian section.

9. Persistent sacro-iliac joint pain

Sacro-iliac pain is common for many months after pelvic fractures which involve hingeing at one sacro-iliac joint, but seldom persists. If it does, a local fusion may be performed.

10. Persistent symphyseal instability

This is a rare complication and an indication for internal fixation: screening may be of help in confirming the diagnosis.

11. Osteo-arthritis of the hip

Central dislocation of the hip is not infrequently followed by this complication. It is dealt with along routine lines. Many cases may come to and are suitable for total hip replacement, and prior reduction of a major displacement will render this easier.

12. Myositis ossificans

Myositis ossificans is seen most frequently after operative intervention or where there is an accompanying head injury. The treatment is along the lines previously indicated.

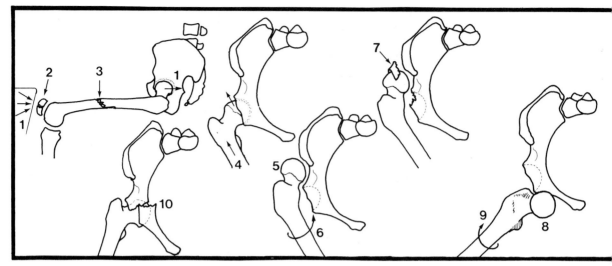

40. *Traumatic dislocation of the hip:* The hip may dislocate as a result of force being transmitted up the femoral shaft. This most commonly occurs as a result of dashboard impact in road traffic accidents (1). Note that this mechanism may be responsible for simultaneous fracture of the patella (2) or of the femoral shaft (3). Force transmitted up the limbs from falls on the foot, force applied to the lumbar region (e.g. in roof falls on kneeling miners) and rarely force applied directly to the trochanter may also cause the hip to dislocate. If the leg is flexed at the hip and adducted (4) at the time of impact, the femur dislocates posteriorly (5) internally rotating at the same time (6). In some cases, the posterior lip of the acetabulum is fractured (7). If the hip is widely abducted, anterior dislocation may occur—even without any axial transmission of force (8). The femur externally rotates (9). Note that the femur is in some other part of the abduction/adduction range, that these mechanisms may be responsible for central dislocation type fractures of the pelvis (10).

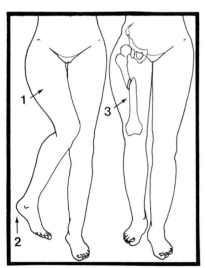

41. *Posterior dislocation of the hip:* *Diagnosis:* In a typical posterior dislocation, the hip is held slightly flexed, adducted, and internally rotated (1). The leg appears short (2). Few other injuries are associated with the agony accompanying posterior dislocation, and this is almost as diagnostic as the deformity. Pain is less severe if the acetabulum is fractured, and the deformity may be concealed if there is an associated femoral fracture (3).

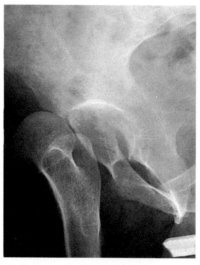

42. *Radiographs* (1) The diagnosis is confirmed by radiographs of the hip; the deformity is usually obvious on the A.P. projection, but dislocation cannot be *excluded* with one view (c.f. dislocation of the shoulder); a lateral projection is helpful in confirming the distinction between an anterior and posterior dislocation, and *essential* if no abnormality is obvious on the A.P. film (ill: obvious posterior dislocation).

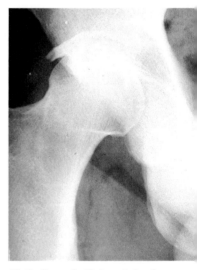

43. *Radiographs* (2) Acetabular rim fractures may be produced by the shearing force of the backward travelling femoral head (40, 7). The fragment may be small (ill.) where it is seldom of consequence. It may be large or comminuted, in which case there is increased risk of sciatic nerve palsy instability in reduction, and later osteo-arthritis.

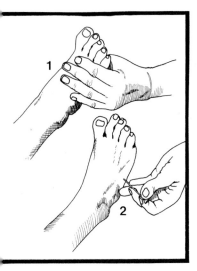

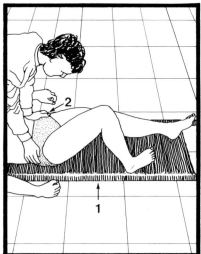

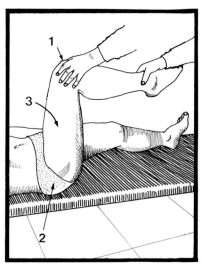

. *Sciatic nerve involvement:* The presence
absence of damage to the sciatic nerve
ould be sought in every case, and
rticularly where an acetabular rim
acture is present. Enquire about numbness
burning sensations in the limb, and as a
inimal screening, test the power of
orsiflexion in the foot (1) and appreciation
pin prick sensation in the leg below the
ee (2).

45. *Reduction* (1) Reduction should be
carried out as soon as a general anaesthetic
can be arranged. The key to success is
complete muscle relaxation: the anaesthetist
should be reminded of this and of the need to
transfer the patient on a stretcher canvas on
to the floor to allow the hip to be
manipulated (1). An assistant should kneel
at the side of the patient and steady the
pelvis (2).

46. *Reduction* (2) When the patient is fully
relaxed (and the administration of
suxamethonium chloride (Scoline) just prior
to manipulation is often invaluable) the
knee (1) and hip (2) are flexed gently to a
right angle, at the same time gently
correcting the adduction and internal
rotation deformities (3). (Note: the
assistant's hands, vital to the reduction, have
been omitted from this and subsequent
drawings for clarity.)

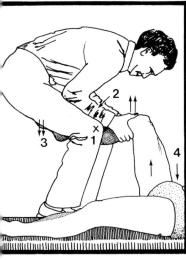

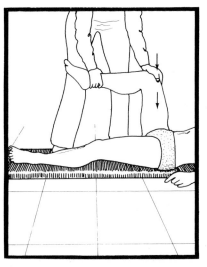

49. *Reduction* (5) Check radiographs should
be taken in two planes. The following
possibilities arise: (a) The dislocation has
been fully reduced. (b) The dislocation and a
rim fracture have both been reduced, and the
hip is stable clinically: *In both (a) and (b)
further treatment is conservative.*
(c) Although the femoral head is concentric
with the acetabulum, the joint space is
increased. This should be elucidated further
with tomography. Persistent displacement of
this type may be due to a trapped bone (rim)
fragment or infolding of the labrum. A
trapped bone fragment should be removed
by surgery, as if left it will lead to rapid onset
osteo-arthritis. Excision of a trapped labrum
is advocated but the grounds for this are less
clear: there would seem some justification
for a 'wait-and-see' approach.

7. *Reduction* (3) The head of the femur
ould now be lying directly behind the
cetabulum and just requires to be lifted
rwards. The force required is variable, but
eat leverage can be obtained by gripping
e leg between the knees (1) resting your
rearms on your thighs (2) and flexing your
nees (3). The assistant keeps the pelvis
om lifting by downward pressure (4).
eduction usually occurs with an obvious
lunk'.

48. *Reduction* (4) Reduction is often less
striking when there is a rim fracture: and
when a rim fracture is present (shown by the
radiographs) the stability of the reduction
should always be checked by downward
pressure on the femur. Gross instability is an
indication for open reduction and internal
fixation of the rim fracture.

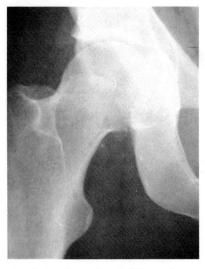

50. *Check radiographs ctd.:* (d) There is persistent displacement of a fracture of the rim and the hip is unstable (ill: note rim fragment situated near upper lip of the acetabulum). (e) There is a displaced fracture of the rim with a persisting sciatic palsy. Operative reduction and internal (screw) fixation of the fragment is indicated in (d) and (e).

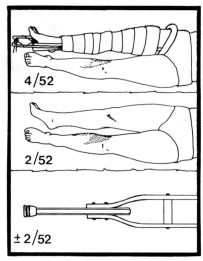

51. *After care:* The hip should be kept at rest for some time to reduce the risks of complications. A common regime is fixed (skin) traction in a Thomas splint for four weeks and bed mobilisation for a further two weeks before weight bearing. If there is a rim fracture, weight bearing should be deferred until about 8 weeks post injury. In some centres, skin traction alone is used.

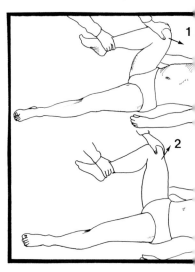

52. *Alternative methods of reduction: Bigelow's method:* Failure to reduce a posterior dislocation of the hip by the method described is uncommon and generally due to insufficient muscle relaxation: nevertheless, if failure occurs, Bigelow's method may be tried. In essence, the hip is reduced by a continuous movement of circumduction which may be broken down into 5 stages: (1) the hip is fully flexed and then (2) abducted.

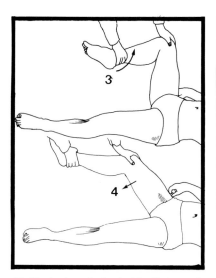

53. *Bigelow's method ctd.:* After flexing and abducting the hip, the joint is smoothly externally rotated (3) and then gradually extended (4).

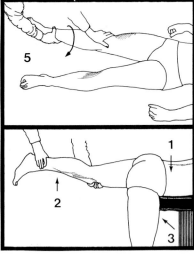

54. *Bigelow's method ctd.:* As extension of the hip progresses, the external rotated limb is turned into the neutral position (5). *Stimson's method:* This is occasionally attempted when a general anaesthetic must be withheld or where there is an associated femoral fracture. The patient is turned into the prone position (1). The end section of the theatre table is removed and the unaffected leg held by an assistant (2). The pelvis is supported by the end of the table (3).

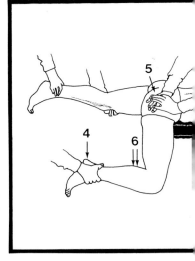

55. *Stimson's method ctd.:* The leg is flexed at the knee and held at the ankle in the neutral position (4). The hip may be reduced by direct pressure over the head of the femur (5) or if the femur is intact, by downward pressure on the upper calf (6). This may be done manually or by the stockinged foot: the latter procedure allows simultaneous application of pressure over the head of the femur as at (5).

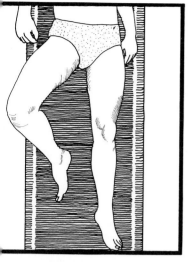

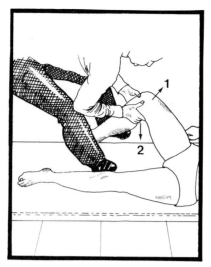

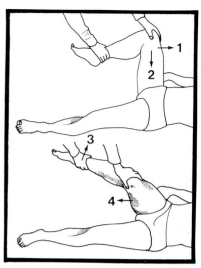

Anterior dislocation of the hip: Anterior ~~l~~ocation of the hip is less common than ~~pos~~terior dislocation. The leg is usually held ~~abd~~ucted and in external rotation. There ~~ma~~y be swelling and later bruising in the ~~gro~~in. Anterior dislocation may be ~~com~~plicated by femoral nerve paralysis or ~~fem~~oral artery compression. (Persistent ~~abs~~ence of the peripheral pulses after ~~red~~uction is an indication for exploration.)

57. *Reduction:* Proceed as for posterior dislocation, with the well anaesthetised patient on the floor, and an assistant steadying the pelvis. Flexing the hip (1) and correcting the abduction and external rotation (2) converts an anterior dislocation into a posterior dislocation. At the end of this procedure the head of the femur is lifted up as before into the acetabulum. (Subsequent management as 51.)

58. *Reduction: Bigelow's method:* This method is less reliable for routine use, but may be tried in the difficult case. Circumduction of the hip is again carried out in the following order of movements: (1) fully flex (2) adduct the hip (3) internally rotate (4) extend (5) bring into the neutral position.

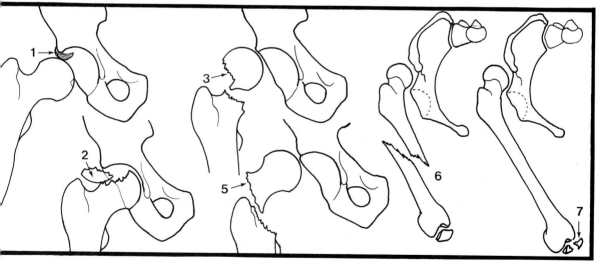

Complications of dislocation of the hip: *Irreducible dislocation:* This may result ~~fro~~m in-turning of the labrum or by bony ~~frag~~ments trapped in the acetabulum. Open ~~redu~~ction is necessary, *but be certain* that ~~the p~~atient has been *completely* relaxed ~~duri~~ng the attempts at closed reduction.

2. *Fracture of the femoral head:* Osteo-chondral fractures of the femoral head may remain displaced after reduction of the hip. Small fragments should be excised, but large fragments (ill.) should be replaced and secured with a cancellous screw or other device. Late osteo-arthritis is common.

3. *Intracapsular fracture of the femoral neck:* The risks of avascular necrosis are extremely high, and the following treatment should be considered: (i) In the elderly, excision of the femoral head, and replacement with a Thomson, Austin-Moore or similar prosthesis. (ii) In the middle aged,

total hip replacement. (iii) In the young, open reduction and internal fixation through a postero-lateral approach.

4. Slipped upper femoral epiphysis complicating hip dislocation: Treat as *3* (iii).

5. Extra-capsular fracture of the femoral neck: (a) The fracture should be dealt with first by open reduction and the insertion of a pin and plate or similar device. This can be taxing due to difficulty in interpreting control films in unfamiliar planes of rotation. (b) The dislocation may then be reduced, usually with ease, by closed manipulation.

6. Fracture of the femoral shaft: (a) It is sometimes possible to treat both injuries conservatively, reducing the hip dislocation by Stimson's method and treating the femoral fracture in a Thomas splint. (b) If Stimson's method fails, it may be possible to apply sufficient traction to the upper fragment by a substantial threaded screw inserted into the greater trochanter percutaneously. (c) It is more satisfactory to expose the femoral shaft and reduce the dislocation by means of a heavy duty bone clamp applied directly to the upper fragment (temporarily insert a large diameter Küntscher nail into the proximal fragment to prevent the bone being crushed with the clamp, and use the linear aspera for orientation). Thereafter the femoral shaft may be internally fixed (e.g. by intramedullary nailing).

7. Fracture of the patella and other knee injuries: The dislocation should be reduced by any of the methods described and the knee injury treated as if isolated (e.g. a comminuted fracture of the patella should be excised).

8. Sciatic nerve palsy: This complicates about 10% of dislocations of the hip.

Fortunately 3 out of 4 are incomplete, and about half recover completely.

If no improvement follows reduction of the hip, exploration is indicated within the first 24 hours of injury *only* if there is a large or comminuted rim fracture which may possibly be causing persistent local pressure on the nerve. Otherwise this complication should be managed conservatively: if the patient is being treated in a Thomas splint, this should be fitted with a foot piece to hold the ankle in the neutral position. When the patient is mobilised, a drop foot splint may be required, and precautions must be taken to avoid trophic ulceration in the foot.

9. Avascular necrosis: The inevitable tearing of the hip joint capsule accompanying dislocation of the hip may disturb the blood supply to the femoral head; in about 10% of cases this may lead to avascular necrosis. Radiographic changes are usually, but not always, seen within 12 months of injury. Clinically, persistent discomfort in the groin and restriction and pain on internal rotation are suggestive of this complication. Avascular necrosis of the head of the femur leads to secondary osteo-arthritis of the hip.

10. Secondary osteo-arthritis of the hip: This is the inevitable sequel to avascular necrosis, but may also occur when dislocation of the hip is accompanied by a fracture involving the articular surfaces. It is also seen as a late complication, sometimes as long as 5–10 years after injury: the cause then is less clear, but may possibly arise from articular cartilage damage concurrent with the initial injury. In the young patient hip fusion may be considered, but generally total hip replacement is the treatment of choice.

11. Recurrent dislocation: This

complication is rare; operative fixation of large acetabular rim fragment in the hip which is demonstrated to be unstable clinically may largely avoid it. Otherwise bone-block type of repair may have to be considered.

12. Myositis ossificans: This is seen mo frequently following exploration of the hip or when the dislocation is accompanied by head injury. It may lead to virtual fusion o the hip. The risk of this complication ensu may be minimised in the following ways: (a) Avoid surgery if possible. (b) Splint the hip following reduction. (c) Avoid passive movements of the hip in the head injury ca with limb spasticity. Late excision (say af one year) of a discrete bone mass may restore function, but the recurrence rate in other circumstances is high.

13. Late diagnosed dislocation: This is euphemism for missed dislocation. Alway suspect dislocation of the hip as a possible accompaniment of fracture of the patella femur. (a) If discovered within a week of injury manipulation may be attempted. (b) After a week and up to several months good results have been claimed by heavy to 18 kg) skeletal traction for up to 3 week under sedation. When radiographs show t femoral head level with or a little beyond acetabulum, the leg is placed in abduction and the traction decreased; this is generall successful in restoring the head to the acetabulum. If this fails, open reduction m be attempted; in either case pessimism regarding the eventual outcome is often unjustified, many cases achieving a good result without avascular necrosis ensuing. (c) After a year open reduction is unlikely be feasible and an upper femoral (Schanz) osteotomy may be considered.

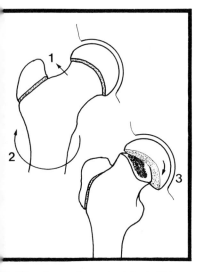

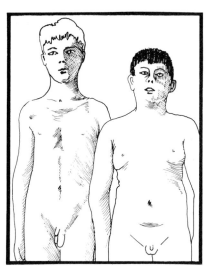

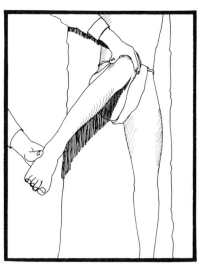

60. *Slipped upper femoral epiphysis:* This condition occurs in adolescence; the term is to some extent a misnomer as in fact it is the femoral shaft which moves proximally (1) and externally rotates (2) on the epiphysis. Only occasionally in advanced cases is there movement of the epiphysis relative to the acetabulum (3). There is never any juxta-epiphyseal fracture (i.e. it is a Salter-Harris Type I lesion).

61. *Aetiology:* Hormonal factors would seem to play an important part in the aetiology for (1) it is commoner in males, (2) it occurs at adolescence, (3) those affected are often adipose and sexually immature, showing features of the Frohlich syndrome, or are very tall and thin, suggesting increased production of growth hormone, (4) the condition is often bilateral, (5) a history of injury is present in less than 30%.

62. *Diagnosis* (1) The condition should be *suspected* in any adolescent with a history of limp and occasional groin or knee pain, especially if belonging to one of the body types described. On clinical examination the leg is usually held externally rotated at the hip, and movements of internal rotation are restricted.

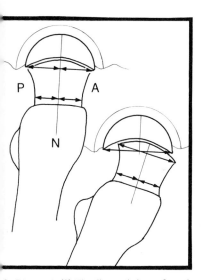

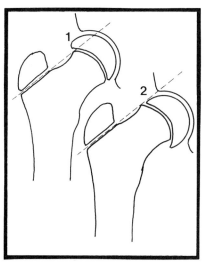

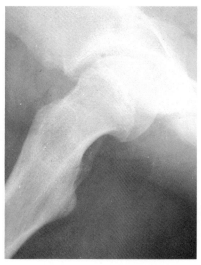

63. *Diagnosis* (2) The diagnosis is confirmed by radiographic examination; and a lateral projection is essential as the earliest signs are more obvious there than in the A.P. A line drawn up the centre of the neck should normally bisect the epiphyseal base of the head; if it fails to do so, slip is present, and the percentage slip should be noted. (Ill. 15–20% slip.)

64. *Diagnosis* (3) In the A.P. view slip is less obvious, but nevertheless may be detected with experience. Radiographs of both hips should be taken to allow comparison and detect early silent slip on the other side. In the normal hip (1) a tangent to the neck should cut through a portion of the epiphysis. When slip is present (2) this is no longer the case.

65. *Diagnosis* (4) Look for radiographic evidence of new bone formation (buttressing) at the inferior and posterior aspects of the neck, i.e. look for evidence of chronicity.

The history, clinical findings and radiographs should allow the case to be diagnosed as (1) an acute slip (2) an acute slip superimposed on a degree of long-standing slip (3) a chronic slip.

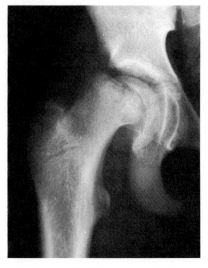

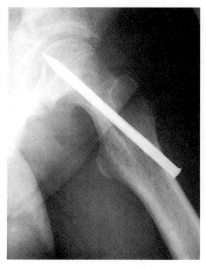

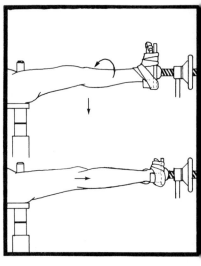

66. *Diagnosis* (5) (1) In an acute slip, the history is short (less than 3 weeks) and the radiographs show slipping without buttressing (ill.). (2) Where an acute slip is superimposed on a degree of chronic slip, there is often a history of intermittent limp and discomfort for several weeks, with recent, sudden deterioration: any buttressing is slight. (3) With a chronic slip, the history is of many weeks duration, and buttressing is a feature.

67. *Treatment* (1) In all cases further slipping should be prevented, and in the first two groups this is done by pinning (which is often followed by rapid epiphyseal closure). As the epiphysis in the child is very dense. Smith-Petersen or similar nails are unsuitable; instead a Nystrum nail (ill.), two or more Moore pins, or a Garden or Howse screw may be used.

68. *Treatment* (2) *Reduction?* (1) If the slip is less than 30% (e.g. as in 67) *the position should be accepted and pinned without manipulation.* (2) If there is an acute slip, or an acute-on-chronic greater than 30%, *gentle* manipulation may be attempted under general anaesthesia by applying *light* traction in the mid abduction/adduction range and turning the leg into internal rotation: thereafter, if the slip is reduced to 30% or less, pin in that position.

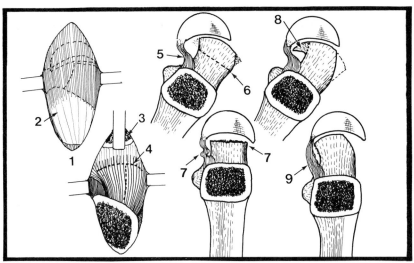

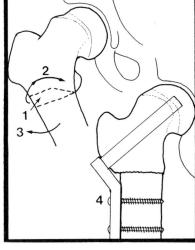

69. *Treatment* (3) *Reduction?* (3) If under the previous circumstances gentle manipulation fails to reduce an acute slip, or an acute-on-chronic slip, to less than 30%, operative reduction should be undertaken: a lateral approach is used (1). The greater trochanter (2) with its abductor insertion is detached and turned upwards (3). The capsule is opened through a T-shaped incision (4) and the vascular bundle to the head (5) teased from the superior and posterior aspects of the neck. The femoral neck is shortened (6) to allow reduction without tension on the bundle (7). Alternatively, it may be possible by excising any buttress (8) to obtain reduction without tension (9). The hip is then pinned and the trochanter re-attached with a screw. (Thereafter, skin traction for 4 weeks and non-weight bearing with crutches till union (3–6 months).)

70. *Treatment* (4) Where there is chronic slipping, manipulation should not be attempted, and slips of under 30% pinned *in situ* (neck re-modelling may make assessment difficult). Where the epiphysis has closed with considerable deformity, functional improvement may be obtained by sub-trochanteric osteotomy, with the base of the wedge to be removed placed anteriorly and laterally (1); this allows correction of rotation (2) adduction (3) and extension. The osteotomy may be fixed with a plate (4) or spica till united.

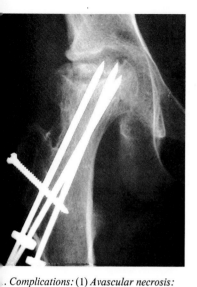

established case is difficult: a choice may have to be made between (i) the uncertain results of osteotomy (ii) the difficulty of hip arthrodesis and the risks of late secondary osteo-arthritis in the knee, other hip, and spine (iii) the risks and long-term uncertainties of total hip replacement.

(2) *Involvement of other hip:* In keeping with the aetiology, the other hip may be affected at any time. This is particularly liable to be missed when the patient is being rested in bed during treatment of the primary complaint. Routine radiography of both hips is advised, particularly in the recumbent patient. If the second hip is involved, treatment is pursued along the lines already described.

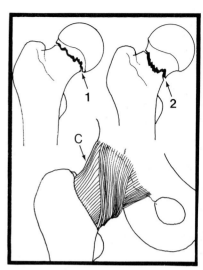

. Complications: (1) *Avascular necrosis:* l.) This is a serious complication in the olescent, and every attempt must be made avoid it by (a) prompt diagnosis rejection of any attempt to reduce the formity by forcible manipulation meticulous handling of the epiphysis and vascular supply during any operative ervention (d) avoidance of unsuitable ernal fixation devices. Treatment of the

72. *Fractures of the femoral neck: Level of fracture* (1) Four sites of fracture are well recognised, the most important being: (1) sub-capital and (2) trans-cervical. The distinction between these two is rather blurred, as rotation in the plane of the X-rays may be misleading. Both, however, lie clearly within the joint capsule (C) and are well described as *intracapsular fractures.*

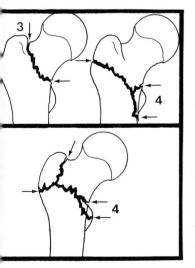

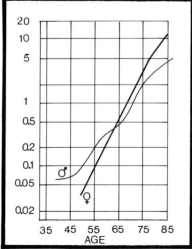

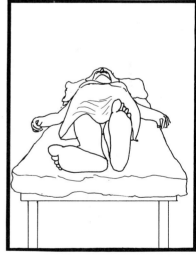

, Level of fracture (2) The other common es of fracture are *extracapsular.* (3) In the er-trochanteric or basal fracture the cture line runs along the base of the noral neck between the *trochanters.* (4) In *trochanteric fractures* the fracture line olves the trochanters, one or both of ich may be fractured or separated, so that effect this is often a comminuted fracture.

74. *Incidence:* The Y-axis of the graph represents the yearly incidence per 1000 population and shows that below the age of 60 the fracture occurs most frequently in men, generally from industrial trauma. The incidence increases with age and in later life is three times commoner in women, where hormonal dependent osteoporosis and a degree of osteomalacia are contributory factors. The fracture is seen from time to time in children.

75. *Diagnosis* (1) Inability to weight bear after a fall, particularly in an elderly patient, with or without pain in the hip, is most likely to be due to this common fracture which must be excluded in every case by radiographic examination: fractures of the pubic rami or distal limb fractures are less common causes of this primary complaint. External rotation of the limb, sometimes with a little shortening, is a valuable (but not invariable) sign.

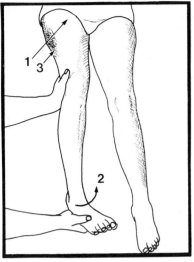

76. *Diagnosis* (2) *Tenderness* will be found over the femoral neck anteriorly (1) and in extracapsular fractures over the greater trochanter. *Pain* is produced by rotation of the hip (2). *Bruising* (3) is a *late* sign in extracapsular fractures only, and is absent in acute injuries. Rarely, with an undisplaced fracture, the patient may be able to weight-bear.

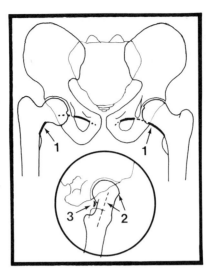

77. *Diagnosis* (3) An A.P. radiograph of the pelvis with a lateral of the affected hip are best for screening of this area. Generally the fracture line is obvious, but if not, look for asymmetry in Shenton's lines (1) and in the lateral, angulation of the head with respect to the neck (2) or fragmentation (3). If there is any remaining doubt, a localised A.P. view should be taken: if this appears negative, repeat the films after 1–2 weeks.

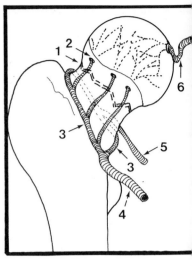

78. *Intracapsular fractures:* These are prone to complications for two clear reasons: (a) the blood supply to the femoral head may be disturbed by intracapsular fractures (1), leading to *avascular necrosis*. The main supply penetrates the head close to the cartilage margin (2) and arises from an arterial ring (3) fed from the lateral and medial femoral circumflex arteries (4 and 5). A small portion of the head is inconstantly supplied via the ligamentum teres (6).

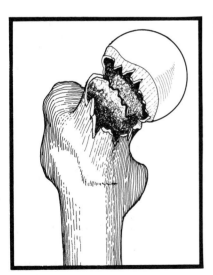

79. *Complications (ctd.)* (b) The head fragment is often a shell containing fragile cancellous bone, and affords poor anchorage for any fixation device. Inadequate fixation may lead to *non-union*. Note that any connection between non-union and avascularity is tenuous—the head is often viable in non-union, and avascular necrosis is seen most frequently in united fractures.

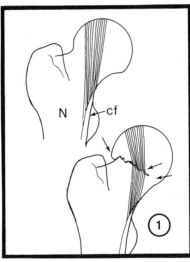

80. *Complications ctd.* It follows that complications are most frequent in proximally situated and displaced fractures. Any displacement should be assessed along the lines laid down by Garden which amongst other things take into account disturbance of the weight-carrying trabeculae radiating from the calcar femorale. *In Garden Type 1 fractures*, the inferior cortex is not completely broken, but the trabeculae are angulated (abduction fracture).

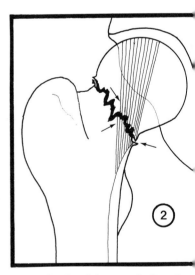

81. *Garden Type 2 fractures:* In Type 2 injuries the fracture line is complete; the inferior cortex is clearly broken. The trabecular lines are interrupted but are not angulated. In both Type 1 and Type 2 fractures there is no obvious displacement of the fragments relative to one another.

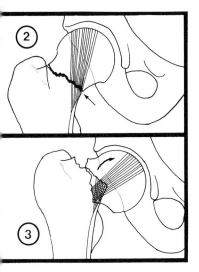

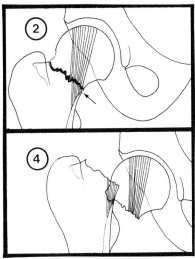

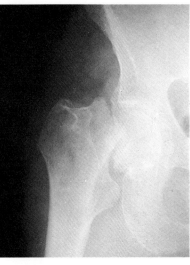

2. *Garden Type 3 fractures:* Here the fracture line is obviously complete. There is rotation of the femoral head in the acetabulum: i.e. the proximal fragment is abducted and internally rotated. This may be apparent from the disturbance in the trabecular pattern. The fracture is *slightly displaced.* (Garden Type 2 injury included for comparison.)

83. *Garden Type 4 fracture:* The fracture here is fully displaced, and the femoral head tends to lie in the neutral position in the acetabulum. (Type 2 injury included for comparison.)
   Garden Type 3 and 4 fractures of the femoral neck carry the worst prognosis.

84. *Garden classification ctd.:* The radiograph shows a typical sub-capital Garden Type 4 fracture. The femoral head is lying in the acetabulum in the neutral position.

Treatment (1) *General principles:* Surgical treatment, generally by internal fixation of the fracture, is the aim in all cases so that the patient may be mobilised as quickly as possible. In the elderly in particular it is important to try to avoid the dangers of prolonged bed rest (e.g. recumbency pneumonia, bed sores, urinary tract infections, muscle wasting, etc.). In addition, unless the fracture is internally fixed, the risks of non-union are extremely high (the so-called impacted fractures frequently displace even whilst on traction).
   (2) *Investigations:* A few days' delay prior to fixation of the fracture seems to have only marginal effect on the prognosis, and this interval may be employed profitably to bring the patient into the optimal medical state. The following investigations may prove invaluable in assessment and are performed routinely in many centres. (i) Chest radiograph, and if there is a productive cough, a sputum film and culture. (ii) Electrocardiograph. (iii) Full blood count, with at some stage grouping and cross matching of blood for surgery. (iv) Estimation of the serum urea and electrolytes. (v) Routine charting of fluid input and output.
   (3) *General treatment:* (i) *Preliminary skin traction* (3–4 kg) may help to relieve initial pain and minimise further displacement of the fracture. (ii) *Analgesics, tranquilisers and hypnotics* appropriate to the patient's pain, age and mental state should be prescribed. (iii) In many units, *intra-venous fluids* are given routinely (with caution where there are concurrent respiratory and cardio-vascular problems) to combat dehydration and minimise the risks of anaemia. (A raised serum urea is clearly associated with a poor prognosis in femoral neck fractures.) Whole blood or packed cells may be required if the patient is markedly anaemic. The type and quantity of replacement is determined by the urinary output, the urea, electrolyte and haemoglobin levels, and the respiratory and cardiac state. Oral fluids are encouraged. (iv) *The physiotherapist* may give valuable assistance in the management of the moist chest. (v) *Nursing* of the highest standard is required if in particular pressure sores are to be avoided, particularly in the heavy patient who is afraid to move because of pain. (vi) *Antibiotics* may be prescribed where there is a heavy purulent spit or frank urinary tract infection; although treatment may be started immediately, bacteriological confirmation must be sought.

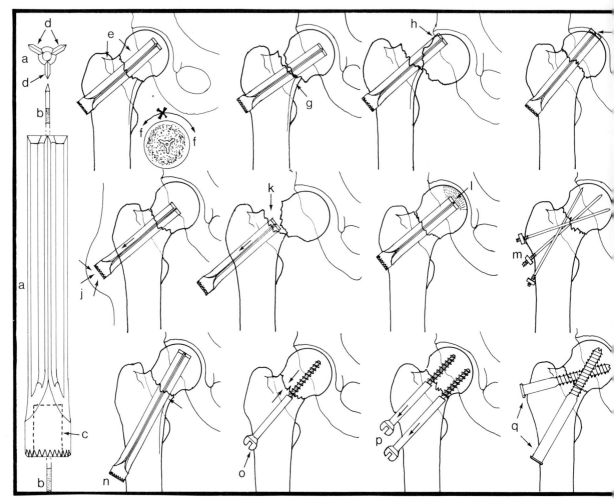

85. *Surgical treatment* (1) Intracapsular fractures may be treated by (i) reduction and internal fixation (ii) primary replacement of the femoral head (iii) total hip replacement. Internal fixation is generally used for all grades of fracture in the young patient, and fractures of grades 1 and 2 at least in the elderly patient. The aim of the internal fixation device is to hold the bone fragments and resist deforming forces in all planes till union occurs. The commonest device is the tri-fin nail or pin (introduced by Smith-Petersen and subsequently extensively modified). In the McLaughlin pattern illustrated (a) the nail is cannulated to let it slide along a guide wire (b), and tapped (c) to take an introducer or hold a plate. The fins (d) are designed to grip both bone fragments (e) and resist axial rotation (f). Although generally reliable, several problems may occur. It may drift in the distal fragment (till it strikes the calcar) with some loss of position (g). It may cut out of the soft bone of the head (h) or penetrate the head following absorption of bone at the fracture site (i). Delay in union may contribute to extrusion (the Escalado effect), with local discomfort (j) or the fracture coming adrift (k). In some cases the volume of bone occupied by the nail may contribute to avascular necrosis (1). To minimise this some surgeons employ Moore pins (m). To combat neck drift (g) a 'long-low nail' may be inserted (i.e. it rests on the calcar from the start) (n). A degree of compression of the fragments may be achieved with a coarse-thread screw (e.g. Howse) (o) but this will not resist axial rotation. Twin screws will overcome this problem, and if laid parallel will accommodate absorption of bone without penetration of the head (p). Garden advocates twin screws placed in the direction of stress forces to resist movement in all planes and obtain an optimal hold on the head fragment (q).

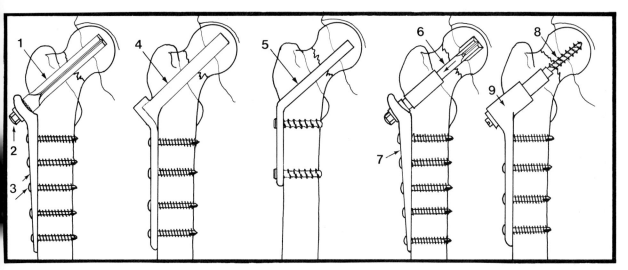

86. *Internal fixation devices ctd.:* To prevent
extrusion of the nail it may be joined to a
plate. This also improves the stability of the
nail in the distal fragment. The McLaughlin
nail plate makes allowance for an infinite
variety of nail plate angles. After insertion of
the nail (1), the plate is attached to it with a
bolt (2); the plate is fixed to the shaft with
self tapping screws (3).

Single piece devices prevent the rare
instance of the components coming adrift.
The pin portion of the fixed angle Honey-
Barnes device (4) is V-shaped. The A.O.
blade-plate (5) is available in a range of
angles, and is channel section. None of these
devices prevent head penetration which the
sliding nail may, by allowing one part to
telescope on a key-way within the other (6).

This may be used on its own, or stabilised
distally with a plate (7). In the Charnley
compression nail, the auger screw in the
head (8) is designed to compress the bone
fragments together by means of a spring in
the box portion (9). All the above devices
necessitate a larger incision and some
increase in operating time than does the
insertion of a simple tri-fin nail.

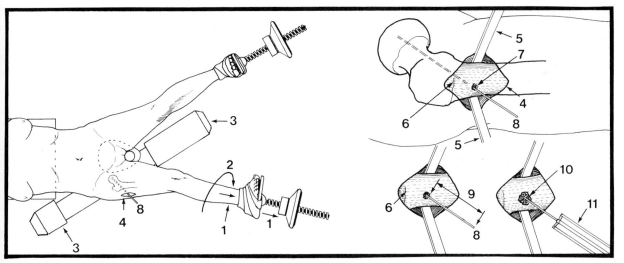

87. *Surgical treatment* (2) Internal fixation
is carried out on an orthopaedic table; if
displaced, the fracture is reduced by
applying traction (1) and internal
rotation (2). The reduction is confirmed in
two planes by radiographs or an image
intensifier (3). (Failure to achieve reduction
may be regarded as an indication for a
replacement procedure.) The operation is
performed blind—i.e.the fracture is not

exposed. A lateral incision (4) is deepened to
bone, and the vastus lateralis reflected and
held with bone spikes (5). The trochanteric
ridge (6) is identified, and a small opening
made in the outer cortex (7) about 3 cm
distal to it. A guide wire (8) is passed
through the opening into the head and the
position checked in two planes. The guide
wire is adjusted until it is in satisfactory
position (ideally lying towards the posterior

and inferior parts of the neck and the centre
of the head). The required length of nail is
calculated by subtracting the length of the
protruding part of the guide wire from its
total length (9). The cortical opening is
widened to take the haft of the nail (10)
which is threaded along the guide wire (11)
and hammered home. The position is
checked. Slight modifications may be
required for other devices.

88. *After care:* One of the aims of internal fixation is rapid mobilisation, and in most cases the patient can be allowed out of bed to sit the day following surgery. Early (i.e. within the first week) weight bearing does not seem to affect the union of intra-capsular fractures in a material way, and should therefore be encouraged as soon as the patient's general condition will permit. After the wound has healed, the patient may often be allowed home, depending on her mobility and social circumstances. An Occupational Therapy Domestic Assessment is often invaluable in making a decision in this respect.

Out-patient attendances, with check radiographs every 4–6 weeks should be arranged until the patient is independent; thereafter, she should be seen at intervals of 6 months to 1 year for a total of 3 years to allow detection of late-onset avascular necrosis.

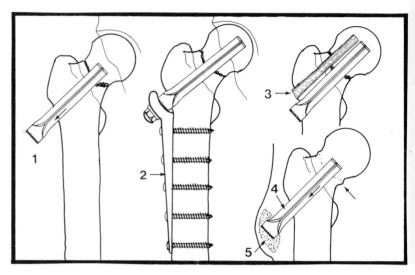

89. *Complications:* (1) *Nail extrusion:* Extrusion of the fixing nail (1) is often the result of persisting mobility at the fracture site and may indicate impending non-union. If it is detected within the first few weeks, the nail should be replaced and something done to prevent recurrence—e.g. the attachment of a plate (2). If extrusion is first noted 5–6 weeks or more after fixation, the chances of non-union are even greater. In these circumstances some surgeons, after re-insertion of the device, would carry out bone grafting (using a trimmed section of the fibula) (3). The addition of a plate would also be desirable. (See also non-union.) Late extrusion after union (4) may cause local discomfort with an overlying bursitis (5) and is easily dealt with by removal of the device (often possible under local anaesthesia).

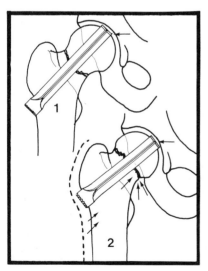

90. (2) *Penetration of the head by the nail:* This may result from a failure of technique (1) or by absorption of bone at the fracture site leading to shortening of the femoral neck (2). In many cases pain is not a problem, and the nail should be left *in situ* until union is sound; it may then be removed to reduce further damage to the acetabulum and the risks of secondary osteo-arthritis.

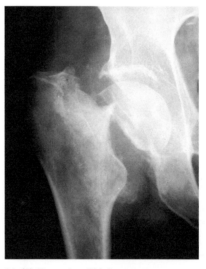

91. (3) *Non-union:* This is seen most frequently in Grade 3 and 4 fractures: this is especially the case if the fracture has not been treated (ill.) or where mechanical fixation has failed. Extrusion or cutting out of the nail, sclerosis or rounding of the bone ends, cystic changes in the neck, or re-displacement of the fracture may be apparent. Prosthetic replacement of the femoral head or total hip replacement are the treatments of choice.

92. (4) *Avascular necrosis:* In most cases, the cause is disruption of the blood supply by the fracture, and the fate of the femoral head is sealed at the time of injury. It seems possible that on occasion a bulky internal fixation device may further disrupt a tenuous blood supply leading to bone necrosis. It is commonest in Grade 3 and 4 fractures.

The patient complains of increasing pain and limp, and of a progressive decrease in functional activity. In some cases there may be a period of many months' freedom from pain after the initial treatment has been carried out, and before the presence of avascular necrosis declares itself. Radiological changes are usually present within the first year, but on occasion may not show for as long as 3 years.

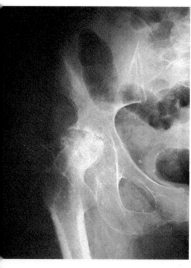
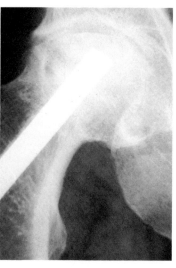

94. *Alternative primary treatment of intracapsular fractures* (1) Where the risks of the patient developing avascular necrosis or non-union are thought to be particularly serious and where it is particularly desirable to avoid surgery, alternative primary treatment must be considered. Adverse factors include the following—(1) A proximally situated fracture line (2) A Grade 3 or 4 fracture (3) A frail and/or elderly patient (say over the age of 75) who is unlikely to survive repeated surgery (4) Marked osteoporosis, or rheumatoid arthritis, where the quality of bony fixation is likely to be poor. (5) Imperfect reduction of the fracture. The two main treatment alternatives are (1) excision of the femoral head and replacement with a Thompson, Austin-Moore or equivalent prosthesis (2) total hip replacement.

. *Radiological changes:* The whole femoral head may be clearly involved, with an increase density; narrowing of the joint space, loss of sphericity of the head, and secondary arthritic ping of the acetabulum may be seen. (See illustration on the left: note that the fixation vice has been removed.)
In many cases avascular necrosis may declare itself in the main weight-bearing portion of e femoral head. ('Superior segmental necrosis'.) In that particular situation it is often fficult to be certain of increased density due to the overlapping acetabular shadow, but the aracteristic double break in the contour of the head should always be sought (see right). ote that in most cases the fracture is united. *Treatment:* Mild symptoms may be controlled th analgesics, but in more severe cases, total hip replacement should be considered.

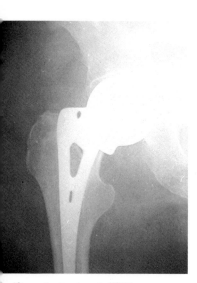
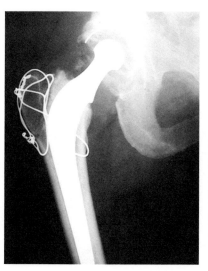
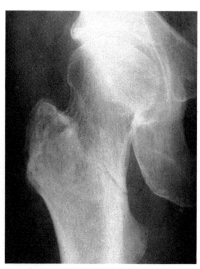

. *Alternative treatments* (2) The ompson prosthesis is cemented in position d is less subject to loosening than the ncemented) Austin-Moore replacement .). The initial morbidity from both these ocedures is appreciable, and is highest en a posterior rather than an anterior proach is used. There is also a later dency to slow erosion of the acetabulum. ey are best reserved for the patient who is t likely to have a long or very active life bsequently.

96. *Alternative treatments* (3) A successful . total hip replacement procedure affords the patient the greatest chance of returning to her pre-fracture state. The most important consideration is the patient's fitness for this more major procedure; it is fully justified in the adverse conditions described if the patient is in good health, physically and mentally active, and the unit's mortality and morbidity figures are low.

97. *Intertrochanteric fractures:* Fractures of this type occurring at the base of the neck have the following points in their favour (a) They are extracapsular, and in the adult are not associated with avascular necrosis. (b) Because of the size of the neck and head fragments, good internal fixation can usually be achieved; non-union is extremely rare, and early weight-bearing after internal fixation is usually possible.

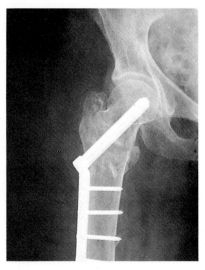

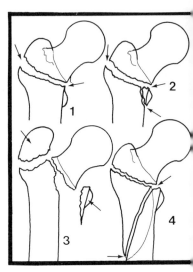

99. *After care:* (a) The patient can usually be allowed to sit out of bed by the second day. (b) Stitches are removed about the 10th day. (c) If, as is usual, good fixation of the fracture has been obtained, the patient can be gradually mobilised during the first week. Full weight bearing is often achieved within the first 3 weeks. (d) The patient is discharged home as soon as a satisfactory level of independence has been regained. (e) Thereafter the patient attends as an out-patient at intervals of 4–6 weeks. (f) As soon as check radiographs show sound union of the fracture, the patient may be discharged from further attendance (again assuming a good functional result). The fixation device is not removed unless the patient is young (e.g. under the age of 45) or the device is giving rise to symptoms.

98. *Operative treatment:* The patient is placed on the orthopaedic table, and if the fracture is displaced, traction in the neutral position will generally achieve reduction. The fracture is exposed through a lateral incision and secured either with a single piece nail-plate (or blade-plate) device; or with a two piece nail-plate (e.g. McLaughlin nail-plate).

100. *Per-trochanteric fractures:* These lie distal to the intertrochanteric line, and several patterns are common. The fracture line may pass through the mass of the greater trochanter and run to the lesser trochanter either with (2) or without (1) its separation. The fracture is often highly comminuted, with separation of the greater and usually the lesser trochanter (3). The fracture may be continuous with a spiral fracture involving the proximal femoral shaft (4).

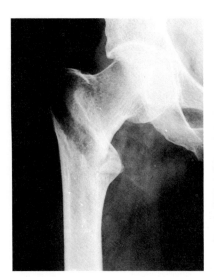

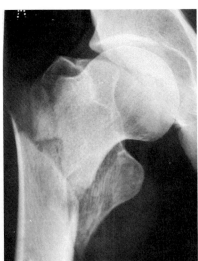

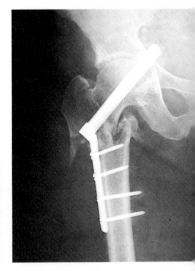

101. *Treatment* (1) Where comminution is absent or slight (Type 1 and Type 2 fractures) stability is not a problem, and nail-plate fixation is adequate. If the fracture requires preliminary reduction, analysis of the radiographs will indicate whether the limb should be internally rotated, externally rotated, or placed in the neutral position.

102. *Treatment* (2) In the unstable Type 3 fracture, it is difficult to achieve strong, reliable fixation. The stresses on any fixation device are high, and mechanical failure is common. The use of a long plate (7 or more holes instead of 5) will give additional security to the distal part, and may give adequate fixation of many Type 4 fractures.

103. *Treatment* (3) Although distal fixation may be good, there is always a tendency for the femoral shaft to drift medially, (or into coxa vara) often with penetration of the femoral head. A sliding nail (or sliding screw) may prevent this. Many surgeons prefer to fix these fractures in the more stable position with the femoral shaft already medially displaced (as in a MacMurray osteotomy).

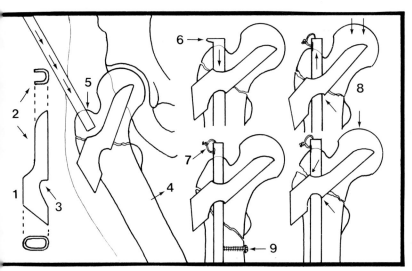

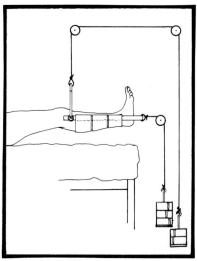

104. *Alternative treatments* (1) All intertrochanteric and many per-trochanteric fractures may be treated with Küntscher Y-nailing. The neck component (1) is manufactured from stainless steel tube cut away at one end to an open U-section (2) and drilled inferiorly. (3) It is inserted under X-ray control; the leg is adducted (4) and with the aid of a jig to ensure alignment, a 10.5 mm Küntscher nail is passed from the greater trochanter downwards (5). Distal migration of the nail must be prevented (e.g. by the use of a flanged nail (6) or a loop of wire passed through the extraction slot (7)). Proximal migration is discouraged by early weight bearing which locks the components together (8). Sometimes rotational deformity may arise if the Küntscher nail is a loose fit distally, although this may be controlled by using short screws keyed into the nail furrow (9).

105. *Alternative treatments* (2) As union is seldom a problem in intertrochanteric and per-trochanteric fractures, they can be successfully treated by bed rest and traction. A Thomas splint may be used if desired for additional support. This form of treatment may be adopted if, for example, the patient is unfit for anaesthesia, or there are problems with other injuries; the risks must outweigh the advantages of early mobilisation.

106. *After care in per-trochanteric fractures:* In stable Type 1 and Type 2 fractures with good quality internal fixation, the patient may be mobilised early with weight bearing at any stage. In the less stable Type 2 and Type 4 fractures, early weight bearing may often be permitted if K-Y nailing is used. In unstable Type 3 fractures, weight bearing should be deferred until callous appears and is seen to be reinforcing the fixation device (i.e. usually after 6 weeks).
Complications: The commonest complication is failure of fixation with drift into coxa vara (usually secondary to cutting out of the fixation device). If this occurs before much callous has appeared, it can usually be corrected by returning the patient to bed and applying skeletal traction (as 105) of 5–7 kg. This is maintained till union is established. If coxa vara is discovered late, the position has usually to be accepted.

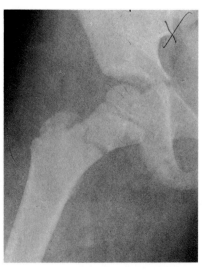

107. *Fractures of the femoral neck in children:* These uncommon injuries result from severe violence, and have been classified by Delbet into 4 Types: Type I: Sub-capital (or trans-epiphyseal): these are fracture dislocations with the capital epiphysis being extruded from the joint.

Avascular necrosis is virtually inevitable. Type II: Trans-cervical: the commonest injury. If undisplaced (ill.) avascular necrosis is uncommon, but if displaced, is very high (60%). In Type III, cervico-trochanteric (basal) and Type IV, per-trochanteric fractures, the incidence of avascular necrosis is lower, but is also related to displacement. Coxa vara and non-union are two further complications of these serious injuries.
Treatment: (1) *All undisplaced fractures* should be treated with a hip spica maintained till union. Complications are low in this group. In displaced fractures, (2) if the child is under 10, manipulative reduction should be tried, and if successful, the fracture secured with Knowles pins. Capsulotomy is sometimes advocated to reduce the incidence of avascular necrosis. (3) Open reduction is undertaken in Type I injuries. In the others, if reduction fails or if the child is over 10, primary sub-trochanteric osteotomy with plaster fixation is advised to reduce the incidence of non-union and coxa vara. (4) Osteotomy may also be advised for non-union. The extent of avascular necrosis is variable and should be treated expectantly. Sometimes hip fusion may be required.

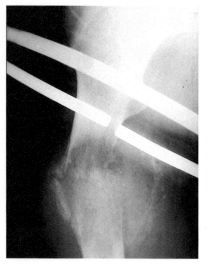

108. *Sub-trochanteric fractures:* Fractures at this level are often pathological (e.g. from metastases). If the patient's general condition is very poor, pain relief may be obtained by traction in a Thomas splint (ill.). In all other cases, internal fixation is advocated by, for example, a McLaughlin nail and 7 or 10 hole plate, or preferably, a Kuntscher nail or Y-nail. Where there is a large osteolytic defect, acrylic cement packed into it will give additional support to a nail and permit immediate mobilisation.

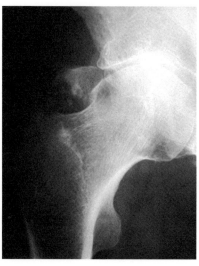

109. *Trochanteric fractures:* Isolated fractures of the greater (ill.) or lesser trochanters may result from sudden muscle contraction (avulsion of gluteus medius, or ilio-psoas insertions). Fractures of the greater trochanter may also result from direct violence. Symptomatic treatment only is required, and the patient may be mobilised after a few days' bed rest.

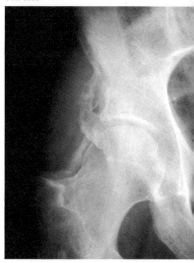

110. Following a head injury and a dislocation of the hip which was reduced by manipulation, this patient complained of persistent pain and stiffness in the hip. What is the cause of this?

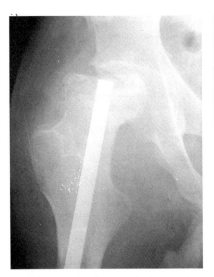

111. Nine months after internal fixation of a femoral neck fracture this patient complained of pain in the hip.
(a) What is the source of his complaint?
(b) What level was the fracture?
(c) Has it united?
(d) What type of internal fixation has been employed?
(e) What deformity of the femoral neck existed before the injury?

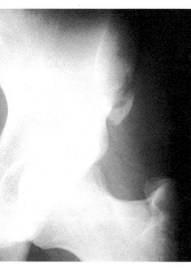

112. This radiograph is of a young man who was complaining of severe pain in the hip and difficulty in weight bearing after a sudden sprint while playing football. What abnormality is present?

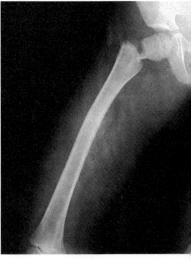

113. This radiograph is of a child who complained of pain in the hip and inability to weight bear after a fall from a tree. What injury is present, and what complications might ensue from this?

10. Myositis ossificans.

11. (a) Avascular necrosis with bone collapse.
    (b) Sub-capital.
    (c) Yes.
    (d) Low angle ('long-low') tri-fin nailing.
    (e) Coxa valga (secondary to poliomyelitis).

112. Avulsion fracture of the anterior inferior iliac spine (rectus femoris).

113. Type III (cervico-trochanteric or basal) fracture of the femoral neck with displacement. Possible complications include avascular necrosis, delayed or non-union, and coxa vara.

12. Fractures of the femur and injuries about the knee

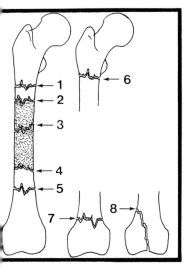

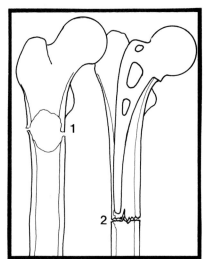

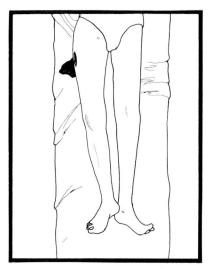

Classification: Fractures of the femoral shaft may involve the upper or proximal third (1), the junction of the proximal and middle thirds (2), the middle third (shaded) (3), the junction of the middle and distal thirds (4), or the distal third (5). In the proximal third, sub-trochanteric fractures (6) are often classified with femoral neck fractures. In the distal third, supracondylar (7) and intercondylar (8) fractures are of importance.

2. *Causes of fracture:* Considerable violence is usually required to fracture the femur, and the common causes include road traffic accidents, falls from a height, and crushing injuries. Pathological fractures may also occur: the commonest cause is senile osteoporosis but metastatic deposits, especially in the sub-trochanteric region are frequently seen (1). Stress concentrations and bone erosions at the stem ends of prostheses may also be responsible (2).

3. *Fluid loss:* In a simple fracture, loss of $\frac{1}{2}$–1 litre of blood into the tissues with accompanying shock is common. Compounding from within-out occurs classically in the upper third. Blood replacement is often required in simple fractures, and normally essential in compound injuries; grouping, cross-matching, and setting up of an intravenous line should be done routinely (except in children). In the transport of patients to hospital, temporary splintage will help reduce local bleeding and shock.

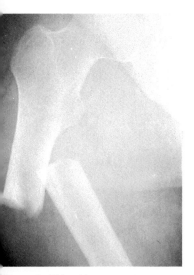

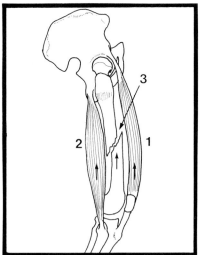

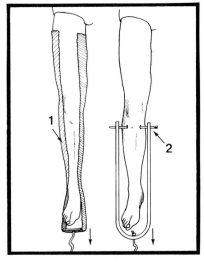

Diagnosis: This seldom presents any difficulty: weight bearing is impossible and there is abnormal mobility in the limb at the level of the fracture. The leg is often externally rotated, abducted at the hip, and shortened. Radiographs confirm the diagnosis. It is most important to exclude fracture of the patella, dislocation of the hip, and fracture of the pelvis of the central dislocation type.

5. *Conservative treatment:* Femoral shaft fractures are frequently treated conservatively, and the first principle to appreciate is that the large muscle masses of the quadriceps (1) and hamstrings (2) tend to produce displacement and shortening (3). Traction can overcome this, and is the basis of most conservative methods of treatment.

6. *Traction methods:* There are two methods of applying traction:
(1) *Skin traction, using adhesive strapping:* This is used in children and young adults. There are occasional problems with skin sensitivity and pustular infections under the strapping.
(2) *Skeletal traction*, using a Steinman pin through the tibial tuberosity. This is preferred in the older patient with inelastic skin and where heavy traction is required. There are occasional problems with pin track infections.

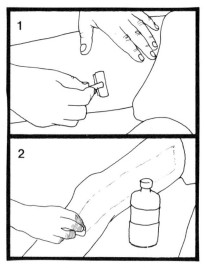

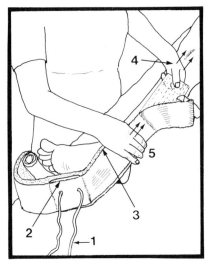

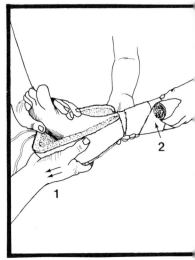

7. *Applying skin traction* (1) With the exercise of care and gentleness this can usually be done without an anaesthetic. (1) Begin by shaving the skin. (2) It is then traditional to swab or spray the skin with a mildly antiseptic solution of Balsam of Peru in alcohol. This may facilitate the adhesion of the strapping.

8. *Applying skin traction* (2) Commercial traction sets use adhesive tapes which can stretch from side to side but not longitudinally. They come supplied with traction cords (1) and a spreader bar (2) with foam protection for the malleoli (3). Begin by applying the tape to the medial side of leg—do this by peeling off the protective backing with one hand (4) while pressing the tape down and advancing the other (5).

9. *Applying skin traction* (3) The leg is internally rotated and the tape applied to the outside of the leg, preferably a little more posterior than on the medial side. The tape should extend up the leg as far as possible, irrespective of the site of the fracture. Now apply traction to the leg (1) and finally secure the tapes throughout their length with encircling crepe bandages (2).

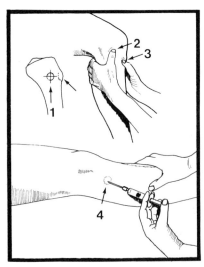

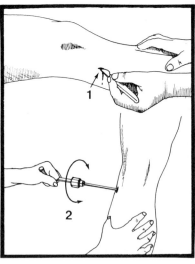

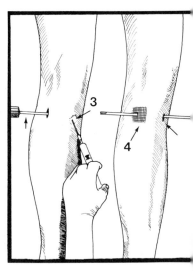

10. *Applying skeletal traction* (1) The preferred site is the upper tibia a little under 1″ (2 cm) posterior to the prominence of the tibial tuberosity (1). It is important to avoid the knee joint: so begin by carefully identifying it by flexing the knee (2), noting its relationship to the tuberosity (3). If a general anaesthetic is not employed, infiltrate the skin and tissue down to periosteum with local anaesthetic (e.g. 2–3 cc of 1% lignocaine) (4).

11. *Skeletal traction* (2) Now make a small incision in the skin (1) enough to take the traction pin only: insert it until the point strikes bone. Drive the pin through the lateral tibial cortex by applying firm pressure and twisting the chuck handle (2). You should feel it penetrate the outer cortex and pass quickly with little resistance till it meets the medial cortex. Stop at this stage.

12. *Skeletal traction* (3) Infiltrate the skin down to periosteum on the medial side, using the lie of the pin to guide you to the expected exit area (3). Drive the pin through the medial cortex, and make a small incision over the tenting skin to allow it to come through. Protect the openings with gauze strips soaked in Nobecutane or a similar sealant (4). Try to insert the pin at right angles to the leg.

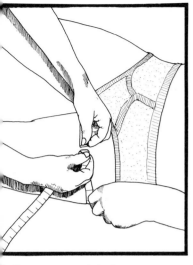

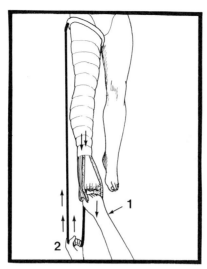

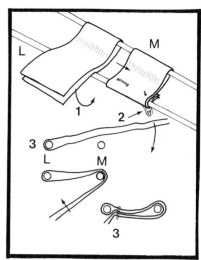

13. *Traction systems* (A) *Skin traction in a Thomas splint* (1) The most important decision in selecting a Thomas splint is the ring size. To save time (e.g. before anaesthesia) the uninjured leg may be measured, and an allowance made for swelling, present and anticipated. It is nevertheless wise to have readily available a size above and below the estimate in case of inaccuracies.

14. *Thomas splint* (2) Applying traction with one hand on the spreader bar (1) the selected splint is pushed up the leg (2). It should reach the ischial tuberosity (or more likely the perineum) and it should be possible to pass one finger beneath the ring round its complete circumference. If the ring is too large or too small, maintain traction while the next size is tried.

15. *Thomas splint* (3) The choice of soft furnishings and their method of application is often made with a fanaticism that may amaze the uncommitted. Slings to bridge the side irons may be formed from strips of 6″ (15 cm) wide calcio bandage (1). It is traditional to secure these with large safety pins inserted from below, close to the outer iron (2). Sometimes spring clips are used. A double bandage thickness ensures greater rigidity (3).

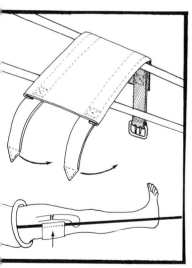

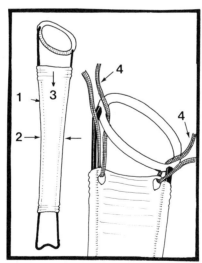

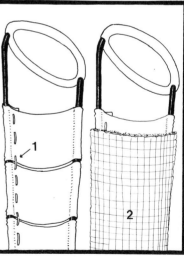

16. *Thomas splint* (4) The sling placed directly beneath the fracture should preferably be unyielding, and one of canvas with web and buckle fastenings is often favoured in this situation. It is customary to apply the splint with the master sling in position; the other slings are then attached and adjusted to the contours of the limb. Less satisfactorily perhaps the splint is applied with all the slings already in position.

17. *Thomas splint* (5) Calico and canvas slings can drift, separate, or ruck, and many prefer the smoothness of an unbroken circular bandage, stretched in double thickness over the splint (e.g. Tubigrip) (1). This has the disadvantage of 'waisting' the splint (2) being less than firm under the fracture, and tending to drift distally (3). The last may be prevented by anchoring it to the ring with ribbon gauze or bandage (4).

18. *Thomas splint* (6) If separate slings are used, their tendency to separate may be minimised by pinning each to its neighbour (1). Nevertheless, a layer of wool should be placed between them and the limb to smooth out any unevenness (2) (not necessary with circular woven bandage). In all cases, a large pad (e.g. of gamgee) should be placed directly beneath the fracture to act as a fulcrum.

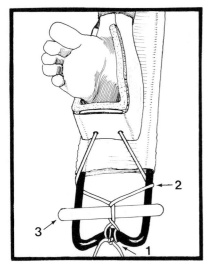

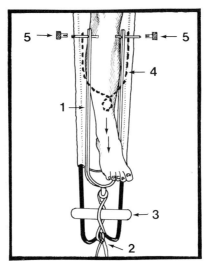

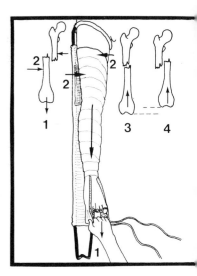

19. *Thomas splint* (7) In long oblique fractures and those with apposition no manipulation will be needed and the traction system may be completed by, for example, tying the cords to the end of the splint (1). The convention of passing the medial cord under the corresponding iron helps to control the tendency to lateral rotation (2). A Chinese windlass (of spatulae or a metal rod) may be used to take up slack (3).

20. *Thomas splint* (8) Where skeletal traction is being used a metal loop (1) (Tulloch-Brown loop) allows a direct pull to be made in the line of the limb. The loop may be tied to the end of the Thomas splint (2) and tensioned with a windlass as previously described (3). A stirrup may be employed to prevent springing of the loop (4). Protect the sharp ends of the pin with caps (5).

21. *Thomas splint* (9) *Manipulation:* With the exception of the young child, manipulation is advisable if there is loss of bony apposition. With the splint in position but unattached, an assistant applies strong traction (1) while pressure is applied in the directions deduced from the radiographs (2). When the traction is eased off, the limb remains the same length if a hitch has been obtained (3) but telescopes if not (4).

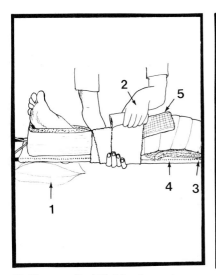

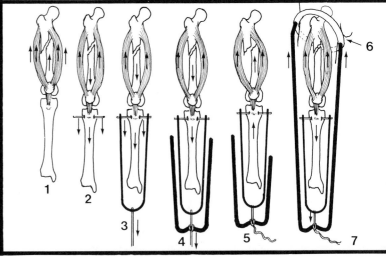

22. *Thomas splint* (10) After the traction cords have been attached, the end of the splint can be raised temporarily on a pillow (1) while the limb is bandaged to the splint, using for example 6″ (15 cm) crepe bandages (2). Note gamgee or wool padding behind the fracture to act as a fulcrum (3), behind the knee to keep it in slight flexion (4), and along the shin to avoid sores (5).

23. *Thomas splint* (11) The system described is normally referred to as fixed traction in a Thomas splint. The basic principles are straightforward, but it is important that they are thoroughly understood. Muscle tension (mainly quads and hams) tends to produce shortening (1); this can be overcome by traction, for example through a Steinman pin (2) aided by a loop and traction cord (3). If the traction cord is tied to a ringless Thomas splint, the reduction is maintained so long as a pull is kept on the cord (4); re-displacement occurs the cord is released (5). This proximal migration is normally prevented by the ring (6) so tha the reduction is maintained even when the traction cord is released (7). Note that muscle tone = tension in traction cord = ring pressure.

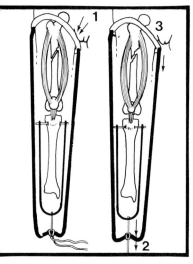

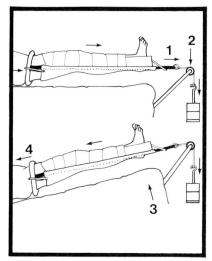

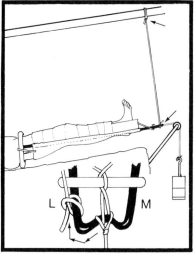

4. *Thomas splint* (12) This pressure of the ring of the Thomas splint tends to produce ores (1) (especially in the perineal, groin and ischial tuberosity regions) and must be relieved. This is done by applying traction (*c.* lb/3 kg) to the anchored cords. If ring ressure is unrelieved, *increase the traction eights*.

25. *Thomas splint* (13) The traction weights have a tendency to pull the patient down towards the foot of the bed (1). This may continue till the splint comes to rest on the traction pulley (2). This may be countered if it becomes a problem by raising the foot of the bed (3), when the traction weight is balanced by the upward component of the patient's body weight (4).

26. *Thomas splint* (14) *Supporting the limb and the splint* (1) To allow the patient to move about the bed and prevent pressure on the heel, it is desirable to support the splint; this may be done most simply by tying a cord from the end of the splint to an overhead bar of the Balkan beam bed. The position of the suspension cord may be adjusted from near the mid-line to either side. (Ill: lateral attachment to control external rotation.)

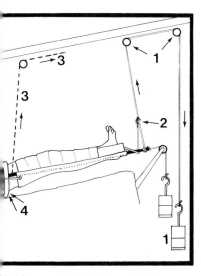

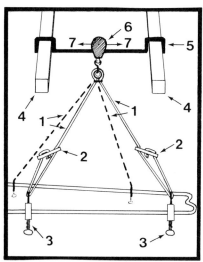

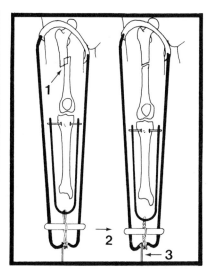

7. *Thomas splint* (15) *Supporting the plint* (2) Some prefer a lively system which an be achieved in various ways, e.g. by eights and a system of pulleys (1). The raction cord may be arranged in Y fashion o straddle both irons of the Thomas plint (2). Support for the proximal end of he splint (3) is less clearly an advantage lthough often pursued—it may cause extra ressure beneath the ring (4).

28. *Thomas splint* (16) *Supporting the splint* (3) Another form of lively splint support ('octopus') consists of elastic Bunjee cord (1) which can be adjusted with tensioners (2). The cords are attached to the splint with G cramps (3) and to cross members of the Balkan beam (4) by means of a bar (5) along which a pulley (6) is free to move, allowing easy movement up and down the bed (7).

29. *Thomas splint* (17) Check radiographs should be taken after the application of a Thomas splint, after any major adjustment, and thereafter at fortnightly intervals till union.
Corrections (a) If there is persistent shortening (1) tighten the windlass in a fixed traction system (2). This will inevitably increase ring pressure, and must be compensated by increasing the traction weight (3). (Soft tissue between the bone ends may nevertheless thwart reduction.)

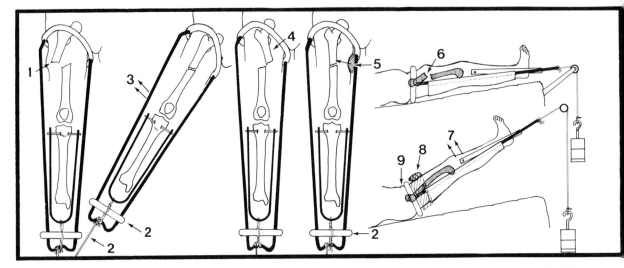

30. *Thomas splint* (18) *Corrections* (b)
Where the proximal fragment is abducted (1)
the position may be improved by increasing
the traction (2) and abducting the leg (3).
The position of the ring traction pulley and
the splint supports will require
corresponding adjustment.

Corrections (c) If the proximal fragment is
adducted (4) increase of traction alone (2)
may lead to an improvement in the position.

It may be helpful to apply side thrust with a
pad (5) between the leg and the medial side
iron.

Corrections (d) Flexion and/or abduction
of the proximal fragment (6) due to
unresisted psoas and gluteal action is
frequently a very painful complication. In
the young patient, raising the splint (7)
and/or abducting the leg and bandaging a
local pad in position (8) may bring the

fragments into alignment, but this
manoeuvre is less certain in the older patient
where internal fixation is frequently
advisable for femoral fractures at this level
and of this type. In any patient in whom this
conservative technique is practised, care
must be taken to avoid pressure in the region
of the anterior superior iliac spine (9).

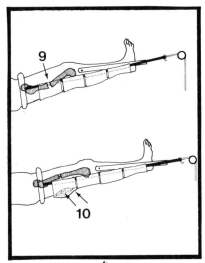

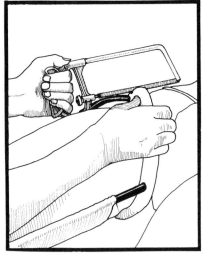

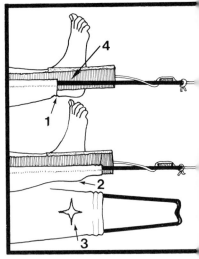

31. *Thomas splint* (19) *Corrections* (e)
Perhaps the commonest residual deformity
requiring and amenable to correction is
backward sag at the fracture site (9). If a
continuous posterior support is used, the
padding behind the fracture should be
increased in thickness. If separate slings are
used, the sling behind the fracture should be
tightened and/or the padding behind the
fracture increased (10).

32. *Thomas splint* (20) *After care* (1) During
the first 72 hours following fracture, swelling
of the thigh from haematoma and oedema
may render the ring tight round its
circumference. (Normally it should be easy
to put a finger under the ring at any point.)
To avoid changing the splint, split the ring
with a hacksaw, ease the ends apart, and
protect them with adhesive strapping.

33. *Thomas splint* (21) *After care* (2) The
following items should be checked daily.
Look for impending pressure sores (and take
appropriate action). (a) *In the Achilles
tendon region* if the slings stop at this
level (1); (b) *Under the heel*, if the heel is
included (2); If a circular woven support is
used, a cruciate incision in it at heel level is
prophylactic (3); (c) *Over the malleoli* (4).

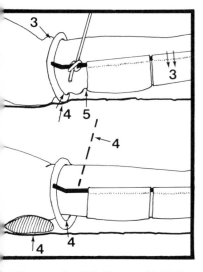

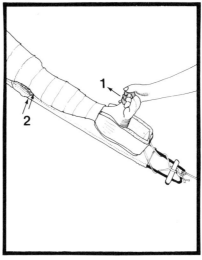

36. *Thomas splint* (24) *After care* (5) In those cases where skeletal traction is employed, look for (i) Loosening of the Steinman pin: this may require re-centring; other treatment is seldom required, so that traction may be continued. (ii) Pin-track infection: a wound swab should be sent for bacteriological examination and the appropriate antibiotic administered. If infection is marked, the traction site may have to be abandoned. (iii) Shifting and digging-in of the loop: adjust with padding.

During the period a patient spends in bed he should practise quadriceps and general maintenance exercises. Splintage in children should be continued till union (6–12 weeks). In adults, mobilisation of the knee joint and/or the patient may be possible before union is complete.

34. *Thomas splint* (22) *After care* (3) (d) *The ing area:* Good nursing care is vital to avoid skin breakdown. In addition, for (1) circumferential tightness—split the ring; (2) perineal pressure—increase the ring traction weight; (3) Anterior spine pressure—lower the splint; (4) Pressure behind the ring—decrease or remove any support weight and place a pillow *above* the ring (4); (e) Pad the edge of the sling if needed (5).

35. *Thomas splint* (23) *After care* (4) Check daily for weakness of ankle dorsiflexion (1) indicative of common peroneal nerve palsy and necessitating careful inspection of the neck of the fibula where the cause is generally felting of the wool padding, transmitting pressure from the side iron (2). Re-pad and fit a Sinclair foot support if the palsy is complete: expect recovery in 6 weeks.

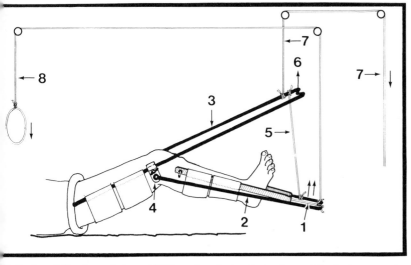

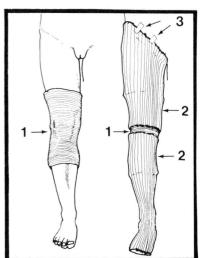

37. *Early mobilisation techniques:* (i) Where there is abundant callus and the fracture cannot be sprung, splintage may be discarded and the knee mobilised till there is sufficient mature callus to allow weight bearing. (ii) *The Pearson knee-flexion piece:* this may be used as soon as some stabilising callus appears at the fracture site.
Method: The traction cord (1) is transferred to the Pearson attachment (2) which is fixed to the Thomas splint (3) and hinges at the level of the knee axis (4). An adjustable cord (5) may be used to gradually advance the range of permissable knee flexion. The end of the Thomas splint is raised (6) and supported (7) while a cord (8) may allow the patient to assist his knee extension manually.

38. *Early mobilisation techniques:* (iii) *Cast bracing* (1) After 4–8 weeks in a Thomas splint, cast bracing may be considered, especially in fractures of the distal half. Many techniques are practised. In a typical procedure the patient is sedated with Diazepam, a sandbag placed under the buttocks, and a cast sock drawn over the knee (1). Circular woven bandages (stockingette) encase the limb in two sections (2) and are taped in position (3).

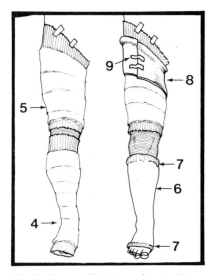

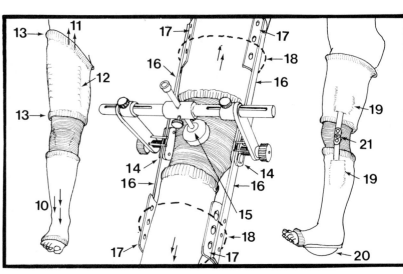

39. *Cast bracing* (2) A layer of wool roll is used to protect the bony prominences below the knee (4) and as a single layer of padding in the thigh (5). A below-knee plaster is then applied (6) and completed by turning back and incorporating the circular woven bandage (7). An appropriately sized bucket top of polythene is selected (8), trimmed as required, and taped in position (9).

40. *Cast bracing* (3) Traction is applied to the leg (10), the bucket is pulled well into the groin (11), a plaster thigh piece applied, moulded in a quadrilateral fashion (to prevent rotation) (12), and completed (13). Maintaining traction in 10° flexion, polycentric hinges (14) are carefully positioned with a jig which is centred on the patella (15). The side-stays (16) are adjusted until the fixation plates (17) lie snugly against the upper and lower plaster components. Large encircling Jubilee clips (18) may be used to hold the hinges in position while the jig is removed and flexion function checked. The hinges are plastered in position (19) and a rocker or boot applied (20). The hinges can be unlocked by removal of 2 set screws (21).

41. *Cast bracing* (4) The cast brace affords moderate support of the fracture, and mobilisation of the patient may be commenced at first using crutches and with the hinges locked. After 1–2 weeks or as progress determines, flexion can be permitted and the crutches gradually discarded. The brace is worn until union is complete.

A number of commercially produced cast-bracing kits are available using materials other than plaster of Paris. (e.g. the bucket may be formed from pre-cut plastic sheet which can be temporarily softened by heating and moulded to shape: resin plaster bandages and polyethylene hinges can be employed.) In many cases these render the technique comparatively simple, with the result that the so-called weight relieving calliper, tubed into the patient's shoe, is now much less frequently employed for early mobilisation than in the past.

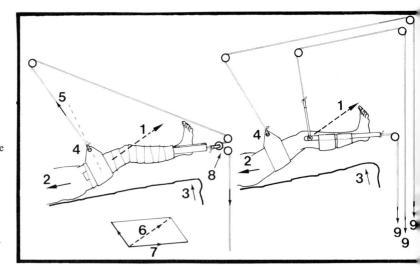

42. *Other methods of treating fractures of the femur:* (1) *Hamilton-Russell traction:* This is particularly applicable in the conservative treatment of bilateral fractures; it is a form of balanced traction where the pull on the limb (1) is countered by the body weight (2) through the bed being raised (3). The fracture and distal fragment are supported by a padded canvas sling (4), angled slightly towards the head (5) to counter a tendency to distal drift. The theory behind the classical arrangement is that the line of pull on the femur is the resultant (6) of a parallelogram of forces, where the horizontal component (7) is doubled because of the pulley arrangement (8). Friction losses spoil the theory, and many prefer direct control of all forces (9). This method of treatment, although often useful, gives restricted support to the fracture. Note that balanced traction can be carried out using a Thomas splint bandaged to the limb, but unattached to any of the traction cords.

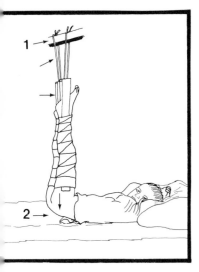

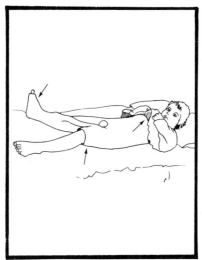

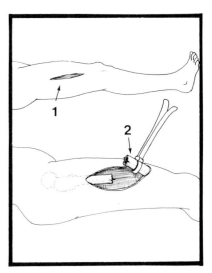

43. *(2) Gallows traction:* Children up to the age of 3 (or 4 if light) are ideally treated by this method. Traction tapes are applied to both legs and fixed to an overhead beam (1) so that the child's buttocks are just clear of the bed (2), making nursing easy. The body weight is responsible for the traction. Gallows traction should not be used in the older child as there is the risk of vascular spasm and peripheral gangrene.

44. *(3) Hip spica:* Stable femoral shaft fractures may be supported by a plaster hip spica: this must include the injured leg to the toes, the other leg to above the knee, and extend to above the nipple line. A hip spica may be used for the fretful child where good nursing care is available at home (with fortnightly out-patient reviews) or for the badly infected compound injury in the adult.

45. *(4) Intramedullary nailing* (1) This is the most reliable of internal fixation methods and is most suitable for fractures of the middle 2/4ths of the femur in adults. It is of particular value in dealing with multiple fractures in the one limb, and where there is a particular need for early mobilisation. The retrograde technique is often employed, and is essential when difficulty in reduction is anticipated. A lateral approach is used (1) and the bone ends are freed and cleared in turn (2).

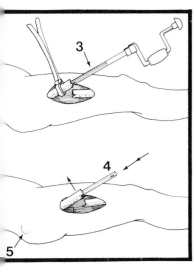

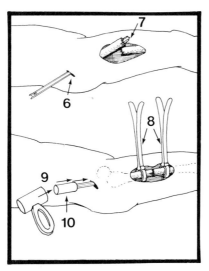

48. *Intramedullary nailing* (4) Nailing may also be carried out, using a guide wire and cannulated reamers, from the trochanter without exposing the fracture. This is dependent on having an undisplaced fracture, or one which can be reduced with an image intensifier. After care is dependent on the quality of fixation. If a tight fitting large diameter nail is used, and interdigitating bone fragments resist torsional displacement, no additional splintage is necessary. The knee may be mobilised and the patient allowed up on crutches.

To avoid the risks of nail bending or fatigue fracture many prefer to defer weight bearing until some callus appears. If fixation is less sound, a period of a few weeks with the leg cradled in a Thomas splint may be thought desirable. After union of the fracture, the nail is removed routinely in all but the very frail (to reduce risk of femoral neck fracture from minor injuries due to local stress concentrations).

46. *Intramedullary nailing* (2) To ensure a clear passage for the nail in the tapered and curved medullary cavity, reamers of increasing diameter (3) are passed, aiming at a compromise between minimal bone removal and maximum nail diameter. A Küntscher (or other pattern) nail is chosen so that the length (gauged by measuring the fragments) is insufficient to penetrate the knee when inserted, and driven up (4), with the hip adducted, till it appears in the buttock (5).

47. *Intramedullary nailing* (3) The nail is delivered through a small incision (6) and driven further up till nearly flush with the proximal fragment (7). The fracture is held with clamps (8) in the reduced position and the nail driven back down (9) across the fracture until it is level with the trochanter. During the driving procedures the sharp ends of the nail are protected with a punch (10).

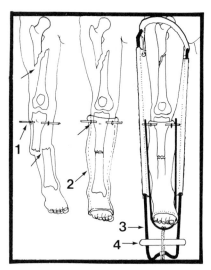

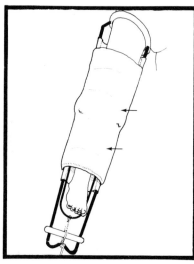

49. *Special situations (1) Fractures of the femur and tibia in the same leg:*
Conservative treatment: A Steinman pin is inserted in the region of the tibial tubercle (or more distal in the child) (1), the tibial fracture is manipulated, and a below-knee plaster applied incorporating the pin (2); a Thomas splint (3) is then used with traction through the pin (4) to control the femoral fracture.
Operative treatment: Generally intramedullary nailing of the femur + tibial plating.

50. *(2) Fractures in the confused patient:*
Where there is an accompanying head injury or a senile confusional state the patient may make frequent (and sometimes successful) attempts to remove the splint. This may be prevented by wrapping one or two plaster bandages round the splint (Tobruk splintage). This technique may also be used to give extra security during patient transportation.

51. *(3) Pathological fracture due to metastatic deposits:* In secondary malignancy, if death is not imminent, intramedullary nailing is advised as a pain-relieving procedure. If there is gross bone destruction, acrylic cement packed into the medullary cavities and around the fracture may give sufficient security to allow the patient to return to weight bearing.

(4) Femoral shaft fractures associated with (acute) ischaemia of the foot: Nearly all simple and the majority of compound fractures will respond to reduction of the fracture. Nevertheless reduction should be carried out under circumstances in which it is possible to carry on with exploration, and if necessary, repair of the femoral artery. If the vessel is, in fact, divided, intramedullary fixation will be required prior to vessel repair.

(5) Shaft fractures associated with nerve palsy: The vast majority are lesions in continuity, and may be associated with temporary ischaemia or nerve stretching. The common peroneal element is most commonly affected. If there is reason to believe that there may be nerve division (e.g. by the nature of a compound wound) nerve exploration and internal fixation may have to be undertaken.

(6) Fracture of the femoral neck and shaft: This combination of injuries is seen as a sequel to high velocity road traffic accidents. If the femoral shaft fracture is a high spiral type, both lesions may be controlled by a nail-plate (with a long plate and if necessary cross screwing of the fracture). In the majority of cases, however, the ideal treatment is a Küntscher Y-nail.

(7) Femoral shaft fracture with dislocation of the hip: See Fractures of the Pelvis, 59.

(8) Fractures of the femoral shaft and patella: The following important points should be noted: (a) Early mobilisation of the knee is essential for retention of function. (b) Avoid excision of the patella where mobilisation of the knee is going to be delayed. (c) Avoid if possible exposure of the femoral fracture and the creation of tethering adhesions between the femur and the quadriceps.

The ideal treatment of the femoral fracture is Küntscher nailing by the trochanteric route (see 67–74 for treatment of patellar fractures). If the femoral fracture must be treated conservatively, it is best to leave even badly displaced or comminuted patellar fractures to unite by fibrous union; the knee should be mobilised as early as possible by one of the methods already described; excision of the patella can then be carried out as a late secondary procedure when no further flexion can be gained.

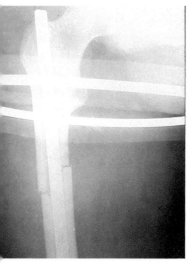

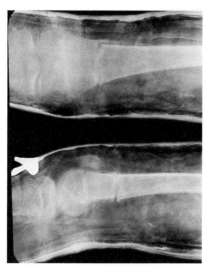

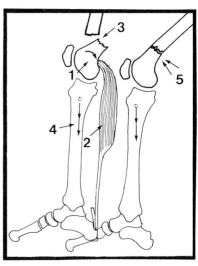

, *Other fractures of the femur: (1)*
actures of the upper third: It is often
ficult to control fractures at this level by
ction and external splintage, although
vation of the splint, abduction and local
dding may be tried (see 30). Pain is a
ther problem due to the psoas and glutei
eatedly and involuntarily flexing or
ducting the proximal fragment. Certainly
the adult intramedullary nailing should be
nsidered for this injury (ill: nailed femur
dled in Thomas splint).

53. *(2) Supracondylar fractures* (1) In
children, fractures in the distal third of the
femur are frequently only minimally
displaced, and may be successfully treated
by the application of a cylinder plaster.
Weight bearing should not be permitted till
evidence of early union appears on the
radiographs, but during this period the
patient may be mobilised with crutches.

54. *Supracondylar fractures* (2) In the adult
especially, supracondylar fractures have a
strong tendency for the distal fragment to
rotate (1) under the continuous pull of the
gastrocnemius (2) into a position of
posterior angulation (anterior tilting) (3).
This cannot be controlled by traction in the
line of the limb (4). It is necessary to flex the
knee and maintain the traction over a
fulcrum (5).

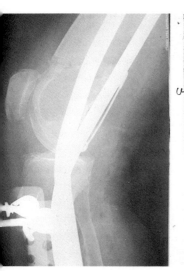

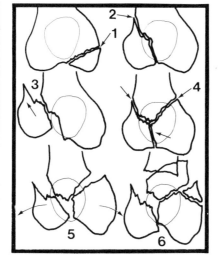

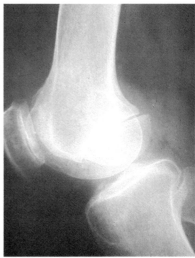

, *Supracondylar fractures* (3) The
cessary degree of knee flexion may be
tained by using a Pearson knee piece, or
tter still by bending the Thomas splint at
 level of the fracture (ill.). Mobilisation of
 knee should be started as early as
ssible, and internal fixation is sometimes
vocated, using an Elliot or A-O blade-
te, or less satisfactorily, bilateral Rush
s.

56. *Fractures involving the condyles (a)*
There are several distinct patterns: (1) Intra-
articular shearing condylar fracture;
(2) Undisplaced unicondylar fracture with a
substantial metaphyseal component;
(3) Displaced unicondylar fracture;
(4) Undisplaced Y (or T) fracture;
(5) Displaced Y-fracture; (6) Highly
comminuted Y-fracture, often with a spiral
fracture of the distal femoral shaft.

57. *Condylar fractures (b) (1) Intra-*
articular shearing fractures: Fractures of
this type frequently fail to unite, possibly due
to disruption of the fracture haematoma by
the synovial fluid. Non-union may be
associated with instability in the knee, and
initial treatment by countersunk cancellous
bone screws and a 6-week period non-weight
bearing in a cylinder plaster would seem
justifiable.

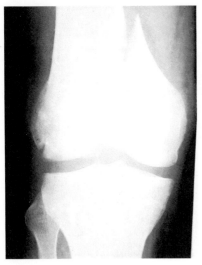

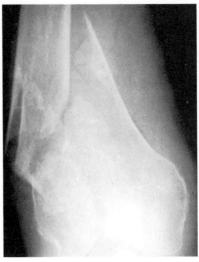

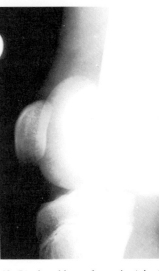

58. *Condylar fractures* (c) (2)
(3) *Unicondylar fractures:* Where
displacement is moderate or slight (2) these
injuries may be treated successfully by
traction. A straight Thomas splint may be
used for the first 1–2 weeks, but thereafter
mobilisation should be commenced, either
with a Pearson knee flexion piece or with
Hamilton-Russell traction. Where
displacement is severe (3), open reduction
and internal fixation with cancellous bone
screws should be undertaken.

59. *Condylar fractures* (d) (4) (5) (6) Where
there is much comminution (6) (Ill.) open
reduction is likely to be unrewarding and the
aim should be early mobilisation, e.g. by
Hamilton-Russell traction for 6–8 weeks till
union is well advanced. Treat Type 4 injuries
as Type 2. In Type 5 injuries, the condyles
should be brought together, either by
traction and manipulation *or* with a
cancellous screw (used with a blade plate) *or*
a length of studding nutted at both ends.

60. *Displaced lower femoral epiphysis:* Thi
injury usually results from hyperextension
and there is risk of vascular complications
reduction should be carried out
expeditiously by applying traction, flexing
the knee to a right angle, and pressing the
epiphysis backwards into position. The kn
should be kept in flexion for three weeks in
plaster slab, and for a further 3–5 weeks in
plaster cylinder in a more neutral position.

61. Complications of fractures of the femur

Among the many complications which may accompany this fracture the
following should be noted:
1. Oligaemic shock (see 3).
2. Fat embolism (see p. 70).
3. Slow or delayed union: These are common complications, and if the
fracture is being treated conservatively, may necessitate prolonged
immobilisation of the knee, with risk of permanent stiffness.
4. Non-union: This is generally treated, as soon as confidently diagnosed, ł
intramedullary nailing and bone grafting. Again there may be problems wi
knee stiffness.
5. Mal-union: Persistent lateral angulation is the commonest deformity in
shaft fractures, and if 25° or more, correction by osteotomy and
intramedullary nailing should be considered. Angulation in the lateral plan
seldom gives rise to much difficulty. Nearer the knee, angulation showing
the A.P. radiographs may give rise to instability, difficulty in walking, and
secondary osteo-arthritis in the knee. Each case must be assessed on its ov
merits, but again corrective osteotomy/osteoclasis should be considered.
6. Limb shortening: Shortening in the adult should be corrected by shoe
alteration to within 1–2 cm ($\frac{1}{2}$″) of the limb discrepancy. In children, any
difference in leg length usually corrects (or indeed over-corrects)
spontaneously within 6–18 months of the injury, and alteration to the sho

is seldom required. Only rarely in epiphyseal injuries is there progressive shortening.

7. Knee stiffness: This is a common complication of femoral and tibial fractures, and of injuries to the extensor mechanism of the knee. Among the factors which are involved are the following:

(a) Quadriceps tethering: If the quadriceps becomes adherent to a femoral shaft fracture, it becomes unable to glide over the smooth distal shaft in the normal fashion, producing as a result fixation of the patella and restriction of movement in the knee. The closer the fracture is to the knee, the more important this effect. Surgical intervention tends to aggravate this tendency (unless it can be followed by rapid mobilisation).

(b) Fractures involving the knee joint: Fractures which involve the articular surfaces may give rise to intra-articular and peri-articular adhesions, or may form a mechanical block to movement. Early mobilisation is especially desirable where a fracture involves the joint.

(c) Prolonged immobilisation: Fixation of the knee for an undesirably long period, for example, by delay in union, may lead to stiffness, and this effect is particularly marked in the elderly.

Treatment

(a) Quadriceps exercises: Stability in the knee and extension power are dependent on a good quadriceps. It is important that the muscle is not allowed to waste, and quadriceps exercises should be started as soon after injury as possible, and intensified on removal of any fixation. (Amongst the few exceptions are injuries to the extensor mechanism where quadriceps exercises are usually delayed for two weeks lest early contraction endanger a repair.)

(b) Flexion exercises: These should also be commenced as soon as possible, provided the means can be devised to support the fracture fully. Flexion should not be permitted unless stress on the fracture can be eliminated, or where healing can be more or less guaranteed (e.g. tibial table fractures).

(c) Discarding walking aids: Walking without the support of sticks or crutches is frequently followed by an improvement in flexion, and such supportive measures should be discontinued as soon as the state of union and the patient's balance will allow.

(d) Physiotherapy: Ideally quadriceps and flexion exercises should be supervised by a physiotherapist with access to aids and facilities such as weights, slings, local heat and hydrotherapy; but basically the patient should be instructed in quadriceps and flexion exercises, and the importance of performing these frequently should be stressed. Passive mobilisation of the patella in appropriate cases may also be helpful.

Physiotherapy should be continued until an acceptable functional range has been achieved (see below) or until a static position has been reached. For this it is necessary to record the range of movements in the knee with accuracy; this should be done initially at weekly and then at monthly intervals. A measurable gain in range, no matter how small, is an encouragement to the patient to further effort; and on the other hand, the absence of any improvement should make it clear to him that to continue treatment is not justifiable.

Notes

Acceptable functional range: What is acceptable obviously varies considerably from case to case, being dependent on the gravity of the injury, the age of the patient, his occupation, athletic or outdoor pursuits, hobbies, etc.; but the basic aim is a stable knee which places little restraint on normal everyday activities. The following factors are important:

Lack of extension: Loss of extension, both active and passive, may be found—e.g. in an angulated supracondylar fracture of the femur, or where there has been previous osteo-arthritis in the knee. Such losses are seldom severe enough to cause appreciable disability, usually being compensated at hip and ankle. If the knee can be passively but not actively extended, this is known as an *extension lag*. Extension lag frequently gives rise to 'giving-way' of the knee. It is common to some degree after most cases of patellectomy, but usually recovers if quadriceps exercises are intensified.

Where extension lag is due to quadriceps tethering, quadriceps exercises should also be encouraged. The patient in most cases of persistent lag learns to compensate for the disability by using the hip extensors to keep the knee straight while standing.

Lack of flexion: Appreciable disability follows if flexion to 100° (i.e. 10° more than right-angle flexion) cannot be obtained, and 100° should be the aim. Flexion to 80°–90° will permit sitting in inside seats (i.e. non-aisle seats) in public transport, cinemas, etc., but will not allow the patient to kneel. Less than 100° will cause difficulty with steps, deep tread and narrow stairs, and if both knees are affected, rising from armless chairs.

Where flexion has just become static at less than 100°, manipulation of the knee under general anaesthesia should be considered. This is best avoided, however, after patellectomy and quadriceps tendon and patellar ligament repairs, because of the risks of secondary rupture. Gains in flexion by manipulation are seldom high, and late manipulations are usually very unrewarding.

Where 80° or less flexion is possible and the position static, the patient's functional disability and functional requirements should be carefully assessed. If there is a marked deficit, quadricepsplasty should be considered. In this procedure the vasti are divided close to the knee so that their tethering effect is eliminated; rectus femoris then becomes the sole extensor of the knee. This often gives a useful gain (often in the region of 40°) although sometimes this is at the expense of an extension lag, and always with some loss of power.

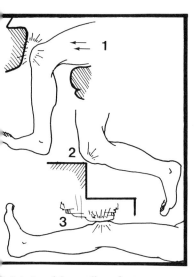

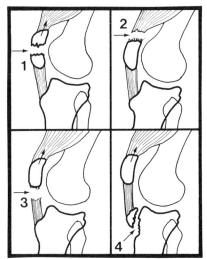

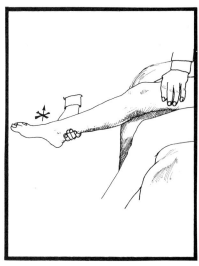

*. Injuries of the patella and extensor *echanism of the knee: Mechanisms* (1) The *tella* may be fractured by direct violence, r example, (a) in road traffic accidents in hich the knee strikes the fascia (1). (Note e association between fracture of the tella, fracture of the femoral shaft and slocation of the hip.) (b) by falls against a rd surface—e.g. the edge of a step (2). (c) heavy objects falling across the knee (e.g. lling rock) (3).

63. *Mechanisms* (2) The patella may also be fractured by indirect violence, i.e. as a result of a sudden muscular contraction (1). This same mechanism may also cause (a) rupture of the quadriceps tendon (2), rupture of the patellar ligament (3), or avulsion of the tibial tubercle (4).

64. *Diagnosis* (1) Fracture of the patella should be suspected when there is a history of direct violence to the knee; fracture of the patella and other injuries to the extensor mechanism should be suspected when there is difficulty in standing after a sudden muscular effort (especially when there is a snapping sensation within the knee). In most cases *there is inability to extend the knee.*

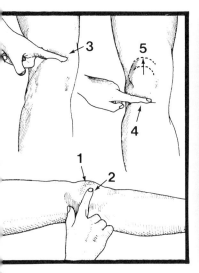

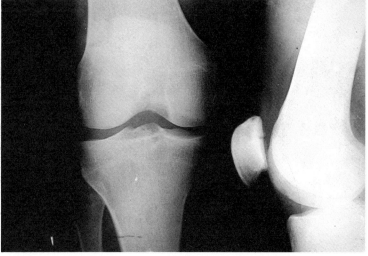

. Diagnosis (2) Note clinically any of the llowing: Bruising and abrasions (1); the esence and site of tenderness (2); any lpable gap above the patella (3) or beneath (4); any obvious proximal displacement of e patella (5).

66. *Diagnosis* (3) In all cases, radiographs are essential to clarify the diagnosis. An A.P. projection and a lateral (preferably in extension) will generally suffice. In the acute case tangential projections cannot usually be obtained because of pain, but these views are often of value in the cases which present late. If there is doubt remaining, oblique projections may be helpful. Do not mistake a congenital bi-partite patella (illustrated) for a fracture. This anomaly most frequently affects the *upper* and *outer* quadrant; it may be obvious in 1 view only. The edges are usually rounded, and this may help to differentiate it from a fracture. Other anomalies, such as tri-partite patella, may also be distinguished by similar rounding and absence of local tenderness.

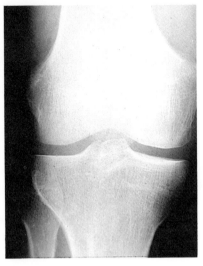

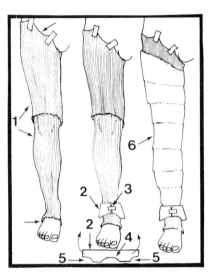

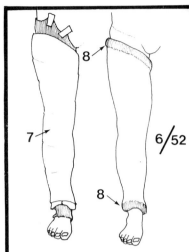

67. *Treatment* (1) *Vertical fractures:* Fractures of this type are usually undisplaced and stable. They do not show in the lateral radiographs. In the A.P. view, the overlapping femoral shadow may make them difficult to detect, and in fact these fractures are frequently missed. Conservative treatment only is required. (See 68, 70.)

68. *Treatment* (2) A 6 week period in a cylinder plaster (plaster cylinder, pipe-stem plaster) is usually advised. *Method:* Apply a layer of stockingette (2 pieces) from the hind foot to the groin (1). Protect the malleoli with a piece of felt(2), butt-joining the ends with adhesive tape (3). Note concavities for the Achilles tendon (4) and dorsum of the foot (5). Pad the leg with wool (6).

69. *Treatment* (3) The knee is normally kep in full extension (but not in recurvatum or hyperextension) while 8″ (20 cm) plaster bandages are applied (7). A slab is not necessary. The edges of the stockingette ar turned back before completion (8). Crutche are usually advised for the first 2 weeks, wi a total of 6 weeks in plaster.

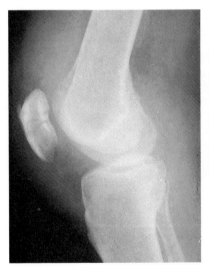

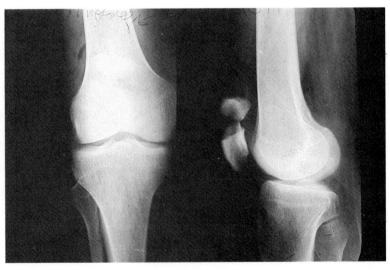

70. *Undisplaced horizontal fractures:* Undisplaced horizontal fractures (even with some comminution) may be treated along similar lines with, however, radiographs at weekly intervals for the first 2–3 weeks to exclude late separation. After removal of the plaster at 6 weeks, physiotherapy will be required, and crutches may be needed again for the first few weeks till confidence is regained.

71. *Displaced horizontal fractures:* Fractures of this type should be explored so that (1) the exact nature of the pathology may be determined and (2) the appropriate treatment carried out.

Knee function after patellectomy is often excellent, but may fall a little short of perfect; although a full range of movements may be regained, there is often a feeling of instability while descending steep slopes, and there may be some weakness in rising from the squatting position. The patella should therefore be preserved, but only if the articular surface can be perfectly restored and maintained in that position until union occurs. In practice, this is onl usually possible when there is no comminution; and although the radiographs (ill.) may suggest that only 2 fragments are present, this can only be confirmed at exploration.

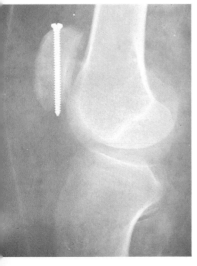

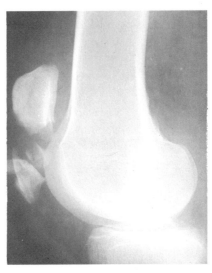

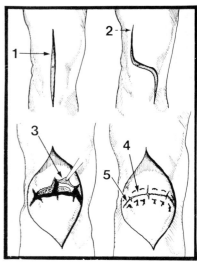

2. *Treatment* (1) If the joint surface can be restored, the fragments may be fixed by (1) one or two vertical screws (2) tension and wiring (3) wiring, through two vertical holes drilled through the patella (U-wire, twisting the free ends) (4) wiring in a figure-of-eight pattern through the quadriceps tendon and patellar ligament, the wire crossing in front of the patella.

73. *Treatment* (2) If the joint surfaces cannot be restored and held, or if as illustrated the fracture is highly comminuted, the fragments should be completely excised and the quadriceps insertion, along with any tearing of the lateral expansions, repaired.

74. For exploration or excision, the patella may be exposed through a mid-line vertical incision (1) or a lazy S (2) with the raising of two flaps. The patellar fragments are carefully dissected free, taking care that every piece is removed (3). The insertion (4) along with the lateral expansions (5) are repaired with mattress sutures and a plaster cylinder applied. Crutches should be used for 4 weeks and mobilisation commenced at 6.

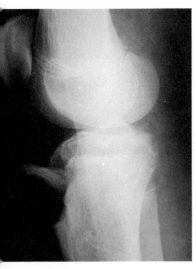

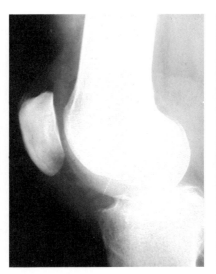

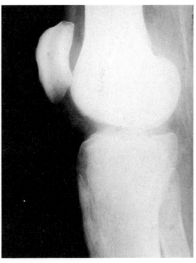

75. *Avulsion fractures of the tibial tubercle:* in the adult, or adolescent near skeletal maturity (ill.) the displacement, if marked, should be reduced and the tubercle fixed with a screw. If displacement is slight, a 6 week period in a plaster cylinder should suffice. In children, surgery should be · avoided if possible because of the risks of premature epiphyseal fusion, but if manipulative reduction fails, open reduction and fixing with a suture may become necessary.

76. *Rupture of the quadriceps tendon:* The diagnosis is essentially clinical, but sometimes may be confirmed by examination of the soft tissue shadows on the radiographs (ill.). The tendon must be re-attached surgically: it is often necessary to drill the patella to provide anchorage for the sutures. Thereafter a plaster cylinder is applied. Quadriceps exercises are commenced at 2 weeks, weight bearing at 4 weeks, and knee flexion at 6 weeks.

77. *Rupture of the patellar ligament:* Again, this is essentially a clinical diagnosis, although proximal displacement of the patella may be suggestive. Surgical repair is as for rupture of the quadriceps tendon. Avulsion fractures of the distal tip of the patella should be treated in a similar fashion after excision of bone fragments (i.e. by re-attachment of the ligament using drill holes for anchorage).

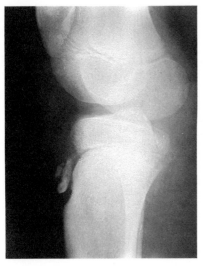

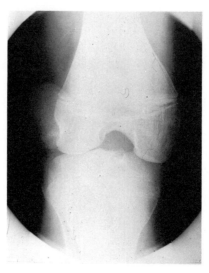

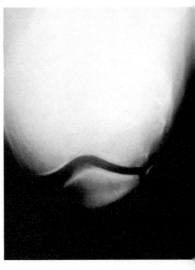

78. *Osgood Schlatter's disease:* In children, sudden or repeated quadriceps contraction may be responsible for this condition which is characterised by recurrent pain, tenderness, and swelling over the tibial tubercle. It may be mistaken for an acute injury. While slow spontaneous resolution is the rule, an acute episode may be treated by 2 weeks in a plaster cylinder. Severe persistent symptoms occasionally merit excision of the detached fragment.

79. *Lateral dislocation of the patella* (1) In this condition the patella dislocates laterally as a result of muscular contraction or a blow on its medial border. It may be reduced (unless of long standing) by applying firm pressure over its lateral aspect (anaesthesia is seldom required). If a first incident, a 6-week period of plaster fixation is advised: if not, apply a pressure bandage for 1–2 weeks.

80. (2) Lateral dislocation commonly occurs as a first or subsequent incident in the course of recurrent dislocation of the patella, a condition seen most frequently in teenage girls. The presence on the tangential projection of the knee of a marginal osteochondral fracture is diagnostic, but may not be obvious until some weeks after a first incident (which may also be overlooked if spontaneous reduction occurs).

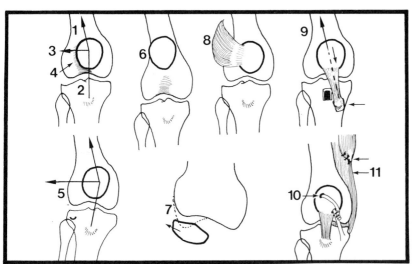

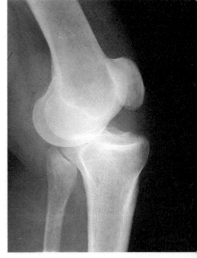

81. (3) Due to the femur meeting the tibia at an angle, the quadriceps (1) and patellar ligament (2) have a lateral component (3) during muscle contraction: this is resisted by the femoral gutter (4) in which the patella usually lies. The tendency to dislocation is increased by genu valgum (5), patella alta (6), hypoplasia of the lateral femoral condyle (7) or an abnormal attachment of vastus lateralis (8). The many methods of treatment include the Hauser procedure, where the tibial tuberosity is transposed medially and distally, correcting patella alta and eliminating the lateral component of quadriceps pull (9). In the Galeazzi repair, more suitable in the adolescent, a semitendinosus tenodesis if performed to stabilise the patella. The tendon is threaded through a hole drilled in the patella (10) and the stump sewn to semimembranosus (11).

82. *Dislocation of the knee* (1) This injury may surprisingly follow comparatively minor trauma. Most commonly the tibia is displaced anteriorly, but medial, lateral, posterior and rotational displacements are also found. There is inevitably major damage to the ligaments of the knee: all or most may be torn along with the joint capsule.

3. *Dislocation of the knee* (2) Sometimes ere is displacement of the menisci, ractures of the tibial spines, common eroneal nerve palsy, and most seriously, opliteal artery damage. *reatment:* Closed reduction appears to give etter results in the majority of cases than ttempts at operative repair. Reduction is enerally easy by traction and the pplication of pressure over the displaced bia. Thereafter the leg should be supported y light traction (6 lb/2–3 kg) in a Thomas lint for 3–4 weeks, followed by a further 4 eeks in a plaster cylinder before obilisation is commenced. Surgery is dicated in the following circumstances:) if closed reduction fails (generally due to utton-holing of the capsule by a femoral ondyle) or (2) if there is persistent rculatory impairment in the limb after duction, when popliteal artery exploration indicated.

84. *Soft tissue injuries of the knee:* When there has been trauma to the knee and the radiographs show little in the way of bony injury, a significant soft tissue injury should be suspected. It would be unrealistic to say that injuries of this type are easy to diagnose: they sometimes are, but often cause much difficulty. There is the common clinical picture of pain in the knee, swelling, and difficulty in weight bearing shared by many lesions. Investigation of each case should aim to exclude (1) Damage to the extensor apparatus (75–78), (2) Lateral dislocation of the patella with spontaneous reduction (79–81), (3) Tears of the ligaments of the knee (85–96), (4) Meniscus tears (99–106).

If there is no hard evidence to implicate these structures (and this is so in the *majority* of cases) a provisional (and rather unsatisfactory) diagnosis of 'knee sprain' or 'sprained ligaments with traumatic effusion' may be made, and the case treated appropriately (e.g. by the application of a crepe bandage support, Jones pressure bandage, or circular woven bandage (Tubigrip)). The case should be re-assessed at weekly intervals thereafter until either the symptoms have settled completely, or a more accurate diagnosis can be established.

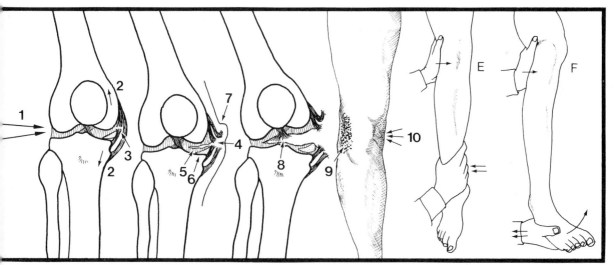

5. *Medial ligament injuries* (1) The ommonest cause is a blow on the lateral de of the knee (1) which forces the joint to valgus (2). With slight force, there is artial tearing of the medial ligament (knee rain) and the knee remains stable on inical testing. With greater violence, the eep portion of the ligament ruptures (partial ar) (3); stressing the knee in 30° flexion ith the foot internally rotated (F) causes ore opening up of the joint than normal, but stressing the joint in extension (E) has no effect. There may be clinical evidence of rotatory instability. With greater violence, superficial *and* deep parts of the ligament rupture (4) and the tear rapidly spreads across the posterior ligament (5). The medial meniscus (6) may also tear. When the knee is stressed in extension (E) slight to moderate opening up will be noted, and if the edge of the ligament rolls over, it may be felt subcutaneously (7). With severe violence, the cruciates (especially anterior cruciate) rupture (8) and the joint opens widely on stressing as at (E). Bruising on the lateral side (9) and medial tenderness (10) are suggestive of medial ligament damage. If there is remaining doubt regarding its integrity, repeat clinical tests after aspiration, or take stress radiographs, comparing one side with the other.

86. *Medial ligament injuries: Treatment* (1)
Sprain: Crepe bandaging or Jones pressure
bandage and crutches till acute symptoms
settle, when the knee may be fully mobilised.
(2) *Isolated tear*, with no evidence of 'rolling
over' of the medial ligament: plaster fixation
with the knee at 45° flexion for 8 weeks.
(3) *Major tear*, and/or where there is a
palpable 'roll over' lesion: operative repair,
meniscectomy and re-attachment of anterior
cruciate ligament if feasible.
Complications of medial ligament injury: (1)
Late valgus instability: It may be possible to
improve stability by reconstruction of the
medial ligament using semitendinosus.
(2) *Persistent rotatory instability:*
Improvement may follow a secondary
medial capsular repair and pes anserinus
transplant.

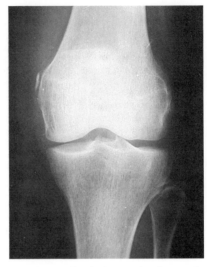

87. *Pelligrini-Stieda disease:* A valgus strain
of the knee may produce partial avulsion of
the medial ligament, with subsequent
calcification in the sub-periosteal
haematoma. There is prolonged pain and
local tenderness, with limitation of flexion,
but no instability. In the acute phase, plaster
immobilisation for 2–3 weeks is advised,
followed by mobilisation. Local
hydrocortisone infiltrations are sometimes
advocated for the chronic case.

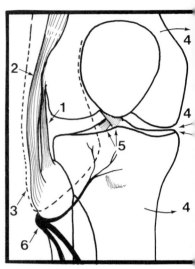

88. *Injuries to the lateral ligament* (1) The
lateral ligament (1) is part of a complex
which includes the biceps femoris tendon (2)
and the fascia lata (3) attached to tibia,
fibula and patella. All these structures may
be damaged if the knee is subjected to a
varus stress (4), and with severe violence the
cruciates (5) will also be torn. The common
peroneal nerve (6) may be stretched or torn.

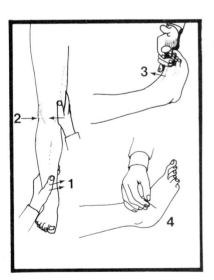

89. *Lateral ligament* (2) Test the stability of
the knee by applying a varus stress with the
knee in extension (1), looking for opening-up
of the joint on the lateral side (2). Test for
common peroneal involvement by looking
for weakness of dorsiflexion of the foot and
toes (3), and/or sensory loss on the dorsum
of the foot and side of the leg (4).

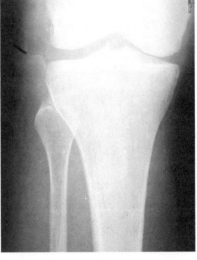

90. *Lateral ligament* (3) In some cases the
radiographs may show tell-tale avulsion
fractures of the fibular head or tibia. (Note in
illustration a small undisplaced fracture of
the head of the fibula, produced by the
lateral ligament, and a large displaced
fragment, indicated by a pointer, avulsed by
the biceps). *Treatment:* (a) If the knee is
clinically stable, symptomatic treatment
only is required (e.g. a crepe bandage and
crutches).

91. *Lateral ligament* (3) *Treatment ctd.:*
(b) If there is instability, operative repair is
indicated, unless there is a definite,
undisplaced fracture which seems likely to
go on to union: in such circumstances a
plaster cylinder should be applied and
retained for 6–8 weeks before mobilisation.
(c) Common peroneal nerve palsy, if present,
is likely to be due either to a lesion in
continuity, or a complete disruption of the
nerve over an extensive area. In neither case
is exploration indicated for the neurological
injury alone, although if the ligament is
being repaired, the opportunity should be
taken to inspect the nerve. In both cases
treatment for drop foot should be started.
With a lesion in continuity, recovery usually
starts within 6 weeks, but a disruptive lesion
carries a poor prognosis.

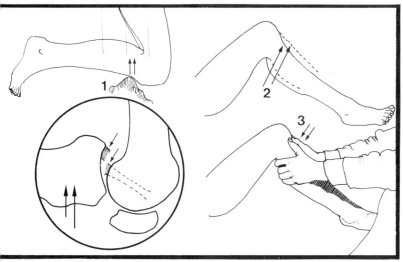

93. (c) Radiographs may show avulsion fractures of the posterior ligament attachments. *Treatment:* If untreated instability persists, disability is considerable, and osteo-arthritis often advances with great rapidity. (a) If there is an undisplaced fracture of the posterior tibial spine representing an avulsion of the posterior attachment of the ligament, the leg should be kept in a plaster cylinder for 6–8 weeks before mobilisation. (b) A displaced tibial spine fracture should be reduced and held with a screw. (c) A detached ligament should be re-attached to bone. As the majority of detachments are posterior, procedures (b) and (c) involve a posterior (popliteal) approach to the knee.

2. *Posterior cruciate ligament injuries:* The mechanism whereby the posterior cruciate ligament is damaged is usually either a fall, in which the tibia strikes a rock or some other object and is forced backwards (1) or from dashboard impact in road traffic accidents. There is often associated damage to the medial or lateral ligaments.

Diagnosis: (a) In most cases there is s striking alteration in the profile of the knee when placed in flexion: the tibia sags backwards (2) and this explains why the anterior drawer test (or the *anterior* cruciate ligament) often gives a false positive: the displaced tibia can be pulled forward to the normal position. (b) The posterior drawer sign may be positive (3). If there is remaining doubt, the knee should be aspirated and examined under anaesthetic.

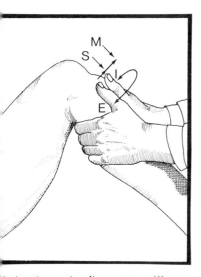

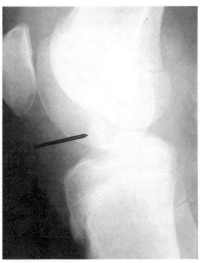

96. *Anterior cruciate ligament tears* (3) *Treatment:* (1) If the anterior tibial spine is undisplaced, treat with a 6–8 week period of fixation in a plaster cylinder. (2) If there is a substantial tibial spine fracture which is displaced, it should be carefully re-positioned at open operation and fixed with a screw. (3) If the anterior attachment of the ligament is avulsed, it should be re-attached to bone at operation. (4) Surgical treatment of the central portion of the anterior cruciate ligament is unrewarding and awaits development. (5) Associated tears of the medial meniscus and medial ligament take precedence in treatment. Any residual antero-posterior drift should be dealt with by intensive quadriceps building.

4. *Anterior cruciate ligament tears* (1) Isolated tears are uncommon (forced flexion or hyperextension injuries); tears of the medial ligament and/or medial meniscus may be associated.

Diagnosis (1) Note variations in the anterior drawer sign: slight slip + internal rotation of the tibia (S + I) = isolated anterior cruciate tear; slight slip + external rotation (S + E) = medial ligament tear; marked slip without rotation (M) = tear anterior cruciate + medial ligament.

95. *Anterior cruciate ligament tears* (2) *Diagnosis* (2) Carefully examine A.P. and lateral radiographs of the knee, looking for tell-tale avulsion fractures (ill: avulsion of the anterior attachment—the anterior tibial spine—indicated with pointer). (3) Independently test the medial ligament, and look for evidence of meniscus injury.

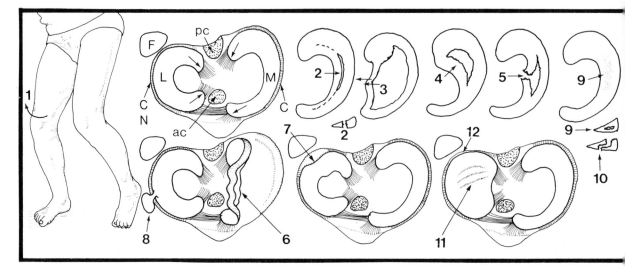

97. *Meniscus injuries:* In the young adult, the menisci are generally injured as a result of a rotational stress applied to the flexed, weight bearing knee (1). Injury can also result from rapid knee extension (anterior horn tears) and direct violence (cysts). The medial (M) and lateral (L) menisci are attached at their anterior and posterior horns to the tibia, and by coronary ligaments (C) to the femur and tibia. The majority of tears commence as vertical splits in the substance of the meniscus

('longitudinal tear') (2); the free edge may displace centrally, forming a bucket handle tear (3) or a racquet tear of the posterior (4) or anterior horns. The central edge may rupture forming a parrot-beak tear (5). In peripheral detachments the whole meniscus may displace centrally (6) or more commonly, the posterior horn only of the lateral meniscus is affected (7). Congenital discoid menisci may also become detached (12) with ridging of their upper surfaces (11), a common condition in

children. Detachments of the anterior horn also occur, but are less common. A meniscus cyst (8) may result from a direct blow (such as a kick) and the lateral meniscus is most commonly affected. Cysts of the medial meniscus must be distinguished from pes anserinus ganglions. In middle age horizontal tears may occur within the substance of the meniscus (9), sometimes without trauma, and may convert to tears with potential for displacement (10).

98. *Diagnosis of meniscus injuries:* Note the following points:

1. Acute tears in the young adult generally result from a clear-cut incident of weight bearing stress, often while engaging in an athletic pursuit such as football. There is immediate pain in the knee and difficulty in weight bearing. Initial disability is usually marked, and if the patient has been playing football, he will be unable to continue. This important aspect of the history should be clarified.

2. Meniscus tears are very uncommon in women. Dislocation of the patella or chondromalacia patellae should always be eliminated before the diagnosis of a torn meniscus is contemplated in women.

3. Absence of knee swelling may be deceptive. After peripheral tears there is certainly usually a rapidly forming haemarthrosis but there may be no immediate swelling after longitudinal tears (the menisci are avascular). Any reactionary synovitis may appear quite late (e.g. several

days) after the initial incident.

4. There is almost invariably joint line tenderness, but as many minor lesions give this finding, this is of little diagnostic value apart from localisation to either side of the joint.

5. A springy block to full extension is however almost diagnostic of a displaced, bucket-handle tear.

6. Some days after the first incident other signs may appear, such as quadriceps wasting and slight oedema in the joint line. When pain subsides, other confirmatory tests such as MacMurray's manoeuvre may give positive results.

7. Radiographs should always be taken to exclude other pathology.

8. In chronic lesions, positive physical signs are often lacking, and further investigation may be required (e.g. by arthroscopy, arthrography, provocative exercises).

Treatment

1. *Locked knee:* Admission at an early date

for meniscectomy. Pending admission, a pressure bandage support, crutches, and analgesics may be prescribed. Attempts to unlock the knee are of questionable value.

2. *Case where the history and findings suggest a fresh meniscus tear:* Treat conservatively. Remember that peripheral detachments can unite, and that many joint injuries may mimic a torn meniscus yet recover completely. A pressure bandage should be applied, the patient given crutches and advised to practise quadriceps exercises. Analgesics may be required. Re-assess thereafter at weekly intervals until the condition fully recovers or until there can be no doubt that the patient is suffering from a torn meniscus and that excision is essential.

3. *Meniscus cysts:* Excise the cyst. In addition, many advocate removal of the associated meniscus which is not infrequently torn.

4. *Horizontal cleavage tears:* Symptoms may resolve with physiotherapy alone, and meniscectomy may frequently be avoided.

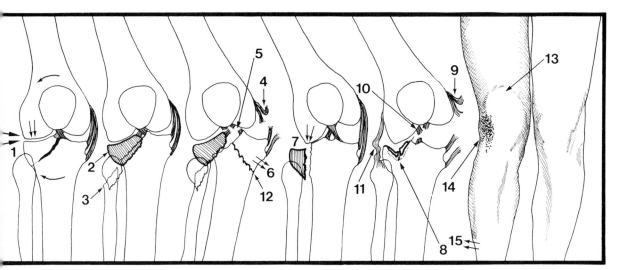

9. *Fractures of the lateral tibial table:* hese generally result from a severe valgus ~~t~~ress, and several patterns of injury are ~~~~und.

~~~~) Impact of the mass of the lateral femoral ~~~~ondyle may be responsible for the 'sliding ~~~~acture' which passes downwards and ~~~~terally from the tibial spine region, the ~~~~ain articular surface remaining intact (1). ~~~~ith increasing violence the tibial fragment ~~~~ depressed (2) and there may be an ~~~~ssociated fracture of the fibular neck (3). In the most severe cases there may be rupture of the medial ligament (4), rupture of the cruciates (5), and medial subluxation of the tibia (6). (b) The 'corner' of the lateral femoral condyle may cause a split fracture (7) or (c) a crush fracture (8) of the tibial table. In either of these cases there may be tearing of the medial ligament (9) or the cruciates (10), relative lengthening of the lateral ligament (11), or crushing of the lateral mensicus. (d) A second fracture line (12) may convert any of these injuries into a bicondylar fracture. (e) Fractures of the medial tibial table are uncommon, but do occur. They may be associated with lateral ligament ruptures and common peroneal nerve palsy. (Their treatment is along similar lines to lateral tibial table injuries.)

Diagnosis: (1) The clinical findings of lateral tibial table fracture include haemarthrosis (13), lateral bruising and abrasions (14), valgus deformity of the knee (15).

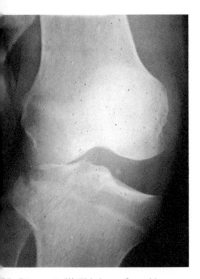

~~~~0. *Diagnosis* (2) This is confirmed by ~~~~diographs, an A.P. view with a 15° tube ~~~~t giving the most information. Measure the ~~~~aximal depression of any fragment relative ~~~~ neighbouring intact bone or a line ~~~~ojected from the (intact) medial table. If ~~~~e medial ligament is suspect (e.g. local ~~~~nderness, etc.) stress films (preferably after ~~~~spiration and under G.A.) may be helpful. ~~~~l:~~ small split fracture with stress films ~~~~owing medial ligament tear.

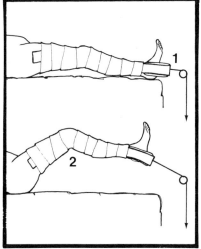

101. *Treatment:* (1) *No ligament damage, no tibial subluxation, and a depression of less than 10 mm:* Apply skin traction of 6–7 lb (3 kg) (1); quadriceps exercises should be commenced immediately and flexion as soon as pain will permit (2). Traction may often be discontinued after 4 weeks; weight bearing may be permitted after 8 weeks. The late results are generally excellent.

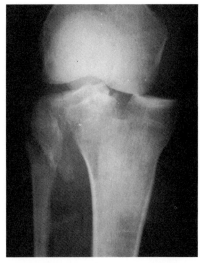

102. *Treatment* (2) *Sliding fracture with 10 mm or more depression:* Unless treated, there will be persistent valgus deformity of the knee, and often some slight residual instability due to relative lengthening of the lateral ligament. Symptoms of weakness, instability, and pain may lead to appreciable disability. (Note medial tibial subluxation in illustration.)

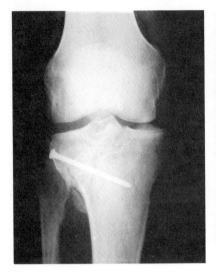

103. *Treatment (2) ctd.:* The fragment should be exposed, coaxed back into position, and fixed with a long screw (ill.) or screws or a piece of studding placed horizontally and nutted at both ends ('bolt fixation'). Any accompanying medial ligament rupture should be repaired.

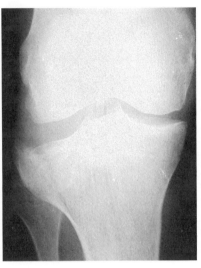

104. *Treatment (3) Split fracture with minimal displacement and any accompanying depression of under 10 mm (ill.):* treat as 101. (4) *Split fracture with marked separation:* Open reduction and internal fixation as in 103. Any accompanying medial ligament rupture should be repaired.

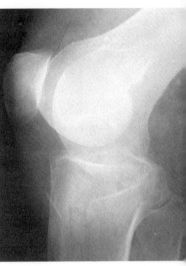

105. *Treatment (5) Crush fracture with depression of more than 10 mm:* With increasing depression, the results of conservative treatment become poorer, and surgical treatment becomes more difficult. On balance, injuries of this type are probably best dealt with by surgery where an attempt is made to elevate the depressed fragments. The intervening space is filled with iliac bone.

106. *Treatment (6) Bicondylar fractures:* If undisplaced, these may be treated by 4 weeks' skin traction in a Thomas splint. The splint can then usually be discarded, and the knee mobilised while traction is maintained (as 101). A longer period may be required before there is sufficient callus to permit weight bearing.

If there is separation of the fragments, they should be approximated using screws or studding (as 103); a supplementary plate may be required to maintain the condylar fragments aligned with the tibia (e.g. a T-plate).

After any of the operative procedures described, mobilisation should be started as early as possible; in many cases traction (as 101) may be used immediately post-operatively. If the quality of fixation is poor, a short (say 3–4 weeks) period in a plaster cylinder may be desirable.

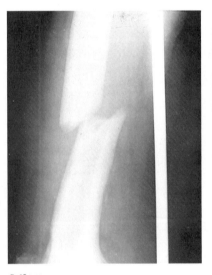

Self test
107. Describe this fracture: how is it being treated? Assuming conservative treatment was being continued, would you make any correction?

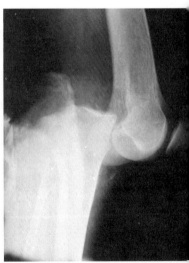

108. What does the radiograph show? What structure is at serious risk?

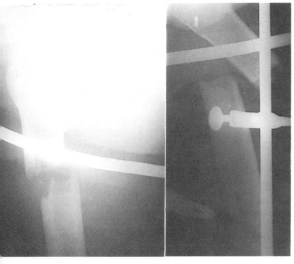
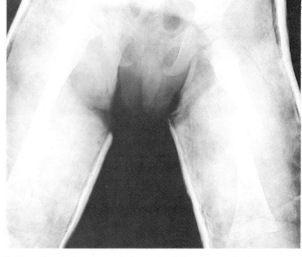

09. What is the level of fracture shown on these radiographs? How is it being treated? Is the position acceptable?

110. Describe the fracture and the method of treatment. Is the position acceptable?

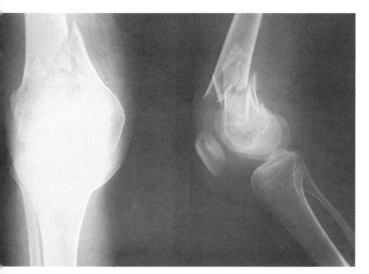
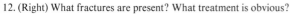
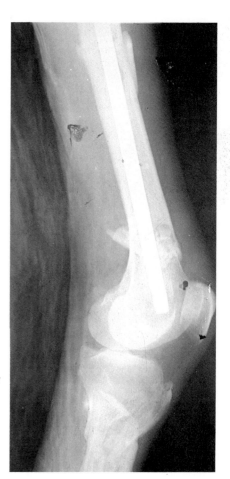

11. (Above) Describe this fracture. What is the unusual feature about the deformity? How might it be treated conservatively?

12. (Right) What fractures are present? What treatment is obvious?

107. Fracture of the femoral shaft at the junction between the middle and distal thirds. It is being treated in a Thomas splint. Traction should be increased, and further padding placed under the fracture to correct the angulation.

108. Dislocation of the knee. (Posterior dislocation with 90° rotational deformity superimposed.) The popliteal artery is in grave danger.

109. Proximal third fracture of the femur being treated in a Thomas splint. The proximal fragment is flexed so that there is no bony apposition, and probably soft tissue between the bone ends. The position is unacceptable, (risk of non-union or mal-union) and internal fixation would be advocated.

110. Oblique fracture of the mid-shaft of the femur (with shortening and angulation) in a child. It is being treated in a plaster hip spica. The position is acceptable: union is likely to be rapid; the shortening will almost certainly resolve spontaneously; any residual angulation is also likely to disappear with re-modelling.

111. Supracondylar fracture of the femur. Angulation is slight, and is in the reverse direction from normal. Traction in a straight Thomas splint might be used and mobilisation commenced at an early date. Alternatively, this fracture might be dealt with by Hamilton-Russell traction and cast bracing.

112. There is a fracture of the mid-shaft of the femur and a supracondylar fracture, both held in alignment with a Küntscher nail. In addition, there is a fracture of the proximal third of the tibia. Such injuries are typical of high velocity road traffic accidents.

13. Fractures of the tibia

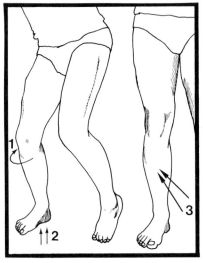

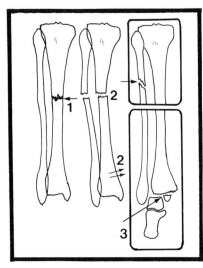

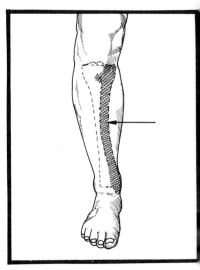

1. *General principles* (1) *Mechanisms of injury:* The tibia is vulnerable to torsional stresses (1) (e.g. sporting injuries), to violence transmitted through the feet (2) (e.g. falls from a height, road traffic accidents), and from direct blows (3) (e.g. road traffic accidents, blows from falling rock, masonry, etc.).

2. *General principles* (2) Isolated fractures of either the tibia or fibula may occur from direct voilence (1) although this is comparatively uncommon. As in the case of the forearm bones, indirect violence leads to fracture of both tibia and fibula (2). Always obtain radiographs of the whole length of the limb to exclude a distal injury accompanying a proximal fracture (3).

3. *General principles* (3) Note that a third of the tibia is subcutaneous. There is little to resist the spiky end of a fractured tibia from penetrating the skin; again, any direct violence to the shin is uncushioned, and the skin is readily split: these factors account for the frequency of both types of compounding in tibial shaft fractures.

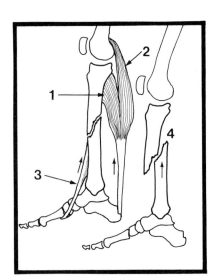

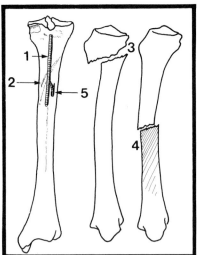

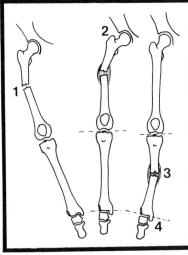

4. *General principles* (4) Partly because of its triangular shape, and partly because of the frequency of injury caused by torsional forces, oblique and spiral fractures of the tibia are common. Muscle tone in the soleus (1), gastrocnemius (2) and tibialis anterior (3) tends to produce shortening and displacement in fractures of this type (4).

5. *General principles* (5) The popliteal artery (1) is anchored as it passes under the origin of the soleus at the soleal line (2). It is susceptible to damage in upper tibial fractures (3) and may cause Volkmann's ischaemia of the calf with permanent flexion contracture of the ankle. Fractures of the tibia may be followed by ischaemia of the distal fragment (4) through interruption of the blood supply through the nutrient artery (5).

6. *General principles* (6) It is particularly important to correct angulation in fractures of this weight bearing bone. Unlike angulation in femoral shaft fractures (1) which can be compensated at the hip (2), residual angulation in tibial fractures (3) will throw inevitable stress at the ankle (4) and/or the knee, leading to pain and secondary osteo-arthritis.

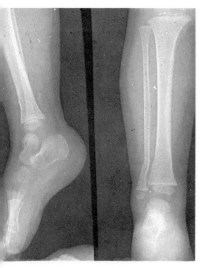

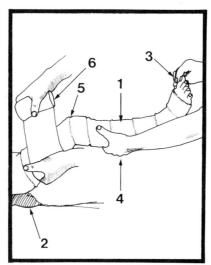

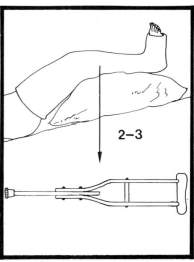

7. *Undisplaced fractures* (1) In children, due to the thickness of the subcutaneous fat and periosteum, and the elasticity of the bones, fractures are often of greenstick pattern and simple. In many cases, too, the fractures are minimally displaced. (Ill: Greenstick fracture distal tibia and fibula, betrayed by fibular kinking and tibial cortical buckling.)

8. *Undisplaced fractures* (2) When deformity is minimal, apply a long leg plaster immediately over a generous layer of wool (1) (mild sedation only may be required). A sandbag under the buttocks (2) may be helpful, while an assistant holds the toes (3) and supports the calf (4). The knee is slightly flexed (5) and the plaster may be applied in one stage with or without a slab (6).

9. *Undisplaced fractures* (3) Elevation of the leg and a regular, careful check of the circulation is essential, and admission for this is desirable. In a child, non-weight bearing with crutches can usually be allowed as soon as there is no circulatory risk (say 2–3 days post injury). Thereafter the child should be seen every 2–3 weeks (the casualty rate in children's plasters is high).

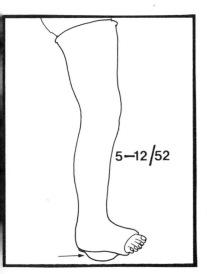

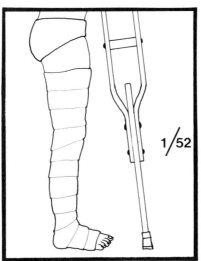

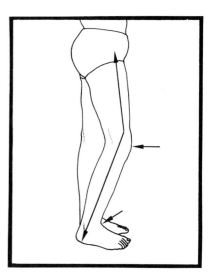

10. *Undisplaced fractures* (4) A walking heel can certainly be applied when there is evidence of early callus on the radiographs (e.g. after 3–4 weeks in a child of 9). Before that a heel may be applied if in your assessment there is no risk of displacement or problems from swelling. Any hesitation may sometimes be dispelled by the appearance of the sole of the plaster which often indicates premature successful weight bearing!

11. *Undisplaced fractures* (5) The fracture may be assessed for union after say 4–5 weeks in a child of 4, 8 weeks in a child of 8, and 8–12 weeks in a child of 12. On removal of the plaster no support for the limb is usually required, but confidence may be raised by a crepe bandage. Crutches for the first few days are advocated as the child often shows timidity in commencing weight bearing: and the parents may require reassurance.

12. *Undisplaced fractures* (6) The child should be reviewed 2 weeks after removal of the plaster. In most cases he will be walking unsupported, the movements in the knee and ankle will have returned, and the limb lengths will be equal. The child may then be discharged. The parents should be reassured that any residual limp will resolve, and that athletic activities may be resumed say in a further 2 months.

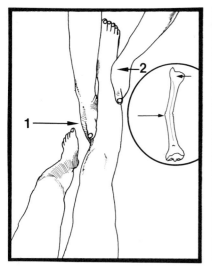

13. *Angled fractures in children* (1) These are reduced under general anaesthesia. One hand is placed over the fracture site (1) while the other, at the ankle (2), is used to correct the angulation. Although the A.P. plane only is illustrated, naturally any deformity in the lateral plane should be similarly corrected.

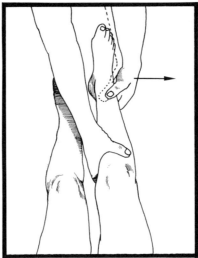

14. *Angled fractures* (2) The pressure of the hand at the ankle should be released, and any tendency for the deformity to recur noted (indicating springy intact periosteum). If this is found, particular care must be taken during the application of the plaster to maintain full correction; alternatively, complete tearing of the periosteum may be obtained by over correction of the deformity.

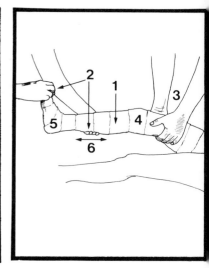

15. *Angled fractures* (3) If there is little tendency to recurrence of angulation, the plaster may be applied as follows: wool roll is wound round the limb from toes to groin (1); one assistant supports the fracture and the toes (2) while the second takes the weight of the thigh (3). The knee is flexed to 15° (4) and the ankle maintained at right angles (5). The supporting hands are moved during the application of the plaster (6). Use a sandbag under the buttocks.

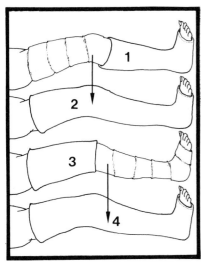

16. *Angled fractures* (4) If there is a tendency to re-angulation, the plaster must be moulded while it sets. Except in the smallest of children it is difficult to apply a full length plaster and mould the fracture within the setting time. A two-stage technique may be used: *either* apply a below knee plaster (1), mould, and complete the thigh (2) *or* apply the thigh cuff first (3), complete the plaster (4), and then mould.

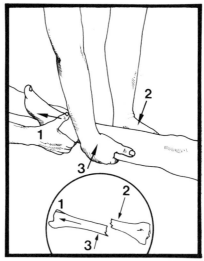

17. *Displaced fractures of the tibia* (1) An assistant applies strong traction in the line of the limb (1) while strong pressure is applied with the heels of the hands above (2) and below (3) the fracture to correct the displacement. The traction is then slackened off to allow the bone ends to engage.

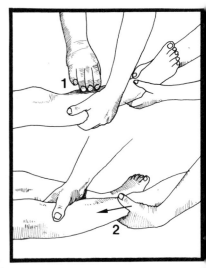

18. *Displaced fractures of the tibia* (2) Checking the reduction clinically can be difficult. Try palpating the fracture line along the subcutaneous border (1) or in the case of a transverse fracture, confirm that a hitch is present by noting resistance to attempted telescoping (2).

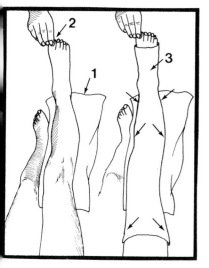

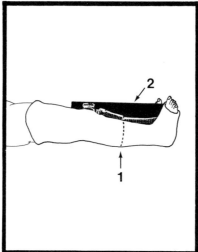

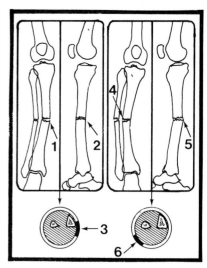

19. *Displaced fractures of the tibia* (3) If the reduction obtained by manipulation is somewhat precarious and it is feared that the fracture might slip during the application of plaster, place the limb on a firm plaster pillow (1), steady the leg by holding the toes (2) and apply a thick, anterior, plaster slab (3) tucking the edges well round the limb. When it has set, the leg can then be carefully bandaged into the slab.

20. *Wedging* (1) Ultimately, if necessitated by circumstance, displacement and even off-ending may be accepted in children. If, however, the radiographs indicate residual angulation, this should be corrected: and this may usually be done by wedging. Begin by marking the plaster circumferentially at the level of the fracture (1) using the radiographs as a guide (2).

21. *Wedging* (2) Now carefully work out where the plaster must hinge to correct the deformity. For example, where there is medial angulation (1) and the lateral projection is normal (2), the hinge should lie medially (3). Where there is lateral angulation (4) along with posterior angulation (5) the hinge should be positioned postero-laterally (6).

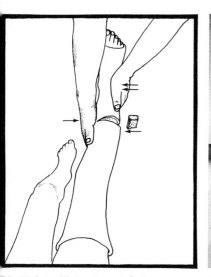

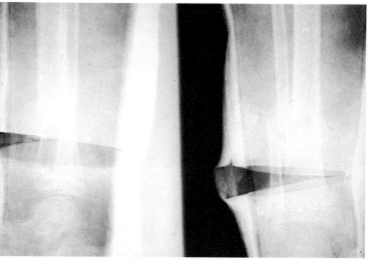

22. *Wedging* (3) Cut through $\frac{7}{8}$ of the circumference of the plaster at the marked level, sparing the hinge; use a plaster saw, or a hacksaw with a fine blade. Now spring the plaster 1–2 cm open; maintain the position temporarily by placing a suitably sized piece of previously prepared cork into the mouth of the wedge.

23. *Wedging* (4) Check radiographs should be taken, and any adjustment made on the result. If a satisfactory correction has been obtained, wool should be packed lightly into the gap on either side of the cork, and the plaster reconstituted locally with a 6″ (15 cm) plaster bandage.

(Ill: A badly angled fracture in the distal third of the tibia has been corrected by wedging. Although the level of the wedge is more distal than it should be, an almost anatomical position has been achieved.) General anaesthesia is not required for wedging, but mild sedation is desirable.

After care should follow the lines described for undisplaced fractures (9–12).

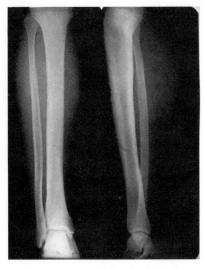

24. *Tibial fractures in the adult* (1) In the adult many tibial fractures may be treated conservatively, and where good results with few complications are the rule, it is unwise to advocate surgery with its additional risks. Conservative treatment may with good reason always be advised for stress, isolated (ill.) and undisplaced fractures, and for slightly displaced stable fractures.

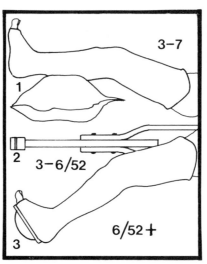

25. *Minimally displaced fractures in the adult* (2) A long leg plaster is applied, check radiographs are taken, and the limb elevated (1) for 3–7 days until swelling subsides. The plaster is checked for slackness and changed if required. As soon as the patient has mastered crutches he may be allowed home (2). A walking heel is applied (3) usually after 3–6 weeks (depending on your assessment of stability) and the plaster retained till union.

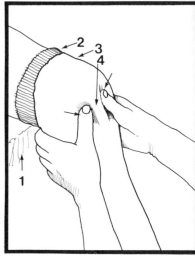

26. *Sarmiento plaster* (1) Alternatively, at 4–6 weeks post injury, the long leg plaster is removed and a Sarmiento cast applied. The patient sits on the edge of the plaster table (1), the foot being steadied by the lap of the operator. Stockingette (2) and wool roll are applied, and the plaster extended over the knee (3). It is firmly moulded (before setting) round the patellar ligament (4).

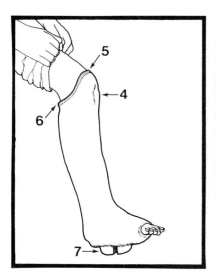

27. *Sarmiento plaster* (2) The plaster is then trimmed from the upper pole of the patella (5) round to the upper part of the calf (6); check that knee movement is free before turning down the stockingette and finishing in the usual way. A rocker sole may then be applied (7) and weight bearing and knee flexion commenced. The plaster is retained until union is sound.

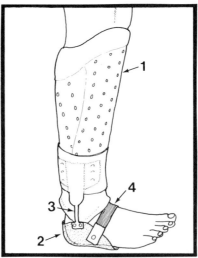

28. *Functional bracing with a gaiter:* In the later stages of fixation, or even as early as 4 weeks when instability is not a problem, a supporting gaiter may be used instead of plaster. The type illustrated may be fashioned from perforated Orthoplast (Johnson & Johnson) thermoplastic sheet (1). For additional support a plastic heel seat (2) may be secured to the brace with polyethylene hinges (3) and a garter strap (4).

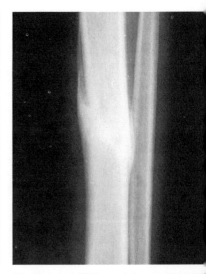

29. *After care:* (1) Intervals between hospital attendances should not exceed 4 weeks, and the fixation—plaster or brace—changed if it becomes unduly slack. (2) Tibial fractures take an average 16 weeks to unite, but union may be sought in 8–12 weeks in the case of a hairline crack, and after 12 weeks in a transverse fracture. Radiographs should be taken (ill: advanced union in tibial fracture) preferably out of plaster.

0. *After care ctd.:* (3) Apparent radiological union should be confirmed by clinical examination. (4) If union is judged sound a crepe bandage support is prescribed for the leg and knee, and full unsupported weight bearing commenced. Sticks or crutches may be required to give confidence over the first few weeks, but the patient should be encouraged to discard these as soon as possible (although the elderly patient may have difficulty in this respect). (5) The patient should be reviewed 2 weeks after plaster has been discarded. The following problems may be encountered:

The knee: pain or discomfort in the knee at the beginning of mobilisation is normal. A small to moderate *effusion* is common. If the period of immobilisation is under 16 weeks, return of flexion is usually rapid.

Physiotherapy is nevertheless advisable in the majority of cases to encourage knee flexion, to develop the quadriceps and to help restore the gait to normal.

(b) *The ankle:* Slight *swelling and oedema* of the foot and ankle are usual for several months after tibial fractures. A crepe bandage or circular woven support is advised until this swelling subsides. Gross swelling with marked stiffness and pain in the foot and ankle should suggest Sudeck's atrophy. Swelling which is maximal over the fracture calls for re-assessment of union. Slight *restriction of ankle movements* is common after tibial fractures, but is seldom incapacitating.

(c) *Athletic activities: Swimming* may be permitted almost as soon as the plaster has been discarded, and should be encouraged.

Cycling can be allowed as soon as knee flexion will allow (*c.* 110°). *Golf* may be allowed as soon as limb swelling is no longer a problem. *Rugby, football and gymnastics* should not be permitted until endosteal callus is sound, till knee flexion is nearly normal (say 130°) and muscle power is restored.

(d) *Return to work:* The patient should be encouraged to return to work as soon as possible, and in sedentary work the patient may do so while in plaster. Factors which may delay return are (a) severe persistent oedema in jobs involving prolonged standing; (b) lack of knee flexion in work involving kneeling; (c) muscle and functional weakness in jobs involving work at heights.

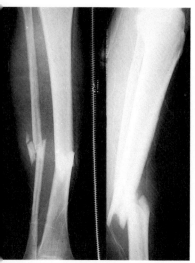 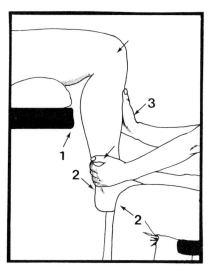 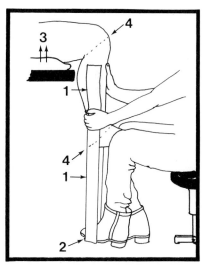

1. *Displaced but potentially stable fractures in the adult:* Transverse fractures of the tibia in particular are potentially stable if good bony apposition can be obtained. Many surgeons like to manipulate this type of fracture; if a good reduction is obtained then conservative treatment is continued along the lines already described; if the position is unsatisfactory, then they may proceed to open reduction.

32. *Reduction techniques:* (a) The fracture may be manipulated as already described for the child (17). (b) It is often helpful, especially if assistance is limited, to let gravity work to your advantage. The patient's knee is flexed over the end of the table (1). Use your own knees to steady or to apply traction to the foot (2). Both hands are free to manipulate the fracture (3).

33. *Reduction techniques ctd.:* (c) Alternatively, it is sometimes possible to apply temporary traction using skin traction tapes (1). The traction may be controlled by the operator's foot on the spreader bar (2) and by elevating the table (3). After manipulation a padded plaster is applied over the tapes from the heel to the knee (4). The tapes are cut, and the foot of the plaster completed.

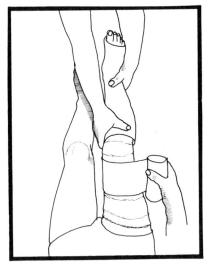

34. *Reduction techniques ctd.:* Once the leg and foot have been encased in plaster in methods (b) and (c), the knee is gently extended to 15°, wool applied to the thigh, and the thigh cuff completed with 8″ (20 cm) plaster bandages. Check radiographs are desirable on completion of the below-knee portion of the plaster, and after the thigh cuff has been added.

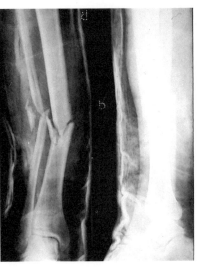

35. *Reduction techniques ctd.:* If manipulation succeeds in bringing the bone ends into apposition, any residual angulation may be corrected within the first few weeks by wedging. (Ill: Post-manipulation radiograph of the previous fracture (31). There is an unacceptable degree of angulation although good apposition has been obtained. The angulation was easily corrected by wedging and union proceeded uneventfully.)

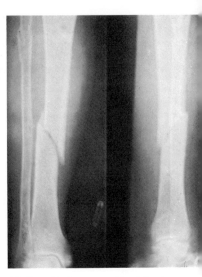

36. *Unstable fractures with minimal displacement:* Oblique and spiral fractures are potentially unstable. Although they may be managed conservatively along the lines indicated, meticulous supervision is necessary during the first 6 weeks. Slackness in the plaster must be promptly dealt with. Slight slipping of the fracture may be accepted, but if evidence of substantial displacement is found, internal fixation should be considered.

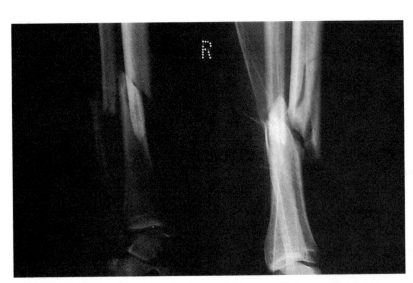

37. *Displaced unstable fractures* (1) Fractures which are unstable because of their pattern may be treated by manipulation to the best position that can be obtained, and by controlling angulation by wedging. Nevertheless this method of treatment requires much experienced supervision; shortening is inevitable, union may be delayed, and stiffness in the knee become a problem: so open reduction and internal fixation are often preferred in the treatment of fractures of this type.

Method: A tourniquet is applied and the fracture exposed and reduced under vision. Some form of internal splintage may then be used to maintain the reduction (e.g. cross screwing, application of a Sherman or Eggar plate, etc.). After wound closure a long leg plaster is applied, with after care along the lines described for the closed treatment of adult fractures.

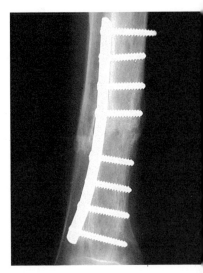

38. *Displaced unstable fractures* (2) Alternatively, some form of rigid internal fixation may be used (e.g. a dynamic compression plate, intramedullary nail, etc.). When the degree of mechanical support is high, a pressure bandage is applied after surgery, and knee flexion commenced. A cast brace may be worn from the time weight bearing starts (2–6 weeks) till there is evidence of union. (Ill.)

39. *Compound fractures of the tibia:* The following points summarise an approach to the management of compound fractures of the tibia: (1) *The skin wound* should be dealt with along the lines suggested on page 49. (2) *The fracture* may be treated by a variety of methods dictated by its pattern, the wound, and the instrumentation available.
a) If the fracture is stable and undisplaced the wound should be dealt with and the limb placed in a padded plaster.
b) If the fracture is stable but displaced, the wound should be extended sufficiently to allow reduction under vision. Plaster is then applied after wound closure.
c) If the fracture is unstable, but the damage to the skin with the risks of infection slight (Grades 1 and 2), open reduction and internal fixation should be considered.
d) If the fracture is displaced and unstable, and damage to the skin severe (and/or the risks of contamination appreciable) it is advisable to avoid internal fixation with the introduction of foreign material into the wound. Several procedures are available to stabilise the fracture without wide stripping of the tissues:

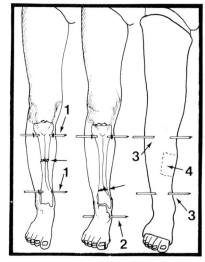

40. The major complication of shortening may be prevented by placing Steinman pins above and below the fracture (1)—the calcaneus may be used in distal fractures (2). The fracture is reduced under vision and the pins incorporated in the plaster (3). (It may be possible to bridge the pins with plaster before the fracture fixation clamp is removed—otherwise use an anterior slab as in 19.) The plaster may be windowed for wound dressing (4).

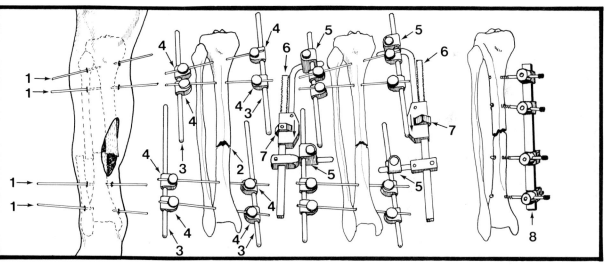

41. *External fixation systems:* The previous method does not prevent undesirable movement at the fracture site, nor does it offer provision for local bone absorption; the incidence of non-union tends to be rather high. Nevertheless two-pin fixation will preserve length until sound wound healing is achieved, and when more radical surgery may be carried out if required.

Better control is possible when two or more pins are inserted into each fragment and linked together mechanically. There are several systems based on these principles (e.g. Hoffman, A.O. External Fixator, Universal Day Frame, etc.). In the Hexcel system illustrated Steinman pins are inserted into each fragment (1). The fracture is reduced (2) and the ends of the pins connected in pairs to rods (3) by split clamps (4). The rods in turn are rigidly connected together by further clamps (5) to square section threaded bars (6) which allow compression of the fragments (7).

Other systems rely on cantilever compression screws—e.g. Oxford system (8).

All these external fixation methods are designed to support the fracture *without* plaster until union, and at the same time to give access to the wound. Their disadvantage is the risk of pin-track infections and loosening.

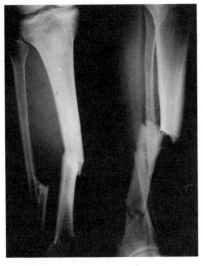

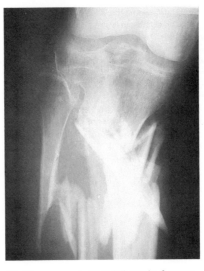

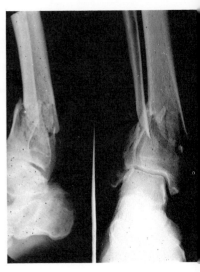

42. *Double fracture:* Plaster fixation gives poor support, and the incidence of non-union at one level is high (although if alignment is maintained, a good result may follow grafting). An intramedullary nail, introduced behind the patellar ligament, is a good method of treatment, and may often be done without exposing either fracture. A long plate is less satisfactory, carrying some risk of devitalising the central fragment.

43. *Gross comminution:* Where the fracture is highly comminuted, the multiplicity of avascular, detached bone fragments are generally impossible to reduce. Conservative management is indicated, and, if after 10–14 weeks there is mal-union or non-union, the appropriate secondary procedure may be carried out.

44. *Fractures in the distal third:* Comminuted fractures in the distal third may also be amenable to treatment by conservative methods; but where a satisfactory reduction cannot be obtained, internal fixation using a plate with cortical screws proximally and cancellous screws distally may be used. *Fractures of the tibia and femur in the same limb:* See Femur, 49.

Self test

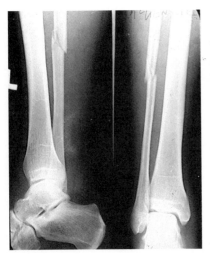

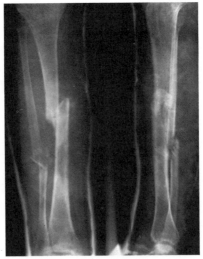

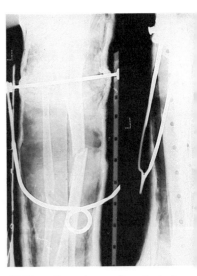

45. *Isolated fractures of the fibula:* The fibula may be fractured by direct violence; symptomatic treatment only is required (e.g. a below-knee walking plaster for 6 weeks). Always ensure, however, that the tibia is not fractured at another level, or that the fibular fracture represents part of a more complex injury to the ankle joint.

46. These radiographs were taken through plaster 10 weeks after injury. Describe the fracture. What further treatment would you advocate? What is the prognosis?

47. The radiographs are of a patient who suffered a fracture of the tibia and femur in the same leg: both injuries are being treated conservatively. Comment on the position of the tibial fracture.

46. The radiographs are of an oblique fracture of the tibia in the middle third, with an associated fibular fracture at the junction of the middle and lower thirds. Both fractures are uniting, and bridging callus is well formed. The general alignment is good. No correction is required: the patient will require to continue with fixation for about another 4 weeks before plaster can be discarded (or a cast brace may be substituted). There will be approximately 1 cm of shortening, but the functional prognosis is excellent.

47. There is an oblique fracture of the tibia in the middle third, with an associated fracture of the fibula. There is a fair degree of persistent medial angulation. The overlying shadow suggests that an attempt has been made to correct this by wedging; it would be desirable to make a further attempt to improve the alignment.

14. Injuries about the ankle

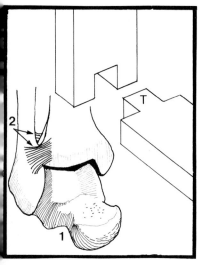

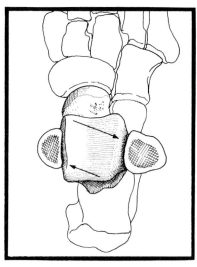

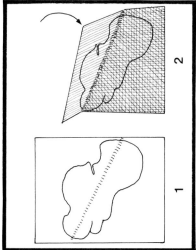

1. *Anatomical considerations (1)* The ankle joint is often fairly compared with the mortise and tenon joint of the woodworker. The talus (1) resembles the tenon (T), and is supported by the two malleoli and the articular surface of the tibia (the ankle mortise).

The lateral malleolus is firmly attached to the tibia by the strong anterior and posterior tibio-fibular ligaments (2).

2. *Anatomical considerations (2)* The talus is held in the mortise on the medial side by the very strong deltoid ligament (1), and on the lateral side by the lateral (external) ligament (2).

The anterior part of the upper articular surface of the talus is wider than the posterior part (3). When the foot is dorsiflexed, the talus pushes the fibula laterally (4) and is more firmly gripped in the ankle mortise.

3. *Mechanics of injury (1)* The *function* of the ankle mortise is threatened if the malleoli are fractured or the tibio-fibular ligaments are torn. The *stability* of the talus may also be reduced by rupture of the medial or lateral ligaments. The commonest injury is when the talus is rotated in the mortise, fracturing one or both malleoli.

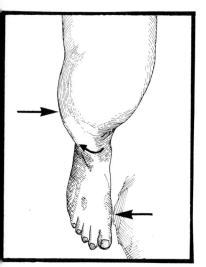

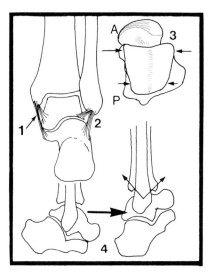

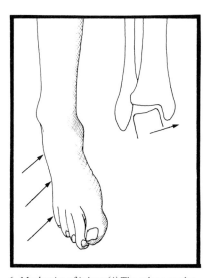

4. *Mechanics of injury (2)* External rotation of the talus may be produced in two different ways. (a) The foot may act as a long lever; any rotational force applied to the inside of the foot is transferred to the talus with a mechanical advantage as in any system of levers. Even greater leverage may occur if, for example, the foot is attached to a ski.

5. *Mechanics of injury (3)* (b) The axis of movement of the sub-talar joint is known to run obliquely in the direction of the crease on this paper model (1).

Inversion of the heel, represented by folding the paper, results in external rotation of the talus (2). (Rose's torque-converter principle.) A common history is of the ankle 'coggling over' on uneven ground.

6. *Mechanics of injury (4)* The talus may be forced into relatively pure adduction as, for example, when the side of the inverted foot strikes the ground heavily. (The external rotation of the talus, produced by inversion of the calcaneus, being countered by the internal rotation of the strike, resulting in net adduction.)

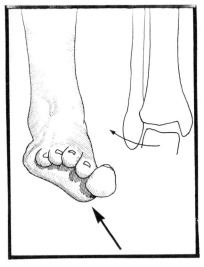

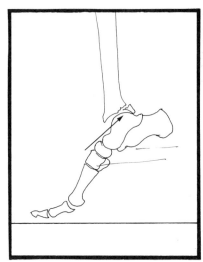

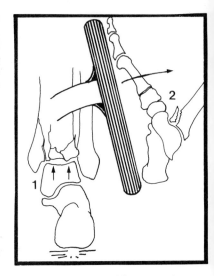

7. *Mechanics of injury (5)* Similarly, if force is applied to the medial side of the heel and foot, the talus will tend to abduct in the ankle mortise.

8. *Mechanics of injury (6)* Many injuries occur during the course of walking or running. Under these circumstances there are additional forces transmitted to the posterior part of the inferior articular surface of the tibia (posterior malleolus).

9. *Mechanics of injury (7)* Compression injuries may be caused by (1) falls from a height, forces being transmitted vertically from heel impact, or (2) following rapid deceleration in car accidents—sometimes aggravated by the pedals being driven into the front compartment and the ankle being forcibly dorsiflexed. Comminution is a feature of this type of injury.

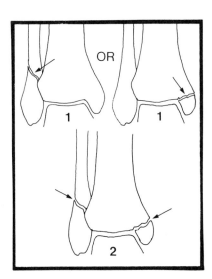

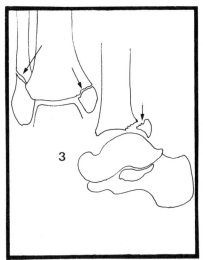

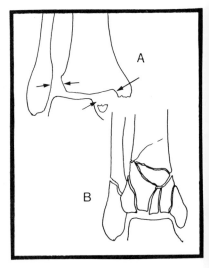

10. *Classification of Potts fracture (1)* Fractures of the distal tibia and fibula involving the ankle joint are loosely referred to as Potts fractures. There are many classifications of these fractures. In the simplest, three degrees of increasing severity are described—(1) Fractures involving one malleolus—first degree Potts fracture. (2) Bi-malleolar or second degree Potts fracture.

11. *Classification of Potts fracture (2)* (3) In third degree Potts fractures, there is a bi-malleolar fracture with in addition a fracture of the posterior part of the inferior articular surface of the tibia—often referred to as the third malleolus. These fractures may also be referred to as tri-malleolar fractures.

12. *Classification of Potts fracture (3)* These fractures may be qualified by noting the presence of diastasis of the ankle or vertical compression.
(A) First degree Potts fracture with diastasis.
(B) Second degree Potts fracture with vertical compression.

Classification of ankle fractures. A fuller and widely accepted classification of ankle fractures is that of Lauge-Hansen which groups these fractures under double-barreled headings. The first word in each group title refers to the position of the foot at the time of injury; the second refers to the direction in which the talus moves within the ankle mortise in response to the causal forces. There are five main groups; they have been arranged here in order of frequency, and a common terminology of usage has been included.

Order of frequency	Lauge-Hansen Classification	Lauge-Hansen Contraction	Position of foot	Direction of talar movement	Common terminology
1	Supination/lateral rotation	S.L.	Inversion	Lateral (external) rotation	External rotation injury without diastasis
2	Pronation/abduction	P.A.	Eversion	Abduction	Abduction injury
3	Pronation/lateral rotation	P.L.	Eversion	Lateral (external) rotation	External rotation injury with diastasis
4	Supination/adduction	S.A.	Inversion	Adduction	Adduction injury
5	Pronation/dorsiflexion	P.D.	Eversion	Dorsiflexion	Vertical compression injury

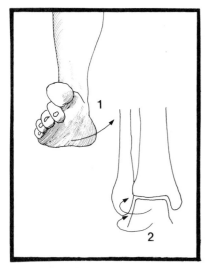

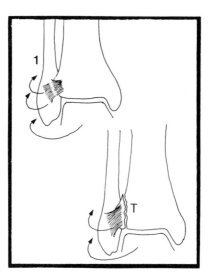

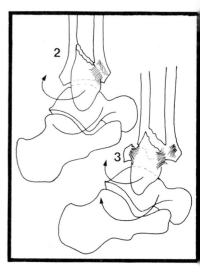

13. *Supination/lateral rotation injuries (1)*
The foot inverts (1). Due to the torque-converter principle, the talus rotates laterally in the ankle mortise (2). The ankle joint structures are thrown under stress and fail in a regular sequence. As each structure fails, the next is stressed. The number of structures involved is dependent on the magnitude of the forces applied to the joint.

14. *Supination/lateral rotation injuries (2)*
The rotating talus carries the fibula with it, leading first to rupture of the anterior (inferior) tibio-fibular ligament (1). Alternatively, the ligament under stress may avulse its tibial attachment (T) (Tillaux fracture).

15. *Supination/lateral rotation injuries (3)*
As external rotation continues, the fibula fractures in an oblique or spiral fashion (2). Note the direction of the spiral.

If displacement continues, the fibular fragment drags off the posterior malleolar fragment (3) to which it is attached by the posterior tibio-fibular ligament (or the ligament tears).

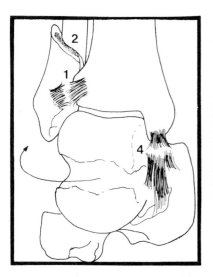

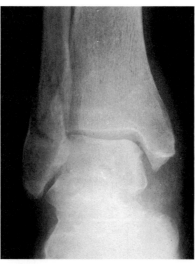

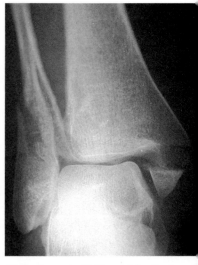

16. *Supination/lateral rotation injuries (4)*
If rotation continues, the fourth structure to fail is the medial ligament or its attachment (the medial malleolus) (4). Such injuries are potentially very unstable and should be carefully distinguished from Stage 1 and 2 lesions.

17. *Radiographs (1)* A spiral fracture of the fibula at the level shown is typical of an S/L injury: in the lateral radiograph the fracture runs downwards and forwards, and there was no evidence of a posterior malleolar fracture. Although there is very slight incongruity between the upper surfaces of the talus and the ankle mortise, absence of tenderness on the medial side of the ankle suggested this was a stage 2 or 3 injury.

18. *Radiographs (2)* The avulsion fracture of the medial malleolus indicates that this is a stage 4 S/L injury. There is lateral shift of the talus in the ankle mortise but the main mass of the fibula maintains its relationship with the tibia, so there is no true diastasis. Nevertheless, this is a very unstable injury.

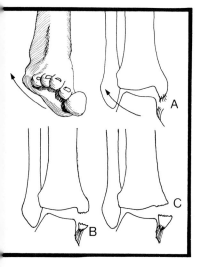

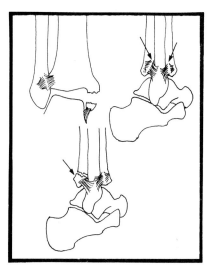

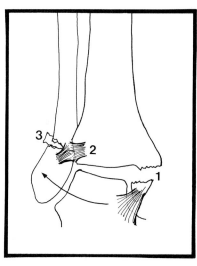

9. *Pronation/abduction injuries (or
abduction injuries) (1)* The foot everts and
the talus swings into abduction. The first
structures to be affected are on the medial
side. Either (A) the deltoid ligament ruptures
(rare) or there is an avulsion fracture of the
medial malleolus. The fragment may be
small (B) or large (C). In either case the
fracture line runs horizontally.

20. *Pronation/abduction injuries (2)* In
second stage injuries of this type, *both* the
anterior and posterior tibio-fibular ligaments
rupture. In the case of the posterior-tibio
fibular ligament, its tibial attachment may be
avulsed instead.

21. *Pronation/abduction injuries (3)* In the
third stage the fibula fractures, often close to
the level of the joint. Comminution may
occur, sometimes with the formation of a
triangular fragment of bone with its base
directed laterally. The distal fibular fragment
is tilted laterally (medial angulation). The
fracture line is often horizontal.

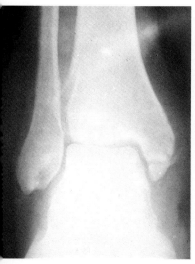

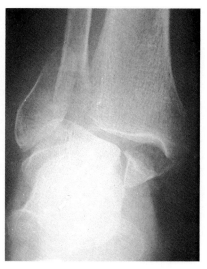

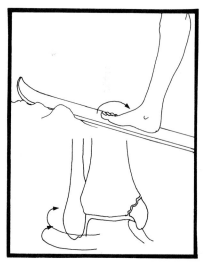

22. *Radiographs (1)* In this example of a
stage 1 abduction fracture, note the small
medial malleolar fragment, the intact fibula,
and the undisplaced talus.

23. *Radiographs (2)* In this Stage 3
abduction fracture, note the direction of
talar tilting, the avulsion fracture of the
medial malleolus with a large fragment, and
the distally situated fibular fracture. The
latter is not strictly horizontal, and its
slightly spiral appearance suggests that there
has been a rotational element.

24. *Pronation/lateral rotation (external
rotation with diastasis) (1)* The talus is
laterally rotated with the foot in the everted
or neutral position (i.e. the foot does not
invert). The rotating talus in the first stage
produces an oblique fracture of the medial
malleolus, or ruptures the deltoid ligament.

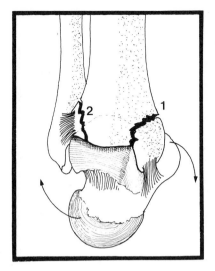

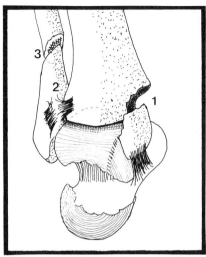

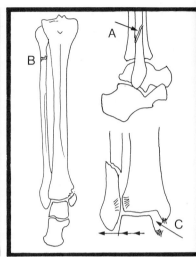

25. *Pronation/lateral rotation (2)* As the talus continues to twist, it impinges on the fibula. The anterior tibio-fibular ligament is put under tension: in the second stage of P/L injuries, its tibial attachment is avulsed (Tillaux fracture) (2) or it ruptures.

26. *Pronation/lateral rotation (3)* In the third stage, the talus continues to rotate, producing a fracture of the fibula (3) spiral or oblique in pattern.

27. *Pronation/lateral rotation (4)* Note that in the lateral projection (A) the obliquity of the fibular fracture is in the opposite direction to that found in S/L injuries. The fibula may fracture proximally at the neck (B)—the Maisonneuve fracture. By Stage 3, the injury is unstable although stress films may be required to demonstrate diastasis (C).

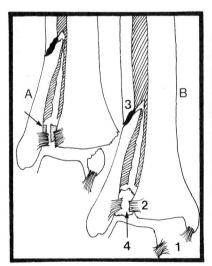

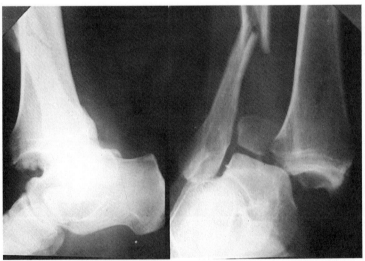

28. *Pronation/lateral rotation (5)* If the talus continues to thrust laterally against the lateral malleolus, the posterior tibio-fibular ligament now ruptures (A) or pulls off its bony attachment (B). The interosseous membrane rips and gross diastasis results (Dupuytren fracture—dislocation of the ankle; Stage 4).

29. *Radiograph.* Note in the lateral projection:
1. The line of the fibular fracture runs in the opposite direction to the fractures of the fibula found in Supination/lateral rotation injuries.
2. The posterior subluxation of the talus.
Note in the antero-posterior projection:
1. The gross lateral displacement of the talus.
2. The obvious disruption which must have occurred in the interosseous membrane.
3. The avulsion of the attachment of the posterior tibio-fibular ligament.

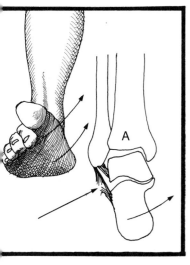

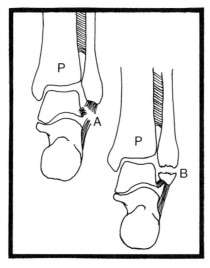

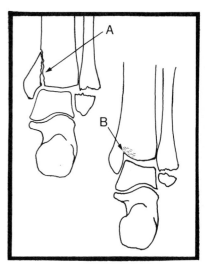

. *Supination/adduction injuries:*
dduction injuries) (1) The foot inverts, but
e tendency to external rotation of the talus
a result of the torque convertor effect is
untered by the direction of forces applied
the forefoot by the impact. The overall
ect is adduction of the talus in the mortise.
the forces are slight, a partial tear of the
eral ligament results (sprain of ankle).

31. *Supination/adduction injuries* (2) With
more severe violence there will be a complete
tear of all three bundles going to form the
lateral ligament (A) or there will be an
avulsion fracture of the lateral malleolus
(with a horizontally running fracture) (B).

32. *Supination/adduction injuries* (3) In the
second stage, the adducting talus strikes the
medial malleolus causing a *vertical or high
oblique fracture* (A). Note i) Instead of the
medial malleolus being pushed off, there
may be a compression fracture of the angle
(B). ii) Occasionally the medial malleolus
may be broken off without damage first
occurring to the lateral ligament.

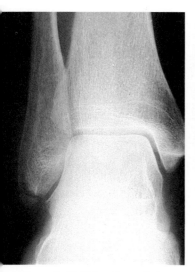

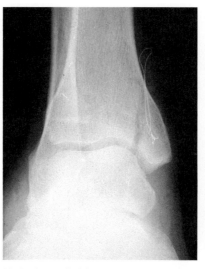

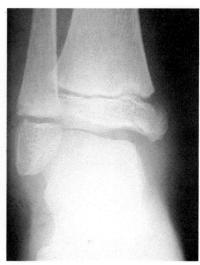

. *Radiographs* (1) This radiograph shows
te clearly an avulsion fracture of the tip
the lateral malleolus, typical of a Stage 1
pination/adduction injury.

34. *Radiographs* (2) Note in a typical Stage
2 injury the fracture line tends to run almost
vertically from the medial corner of the
ankle mortise. There is some rotation in the
radiographic projection so that the fibular
shadow overlaps the tibia. The linear opacity
near the medial malleolus dates from a
previous Achilles tendon repair.

35. *Radiographs* (3) In this child's ankle
there is a greenstick-type fracture of the
medial malleolus with some compression of
the angle between the medial malleolus and
the inferior articular surface of the tibia.

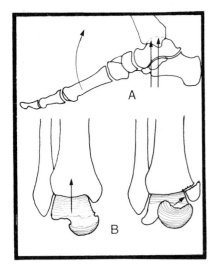

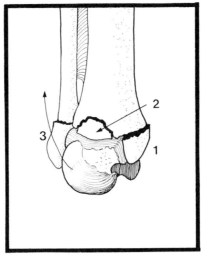

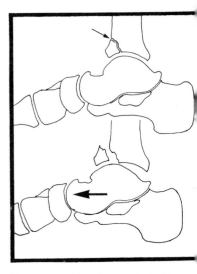

36. *Pronation/dorsiflexion (compression injuries)* (1) Commonly the foot is dorsiflexed at the ankle in association with an upward compression force—usually from a fall from a height or from a road traffic accident (A).

As the talus dorsiflexes, its wide anterior part is forced between the malleoli, shearing off the medial malleolus (B).

37. *Pronation/dorsiflexion injuries* (2) As violence continues, the anterior tibial margin (2) is fractured, to be followed by the lateral malleolus (3).

38. *Pronation/dorsiflexion injuries* (3) Fractures of the anterior tibial margin show quite clearly in lateral projections of the join and help to identify quite clearly this class of fracture. The talus may sublux anteriorly, carrying the marginal fracture with it.

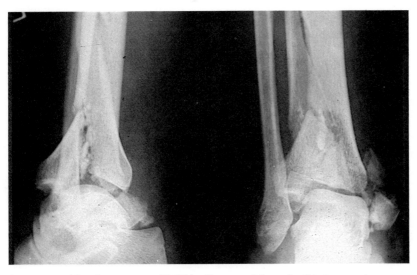

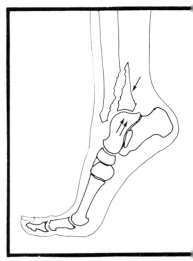

39. *Pronation/dorsiflexion injuries* (4) With still greater violence the tibia fractures in an irregular fashion, often with great comminution. There may be great irregularity of the inferior articular surface of the tibia. Note in the lateral radiograph the large anterior marginal fracture. In the antero-posterior view note the typical medial malleolar fracture, the gross comminution, and the disruption of the inferior articular surface of the tibia. In this case the fibula has remained intact.

40. *Other compression injuries:* If a fall occurs on to the plantar-flexed foot, the posterior articular surface of the tibia may be fractured. In addition, fractures of both malleoli (as in typical pronation/dorsiflexion injuries) may occur when the broad anterior portion of the talus is driven between them.

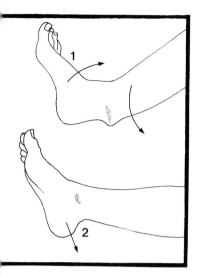

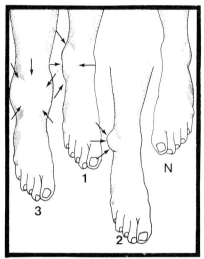

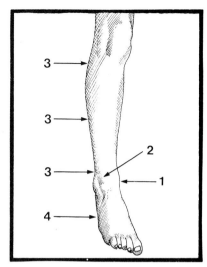

. *Deformity:* Note the presence of any
formity. Look for (1) External rotation of
e foot relative to the leg. If the medial
alleolus is fractured and laterally
splaced, the distal end of the tibia may
come quite prominent under the skin.
) Posterior displacement of the foot, a
mmon feature of posterior malleolar
ctures.

42. *Swelling:* Note the site and distribution
of swelling and bruising. e.g. (1) Diffuse
swelling in front of the lateral malleolus in
many ankle injuries. (2) Egg-shaped swelling
over the lateral malleolus shortly after
complete lateral ligament tears or lateral
malleolar fractures (MacKenzie's sign).
(3) Gross swelling and bruising in many tri-
malleolar and compression fractures.

43. *Tenderness:* Try to localise tenderness if
at all possible. In particular, check:
1. Medial malleolar area.
2. Anterior tibio-fibular ligament area.
3. The whole length of the fibula.
4. The base of the fifth metatarsal.
   (Avulsion fractures following inversion
   injuries are often confused with ankle
   fractures.)

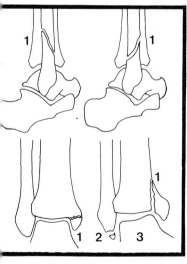

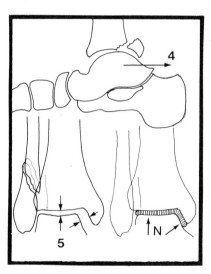

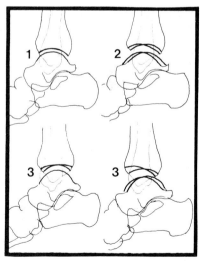

. *Interpreting the radiographs* (1) In
ouping and staging these injuries, note:
) The site and slope of any fracture. (If in
ubt, note the soft tissue shadows, or
amine an oblique (Cobb) projection.)
) Small fragments suggesting avulsion
uries. (If in doubt about ligament
egrity, stress films may be helpful.)
) Talar tilting.

45. *Interpreting the radiographs* (2) Note
also any shift of the talus relative to the
tibia: for example, (4) posterior subluxation,
associated with a posterior malleolar
fracture (5) lateral subluxation: note that the
'gap' above the talus should be the same as
between the medial surface and the medial
malleolus.

46. *Interpreting the radiographs* (3) Note
the following possible appearances in the
lateral: (1) Tibia and talus congruent: true
lateral projection. (2) Tibia and talus
congruent: slight rotation in lateral
projection: two pairs of parallel articular
shadows. (3) Tibia and talus not congruent.

Principles of treatment of ankle injuries

The first considerations in treatment are:
1. The restoration and maintenance of the normal alignment of the talus with the tibia.
2. Ensuring good conditions for union or repair in the injured structures, so that there is no problem in the future with instability.
3. Ensuring optimum restoration of articulating surfaces to lessen the chances of osteo-arthritis in the joint.

Excellent results can be obtained by conservative methods in the majority of Potts fractures. Results are almost universally good in certain types—for example, the stable lateral malleolar fracture—so that in these surgery would not normally be considered. The unstable bi-malleolar or tri-malleolar fracture, however, requires precision in reduction, great care in the techniques of plaster fixation, and above all skilled surveillance for many weeks following injury. Many surgeons prefer to avoid these uncertainties by accurate open reduction and internal fixation. In a number of fractures, especially where there has been soft tissue interposition, reduction can only be achieved by open methods.

For the sake of simplicity, treatment has been divided into the following:

1. Fractures of one malleolus without talar shift.
2. Fractures of two or three malleoli (where there is actual or potential talar shift).
3. Injuries with diastasis and summary of post-operative care.
4. Compression fractures.
5. Lateral ligament injuries.
6. Epiphyseal and miscellaneous injuries.

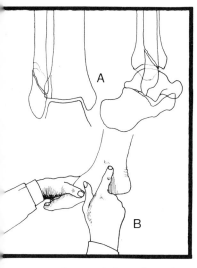

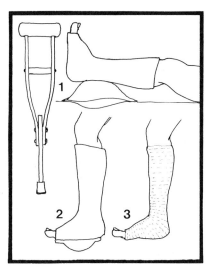

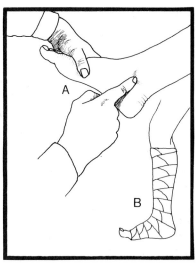

7. *Fracture of one malleolus without talar shift* (a) The commonest ankle fracture is the S/L Stage 2 lesion, a stable injury (A). Associated tenderness over the medial aspect of the joint (B) is indicative of potential instability (S/L 4). Assuming that deformity has not occurred, the latter injury is usually treated by a below-knee plaster.

48. *Fracture of one malleolus with potential instability* (b) The leg should then be elevated (1) and crutches used for 2–3 days till swelling has subsided. (2) A walking heel may then be applied and the plaster retained for about 6 weeks. A circular woven bandage or similar support may then be worn till any tendency to swelling settles. Physiotherapy is seldom required.

49. *Stable fracture of one malleolus:* If there is no medial tenderness (A) symptomatic treatment only is required: adhesive strapping, crepe bandaging or other support (B) may suffice, and should be retained till all swelling has subsided. In many stable injuries, however, symptoms can only be adequately controlled by plaster, and a regime similar to (a) and (b) above may be followed.

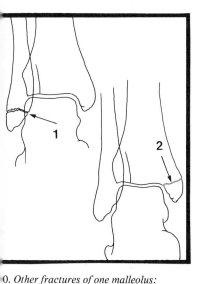

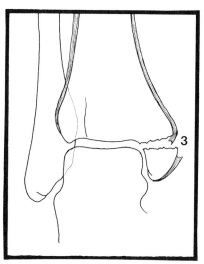

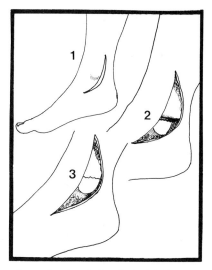

0. *Other fractures of one malleolus:*

. Avulsion of the tip of the lateral malleolus (S/A Stage 1) may also be treated successfully by 6 weeks' plaster fixation.

. Hair-line crack fractures of the medial malleolus (e.g. P/A Stage 1, P/L Stage 1) may be treated in a similar manner.

51. *Displaced medial malleolus* (a) Non-union of the medial malleolus is comparatively common and a frequent source of persisting pain and instability after ankle injuries. This is likely to occur if there is any persisting separation of the fragments (3). This is usually due to soft tissue interposition (periosteum, extensor retinaculum, tibialis posterior tendon) and is an indication for open reduction and internal fixation.

52. *Displaced medial malleolus* (b) (1) A J-shaped incision is made under a tourniquet. (2) The medial malleolus is exposed, and any soft tissue between the fragments removed. (3) The fracture is then reduced under vision and held temporarily with a Charnley malleolar clamp or other device.

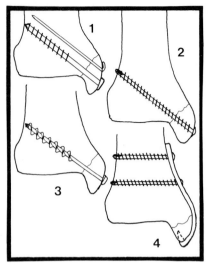

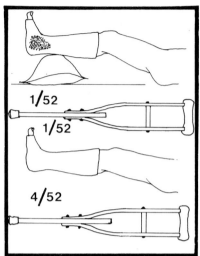

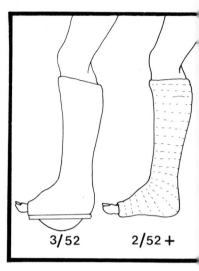

53. *Displaced medial malleolus* (c) The malleolus is then secured, with for example: (1) A.O. cancellous screw with a Kirschner wire (to prevent rotation of the fragment). (2) A long self-tapping screw penetrating the lateral cortex. (3) A lag screw and washer. (4) A Zuelzer plate.

54. *Displaced medial malleolus* (d) After closure of the wound, a padded below-knee plaster is applied, and the tourniquet released. The leg is elevated until swelling subsides (about 1 week). Non-weight bearing with crutches may then commence. The plaster is changed at about 2 weeks and the stitches removed. (The times indicate the approximate duration of each phase of treatment.)

55. *Displaced medial malleolus* (e) A walking heel may be applied at about 6 weeks, and this is retained until union is considered sound (usually at about 8 or 9 weeks). A circular woven bandage or crepe support is then worn until swelling subsides Physiotherapy may be required.

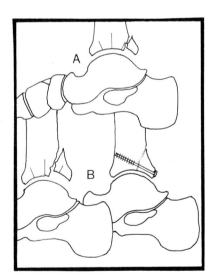

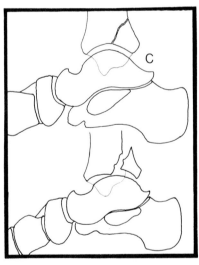

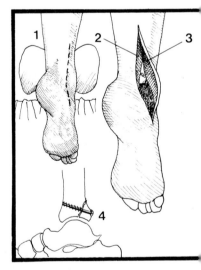

56. *Posterior-malleolar fractures* (1) Isolated fractures of the posterior malleolus are uncommon and do not fit neatly in the Lauge-Hansen classification. Assess on the basis of size and displacement: (A) If 25% or less of the articular surface, accept any displacement and treat as an S/L Stage 2 injury. (B) If more than 33%, and displaced, internal fixation is desirable.

57. *Posterior malleolar fractures* (2) (C) If 33% or more of the articular surface is involved and *undisplaced*, the injury may be treated conservatively by 8 weeks in a below-knee plaster. Nevertheless, there must be most careful surveillance, with radiographs being taken weekly in case there is some late slip (which would require internal fixation).

58. *Posterior malleolar fractures* (3) If a large posterior malleolar fragment is the sol injury, it may be exposed by the postero-*lateral* approach of Henry. (Ref: Henry, A. K. (1973) *Extensile Exposure* Edinburgh: Churchill Livingstone.) The patient is prone, with the ankle on a sandbag, and the foot over the end of the table. The fracture is found between the Achilles tendon and flexor hallucis longus medially (2) and peroneus brevis laterally (3). It is fixed by one or two screws (4).

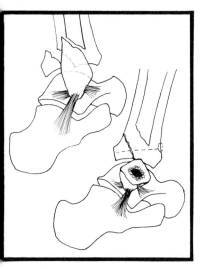

Bi-malleolar and tri-malleolar fractures: Bi-malleolar fractures are unstable injuries, and where the posterior margin of the tibia is involved, instability is increased. Accurate reduction is essential for a good functional result. Conservatively treated cases must be most carefully supervised for the early detection of late displacement which may demand repeated manipulation or internal fixation.

Where internal fixation is employed, a decision must be made on its extent. Whatever procedure is contemplated, the medial malleolus should be fixed, for reasons already given. If the posterior malleolus is intact, fixation of the medial malleolus often restores very reasonable stability to the joint; this may be tested on the table. Nevertheless, any stability achieved remains dependent on the single screw usually employed for fixation: the additional support of a plaster is required until malleolar union is well advanced.

If both malleoli are adequately fixed, stability is guaranteed, and immediate plaster fixation is not required.

If the posterior malleolus is fractured, and the fragment is large, all three malleoli should be fixed if internal fixation is being carried out. If the fragment is small, and only two malleoli are fixed, immediate additional plaster support is desirable.

59. *Posterior malleolar fractures* (4) In more extensive ankle injuries, advantage may be taken of medial and lateral malleolar exposures to visualise and reduce any posterior malleolar fragment. Where the fibula has been fractured, excellent access may be obtained by turning it downwards. The posterior malleolus may then be fixed by backwardly directed screws.

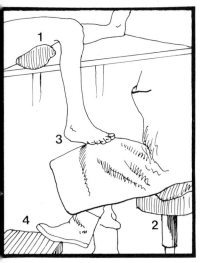

60. *Conservative treatment: manipulation* (1) Conservative treatment may be proposed if the patient is frail, a poor anaesthetic risk, or the skin and circulation poor. The patient is anaesthetised and the leg abducted over the edge of the table with a sandbag behind the thigh (1). The surgeon's stool (2) or the table should be adjusted until the toes can be steadied with the knee (3). A footstool may be helpful (4).

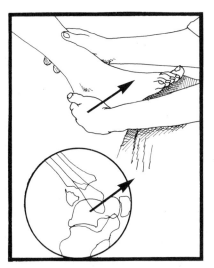

61. *Manipulation* (2) Carry out a reduction rehearsal. The malleoli generally preserve their relationship with the talus and the foot, so that *in essence it is a case of re-aligning the foot with the tibia.* In most cases, three elements require correction. (a) Begin by correcting any posterior subluxation by grasping the heel and lifting it anteriorly.

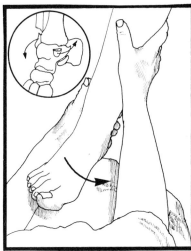

62. *Manipulation* (3) (b) Still grasping the hind foot, correct any external rotation. It should be noted that little force is required for these corrections, and in many cases re-alignment is completed by sensations similar to those experienced when reducing a dislocation.

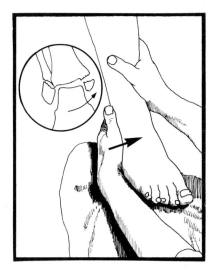

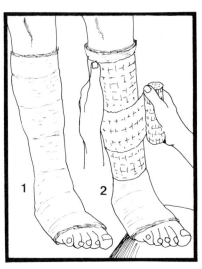

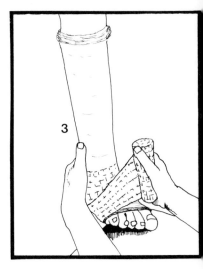

63. *Manipulation* (4) (c) Finally correct any abduction deformity. Note (1) The appearance of the ankle should be restored to normal. (2) Over-correction is difficult or impossible. Repeat the procedure until you can remember the movements and force required for reduction.

64. *Manipulation* (5) Now apply wool roll to the limb making sure that the malleolar prominences are well covered (1). Without hurry follow this with two to three 6″ (15 cm) plaster bandages from the level of the tibial tubercle to just above the ankle (2).

65. *Manipulation* (6) Smooth the plaster well down and then quickly apply two 6″ (15 cm) plaster bandages to the foot and ankle. The toes may be steadied with your knee (3). On completion, you should be left with a plaster which is setting at the calf, but is quite soft and mouldable at the foot and ankle.

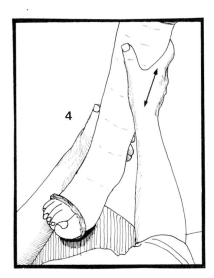

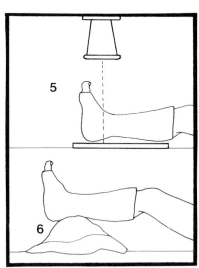

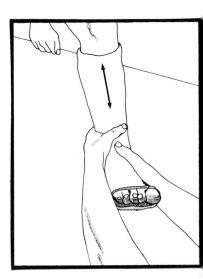

66. *Manipulation* (7) Now repeat the reduction manoeuvre and hold the limb in the reduced position until the plaster has set (4). Steady the forefoot with the knee (to keep the ankle at right angles) and ease the hands slightly upwards and downwards to prevent local indentation of the plaster. Extend it above the knee if the fracture is very unstable.

67. *Manipulation* (8) Check the position of the fracture with radiographs before the anaesthetic is discontinued, and if necessary, repeat the procedure (5).

Precautions should be taken over swelling—e.g. elevation, splitting of the plaster (6).

68. *Manipulation* (9) The plaster should be examined for slackness as swelling subsides. If it becomes slack, it must be changed with care to prevent slipping, and general anaesthesia may be necessary. Radiographs should be taken weekly: re-manipulation under anaesthesia or internal fixation may have to be considered if there is any slip.

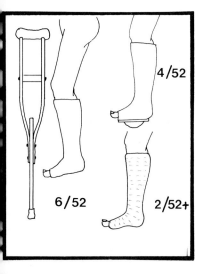

69. *After care* (2) A walking heel should not be applied before 6 weeks: prior to that the patient may be mobilised, non-weight bearing, with crutches. Plaster fixation should be maintained until union (usually 9–10 weeks). Confirm clinically and radiologically. Thereafter bandage supports should be worn till swelling subsides. Physiotherapy is often required.

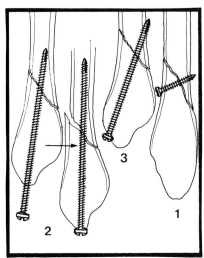

70. *Internal fixation* (a) Indications for internal fixation and methods of fixing the medial and posterior malleoli have been discussed. Various techniques are used for the fibula. (1) One or two screws across the fracture (e.g. using A.O. small fragment set). (2) A long intermedullary screw is sometimes used, but may tilt the fibula (the tip lies lateral to the axis). (3) A low oblique screw penetrating the medial cortex.

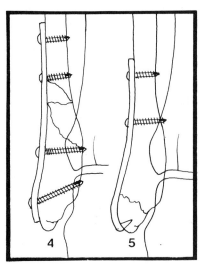

71. *Internal fixation* (b) (4) In the case of a comminuted fracture, a small well-contoured plate and screws may be used. (5) Where an avulsion fracture has left a fragment which is rather small for direct screwing, a Zuelzer hooked bone plate may be used.

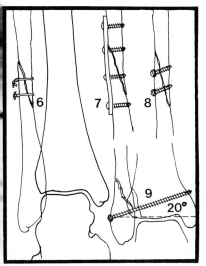

72. *Internal fixation* (c) (6) High spiral fractures may be treated by cerclage, although a plate and screws (7) or cross screwing (8) may be more surely followed by union. (7) Especially where there is a tendency to diastasis, an oblique screw may be used: this should be inserted at the level of the joint and angled at 20°. *It should be removed as soon as union occurs.*

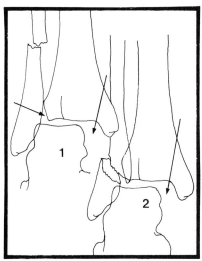

73. *Diastasis* (1) Wide separation of the tibia and fibula is a feature of P/L injuries (1). In many other fractures the basic problem of talo-tibial misalignment may be present although there is no true diastasis (e.g. 2). In most cases diastasis is fully corrected if the malleolar components are fixed, and treatment should proceed along the lines detailed for malleolar fractures.

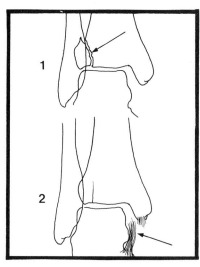

74. *Diastasis* (2) Persistence of diastasis may be due to (1) imperfect reduction of a Tillaux fracture or (2) an invaginated deltoid ligament. If attention is paid to these areas and diastasis still persists, cross screwing as detailed above may be carried out. This must be done with the ankle in dorsiflexion, otherwise dorsiflexion may be permanently restricted.

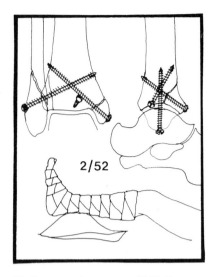

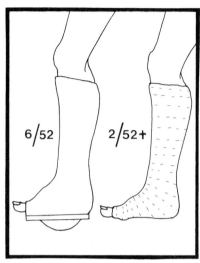

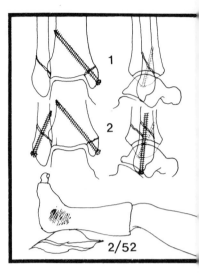

75. *Post-operative treatment* (1) If all fragments are well held with screw fixation, a light pressure bandage may be applied, and immediate non-weight bearing exercises commenced with the limb elevated. Crutches may be used after any swelling has subsided.

76. *Post-operative treatment* (2) After two weeks the stitches are removed and a close fitting plaster is applied; assuming that swelling is not a problem, weight bearing can begin. Plaster is retained for about 6 weeks (after removal of the stitches) until there is evidence of union; thereafter a circular woven or crepe support is applied till any swelling subsides.

77. *Post-operative treatment* (3) If the medial malleolus only is fixed in a bi-malleolar fracture (1) or the posterior malleolus not fixed in a tri-malleolar fracture (2), plaster fixation is usually advised from the outset.

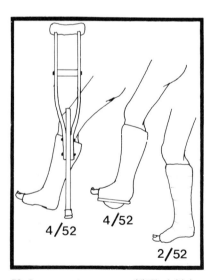

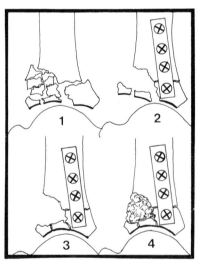

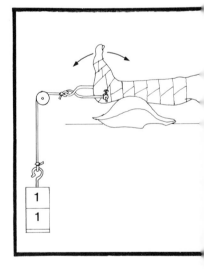

78. *Post-operative treatment* (4) The initial plaster is changed after two weeks to allow removal of stitches. A walking heel can usually be applied about the 6th week. Union is usually sound after a further 4 weeks when a crepe or other bandage support may be substituted.

79. *Compression fractures* (1) The main problem is comminution (1). If there is one substantial articular fragment intact, a reconstruction may be possible: a plate and screws are used to hold the main fragment (2). The remaining articular fragments are assembled on the talus (3). Any defect is packed with bone chips (4). This is seldom an easy procedure and may prove impracticable.

80. *Compression fractures* (2) Conservative treatment is necessary if comminution is too great: e.g. (a) Approximately 2 kg of traction is applied through a calcaneal pin to maintain alignment. (b) Active exercises are commenced as soon as pain will permit. (c) Weight bearing is deferred till union is sound (to avoid compression). (d) If O.A. becomes a problem, ankle fusion may be required.

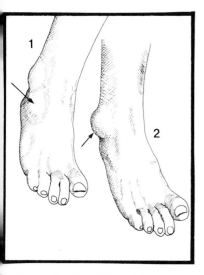

81. *Diagnosis* (1) A soft tissue injury is diagnosed where there is a history of trauma and the radiographs are normal. A history of an inversion injury is obtainable in most lateral ligament injuries. In sprains, swelling and tenderness follow the fasciculi of the lateral ligament (1). In complete tears of the lateral ligament, swelling at first lies over the lateral malleolus (2).

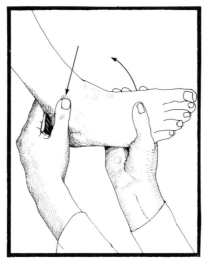

82. *Diagnosis* (2) If the findings suggest a more substantial injury, grasp the foot and gently adduct the talus in the ankle mortise, feeling for any gap opening up at the outer corner of the joint. Compare with the other side. Excess movement of the talus on the injured side suggests a complete lateral ligament tear.

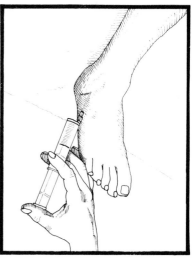

83. *Diagnosis* (3) If the manoeuvre cannot be performed adequately because of pain, infiltrate the fasciculi of the lateral ligament with local anaesthetic (e.g. 20 ml of $\frac{1}{2}$% Lignocaine) or administer a general anaesthetic. Repeat the manoeuvre, and for further confirmation, take A.P. radiographs under stress.

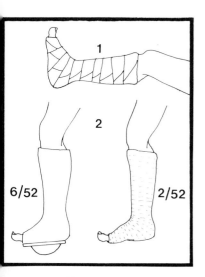

84. *Treatment* (1) Simple sprains resolve in a few days with local supportive measures (adhesive strapping, crepe bandaging, etc.) rest and elevation (1).
  Complete lateral ligament tears should be treated either by surgical repair or by plaster fixation for 6 weeks (2), followed by a lighter support till free from discomfort.

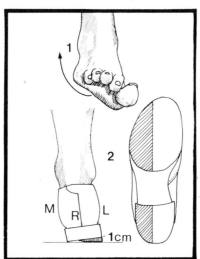

85. *Treatment* (2) Chronic instability should be investigated by plain and inversion films (assuming clinical examination has not revealed any muscular or neurological cause).
  Conservative treatment may be tried, using physiotherapy to develop the evertors of the foot (1) and by lateral wedging of the heel and sole of the footwear to maintain the foot in eversion. (2)

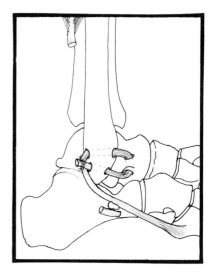

86. *Treatment* (3) Surgical reconstruction may be required if simple measures fail, and instability has been demonstrated. In the Watson-Jones reconstruction, the peroneus brevis tendon is threaded through holes drilled in the fibula and talus and sewn to itself. The upper stump is sewn to peroneus longus. The tendon replaces the torn ligament, and the success rate of the operation is high. Failure may indicate sub-talar laxity.

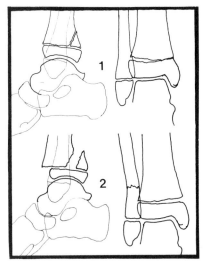

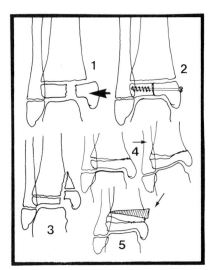

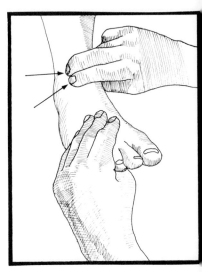

87. *Epiphyseal injuries* (1) (a) Salter/Harris Type 1 injuries are rare. (b) The commonest injury is sup./lateral rotation producing a Type 2 lesion. In many, displacement is minimal (1) and can be treated in a below-knee plaster for 4–6 weeks.

Where displacement is appreciable (2) the ankle should be manipulated as described for bi-malleolar fractures.

88. *Epiphyseal injuries* (2) (c) A Salter/Harris Type 3 injury may sometimes be reduced by applying firm local pressure under G.A. (1). If unsuccessful, cross screwing may have to be considered, taking care to avoid damaging the epiphyseal plate (2). (d) Type 4 injuries (3) should be treated by open reduction. (e) In Type 5 injuries (4) late corrective osteotomy may be needed (5).

89. *Sprain of inferior-tibio fibular ligament:* Inversion injuries of the ankle may lead to a first stage sup./lateral rotational tearing of the inferior tibio-fibular ligament. Pain may be quite severe, and tenderness well localised over the ligament. A 6-week period of plaster fixation is advised, although in cases of chronic disability hydrocortisone injections and even cross screwing are advocated.

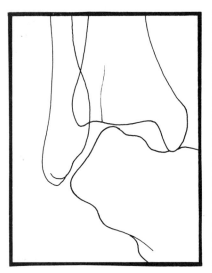

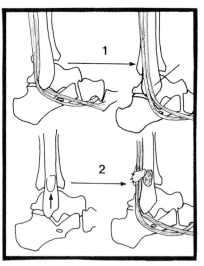

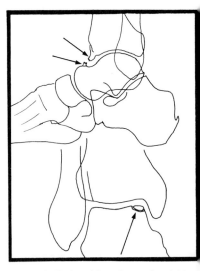

90. *Ankle dislocation without fracture:* Rarely the ankle may dislocate without fracture. Although rupture of both medial and lateral ligaments must take place, conservative management by closed manipulative reduction and plaster fixation may achieve a good result. Avascular necrosis of the talus is a minor risk in this situation.

91. *Recurrent dislocation of peroneal tendons:* A rare condition in which eversion causes painful clicking sensations as the peroneal tendons repeatedly snap over the lateral malleolus (1). The condition is associated with a defect in the superior peroneal retinaculum. A flap of bone and periosteum can be used to reconstruct the defective ligament (2).

92. *Footballer's ankle and osteochondritis tali:* Tibial and/or talar osteophytes (1) may arise in footballers from repeated anterior capsular tears, and limit dorsiflexion. Excision for this is seldom indicated. Pain may follow a fresh tear (treat symptomatically by P.O.P. fixation) or from early ankle joint osteo-arthritis.

Osteochondritis tali (2)—See under Foot 22.

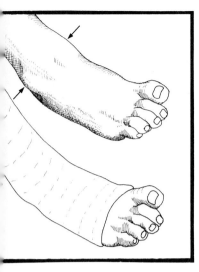

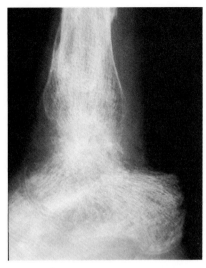

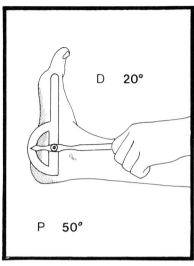

3. *Swelling:* Swelling persisting for weeks or even months after fixation has been discarded is so common as to be an almost normal occurrence. Assuming that the fracture has united in good position, local supportive measures should be continued to resolution. The patient should be reassured and advised regarding elevation and activity.

94. *Sudeck's Atrophy:* Where swelling is gross, and especially if the toes are involved, suspect Sudeck's atrophy. There may be glazing of the skin and pain. Radiographs may show typical porotic changes, and confirm union of the fracture. Intensive physiotherapy and continued use of supports will be required. Convalescence may be expected to be slow with occasionally some permanent functional impairment.

95. *Stiffness, 'weakness' and disturbance of gait:* Again, assuming sound union, these symptoms generally respond rapidly to appropriate physiotherapy and occupational therapy. Progress may be assessed by charting the range of ankle joint movments. (The normal range is indicated, but compare the sides.) Note also the range in the sub-talar joint.

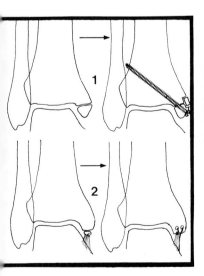

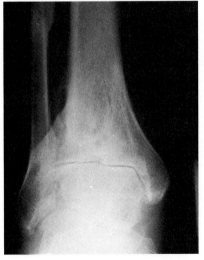

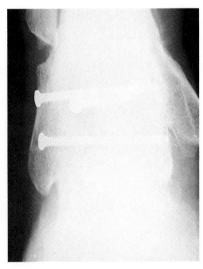

6. *Instability:* Instability due to lateral ligament damage has been described; instability may follow damage to the medial structures.

Non-union of a large medial malleolar fragment should be treated by internal fixation: additional grafting may be necessary (1). When the tip only is involved, it may be excised and the lateral ligament sutured to the stump (2).

97. *Osteo-arthritis* (1) Considering the incidence of ankle fractures, osteo-arthritis is an uncommon complication. It is most likely to follow compression fractures, and fractures with residual diastasis or talo-tibial incongruity. Note in this example of an old compression fracture the central split in the tibial surface, the broadening of the mortise and the narrowed joint space.

98. *Osteo-arthritis* (2) If symptoms of pain, swelling, stiffness and disturbance of gait are troublesome, then fusion may be advised. In the Crawford-Adams fusion, the articular surfaces are cleared, the fibula is inlaid in the talus and tibia and held in position with cross screws. Late function is generally good due to persistent mid-tarsal movement.

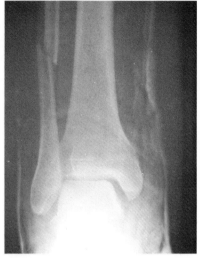

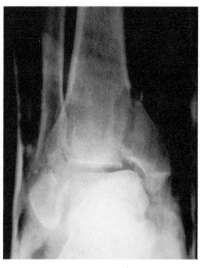

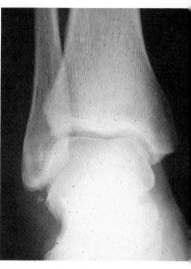

Self test

99. This A.P. radiograph shows the position achieved by closed manipulation of a Dupuytren fracture-dislocation of the ankle. (Pronation/lateral rotation Stage 4 injury.) Is reduction complete?

100. Classify this injury. Is the reduction satisfactory?

101. This radiograph was taken of a patient complaining of pain in the ankle after an inversion injury. Do you detect any abnormality?

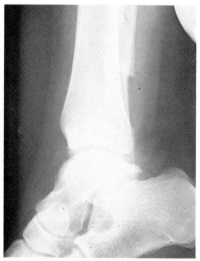

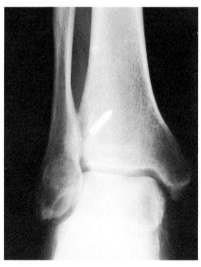

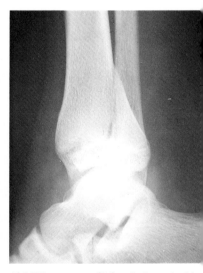

102. On the information available on this lateral radiograph, classify this injury. Is the talus congruent with the tibia?

103. What is the most likely explanation for the broken screw showing on this radiograph?

104. What pattern of injury is shown in this lateral radiograph?

99. No: there is persistent lateral talar shift (Note the gap between the talus and the medial malleolus) due to slight persistent diastasis. This position would be accepted by a number of surgeons, while others would prefer to correct this by cross screwing.

100. The vertical fracture of the medial malleolus is typical of a supination/adduction stage 2 injury (Adduction fracture.) Reduction is incomplete, and there is disturbance of the inferior articular surface of the tibia. Open reduction is indicated.

101. A small opacity is present distal to the tip of the lateral malleolus, and probably represents avulsion of the fibular attachment of the lateral ligament. The fragment is small, and clinical confirmation would be desirable.

102. The direction of the spiral fracture of the fibula suggests that this is a P/L injury. The talus and tibia are not congruent (double talar shadow, single tibial shadow.)

103. The original pathology has been a fibular fracture or a diastasis treated by an oblique screw. Ankle movements have been permitted before removal of the screw. This has resulted in distortion of the inferior tibio-fibular joint, and fracture of the screw, the lateral portion only of which has been accessible for removal.

104. This is an epiphyseal injury, in which there is slight backward displacement of the distal tibial epiphysis, along with a small fragment of metaphysis (juxta-epiphyseal fragment), i.e., a Salter and Harris Type 2 injury. There is some evidence on this lateral view of talo-tibial incongruity, and manipulation would be indicated.

15. Foot injuries

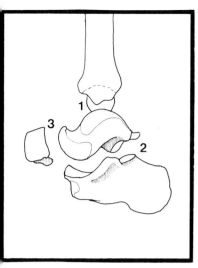

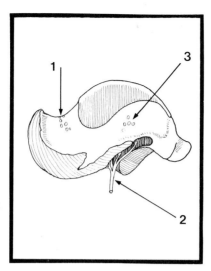

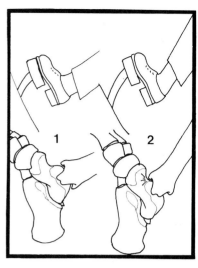

1. *Anatomical considerations* (1) The talus plays a key role in no less than 3 joints: (1) The ankle joint—articulating with the tibia and fibula. (2) The sub-talar joint—articulating with the calcaneus. (3) The talo-navicular joint: along with the calcaneo-cuboid joint, this forms the *mid-tarsal* joint. Secondary osteo-arthritic changes may occur following fractures which cause articular irregularity.

2. *Anatomical considerations* (2) Secondary osteo-arthritis may also follow avascular necrosis which occurs in half of all talar neck fractures. The blood supply of the talus enters at three sites: (1) The neck. (2) The sinus tarsi area. (3) The medial side of the body. The more sources disturbed, the greater the risk to the blood supply.

3. *Mechanisms of injury:* The commonest fracture is of the neck. This may occur in car accidents, when pedal impact (1) forces the talar neck against the tibial margin (2). (There is a long association between this injury and light aircraft crashes where the feet are violently dorsiflexed against the rudder pedals—'aviator's astragalus'.) The injury may also follow falls from a height in a crouching position.

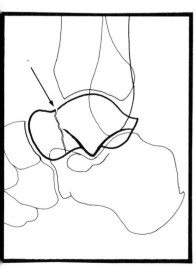

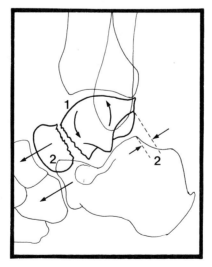

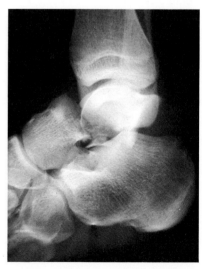

4. *Classification of talar neck fractures* (1) Talar neck fractures have been classified into 4 types of increasing severity. *In Type 1* the talar neck is fractured without displacement. Incomplete hair-line cracks are not uncommon. Only the blood supply through the neck is affected, and the incidence of avascular necrosis is under 10 per cent.

5. *Classification* (2) *In Type 2* fractures there is an accompanying sub-talar subluxation. The proximal portion of the talus adopts a position of plantar flexion (1). The *head* of the talus maintains its relationship with the navicular and calcaneus, (and the rest of the foot) which sublux forwards (2).

6. *Classification* (3) Note in the radiographic example a more severe degree of plantar flexion of the proximal fragment, and greater subluxation. The blood supplies through the neck and sinus tarsi are both interrupted, and the incidence of avascular necrosis rises to 50 per cent in fractures of this type.

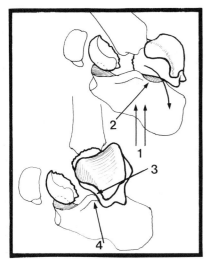

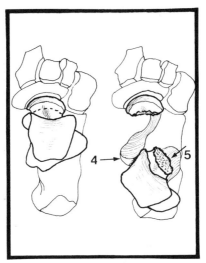

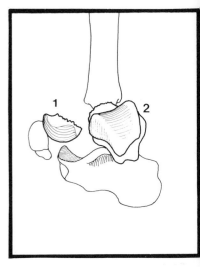

7. *Classification* (4) *Type 3 Injuries:* With further dorsiflexion and upward force (1) the tibia is driven between the two talar fragments. The posterior fragment is extruded backwards, while at the same time the convex posterior articular surface of the calcaneus (2) guides it medially. It comes to rest with its medial surface (3) caught on the sustentaculum tali (4).

8. *Classification* (5) In its final position (ctd.) the main portion of the talus lies on the medial side of the ankle, with its fractured surface (5) pointing laterally. All three sources of blood supply are disturbed. The risks of avascular necrosis are high, rising to 85 per cent.

9. *Classification* (6) In the rare *Type 4 injury*, the head of the talus dislocates from the navicular (1) in association with a Type 3 (2) or a Type 2 injury. The incidence of avascular necrosis here is also high.

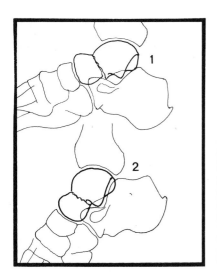

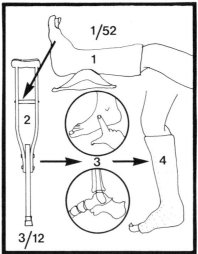

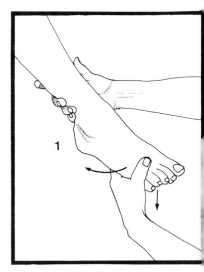

10. *Diagnosis:* The diagnosis may be suspected from the history, but is made radiologically. Care must be taken to differentiate between Type 1 and Type 2 injuries. If doubt exists, two laterals, one in dorsiflexion (1) and one in plantar flexion (2) should be taken and compared. These will reveal any subluxation (Type 2 illustrated).

11. *Treatment of Type I injuries:* (1) Padded plaster with toe platform and elevation for about a week. (2) Non-weight bearing with crutches for 3 months. (3) The fracture is then assessed out of plaster for union and absence of avascular necrosis. (4) If there are no complications, weight bearing may commence with a light support. Physiotherapy will be required for ankle, sub-talar joint and calf.

12. *Treatment, Type II injuries* (1) Reduction may be attempted by closed methods: (1) The foot is plantar flexed and everted. (2) A padded plaster is applied in this position and check radiographs taken. If a satisfactory reduction has been obtained, then conservative treatment may be continued.

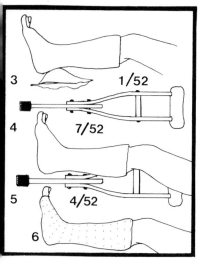

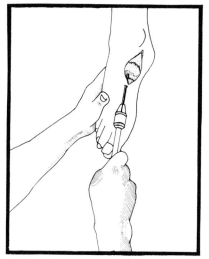

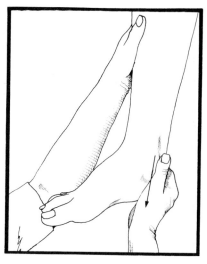

13. *Treatment, Type II injuries* (2) (3) The limb is elevated for a week before (4) non-weight bearing with crutches is permitted. After 7–8 weeks the plaster is changed and the foot brought up to a right angle (5). Non-weight bearing is continued for a further 4 weeks. Thereafter, if the fracture is united and there is no evidence of avascular necrosis, weight bearing may be allowed (6) with a support. Physiotherapy will almost certainly be needed.

14. *Treatment, Type II injuries* (3) If closed methods fail in obtaining a reduction, open reduction will be required. The fracture may be secured with a Kirschner wire passed backwards from the head of the talus into the body. The after care is as in 13; the Kirschner wire may be removed at the change of plaster.

15. *Treatment, Type III injuries* (1) The displaced portion of the talus is situated subcutaneously, and there should be no delay in reducing it as the overlying skin is tightly stretched over the bone and likely to slough. Facilities for open reduction should be available, but closed methods should be attempted first. 1 Begin by gripping the heel and applying traction to it.

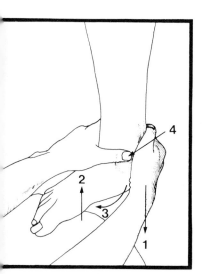

17. *Treatment, Type III injuries* (3) (f) After reduction, proceed with elevation and gradual mobilisation as described in 13 above. If closed reduction fails (and this is frequent) open reduction will be necessary. The best access is gained by a postero-medial incision, but the condition of the skin may dictate a less direct approach.

   Treatment of Type IV injuries: These uncommon injuries are likely to require open reduction. All fragments should be retained, even if completely detached and obviously avascular. On no account should the talus be excised.

   Complications of talar neck fractures: (1) *Skin necrosis.* The skin may become tightly stretched over a displaced talus and undergo necrosis with late sloughing. *Early reduction is imperative to avoid this complication.* (2) *Compound injuries.* Thorough debridement of the wound is essential, but again every effort must be made to retain the main fragments. Treatment should follow the usual lines established for the management of compound fractures. If sepsis occurs *in conjunction with avascular necrosis*, healing may only be obtained after excision of the avascular fragments.

16. *Treatment, Type III injuries* (2) Dorsiflex the foot with the knee. Maintaining traction, pull the heel slightly forward and evert it to open up the space for the talus. 4 Apply strong pressure over the displaced body of the talus: press laterally, but also slightly anteriorly and downwards. Plantar flex the foot. If purchase on the heel is poor, a Steinman pin through the heel and a calliper may be used.

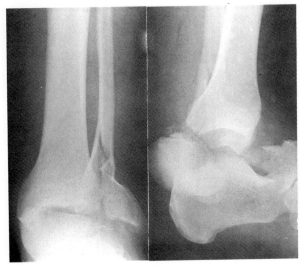

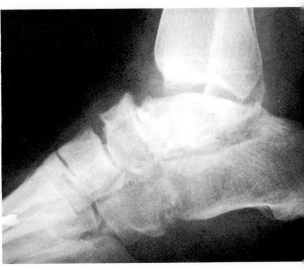

18. (3) *Potts fracture:* Rarely, malleolar fractures may be found complicating talar neck fractures. Closed reduction is here unreliable, and open reduction with internal fixation of the malleolar fracture is desirable. (Illustrated: Type 3 fracture with fracture of the lateral malleolus.)

19. (4) *Avascular necrosis:* The diagnosis is made from the radiographs. *Increased density* is often apparent by 6 and usually by 12 weeks: but do not be confused by the dense shadows cast by the overlying malleoli in the lateral. Re-vascularisation always occurs in closed injuries and is usually advanced by 8 months. (Check progress by monthly radiographs.) *Weight-bearing before re-vascularisation is complete is likely to cause marked flattening of the talus.* (Ill.) Local supports and physiotherapy will be required. Secondary osteo-arthritis is common and should be kept in mind. Because of its key position, avascular necrosis of the talus may lead to osteo-arthritis of the ankle, sub-talar or mid-tarsal joints (or any combination of these).

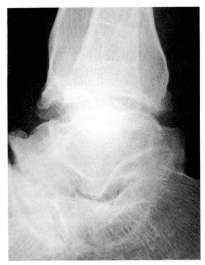

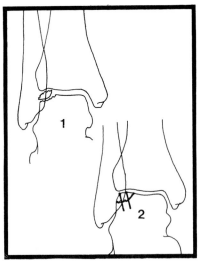

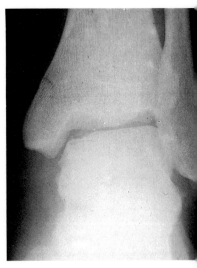

20. (5) *Osteo-arthritis:* This may occur secondary to avascular necrosis or mal-union. Determination of the joints involved is important, and this may be facilitated by the site of the pain and the clinical and radiological appearances. Local anaesthetic infiltration of suspected joints is occasionally helpful. Thereafter the appropriate fusion may be advised. (Where all three joints are involved, as here, all will require fusion.)

21. *Other talar lesions:* (1) *Dome fractures:* A portion of the upper articular surface of the talus may be detached as a result of a shearing injury: occasionally the fragment is inverted, effectively preventing union (1). If the fragment is substantial, it should be replaced and secured with, for example, Smillie pins (2); if the fragment is small, it may be excised. Thereafter, plaster fixation for 6 weeks is advisable.

22. (2) *Osteochondritis tali:* This may occur as a sequel to a non-displaced shearing fracture, although frequently there is no history of injury. (Note the lesion on the medial side of the upper articular surface.) Where there is appreciable pain and swelling, it is usual to place multiple drill holes through the base of the lesion in an attempt to encourage re-vascularisation.

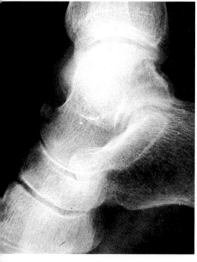

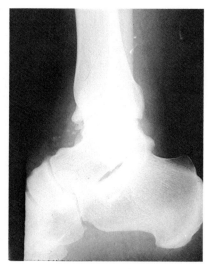

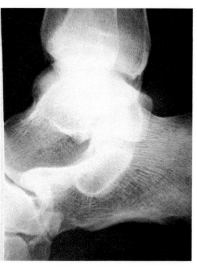

23. (3) *Avulsion fractures:* Minor avulsion fractures of the talus may result from inversion, eversion, plantar flexion and rarely dorsiflexion strains of the ankle—when flakes of bone are pulled off by ligamentous or capsular attachments. These injuries require symptomatic treatment only e.g. 2–4 weeks in a below knee walking plaster).

24. (4) *Footballers' ankle:* Repeated forced plantar flexion may lead to avulsion of the anterior capsular attachments of the ankle with calcification developing in the haematomata. This produces exostoses of the tibia and talus and sometimes, as here, patchy areas of calcification in the anterior capsule. (See also ankle, 92.)

25. (5) *Fractures of the body of the talus:* (1) The upper articular surface of the talus may be fractured by the same mechanisms which produce compression fractures of the ankle. Vertical splits without significant disturbance of the ankle or subtalar joints (ill.) may be treated as Type 1 talar neck fractures. (2) If displacement has occurred, accurate reduction and cross screwing should be carried out.

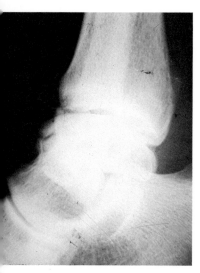

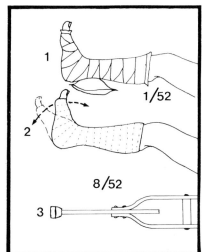

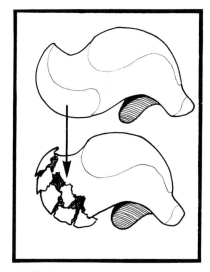

26. *Body fractures:* (3) Often there is a high degree of comminution. The convexity of the body may be flattened and the talus compressed as it is squeezed between the tibia and calcaneus. Such fractures may also involve the sub-talar joint, and there is invariably extensive damage to the cartilaginous surfaces of the ankle joint. Surgical reconstruction is seldom possible.

27. *Treatment:* A typical conservative line of treatment might be: (1) Initial pressure bandaging and elevation. (2) Intensive active exercises as soon as pain and swelling will permit. (3) Avoidance of weight bearing until union is well advanced (about 8–10 weeks). Persistent pain and functional restriction would be indications for ankle fusion.

28. (6) *Compression fractures of the head of the talus:* These fractures are uncommon, but usually highly comminuted and unsuitable for attempts at reconstruction. Early mobilisation of the foot should be the aim, and a regime similar to 27 may be followed.

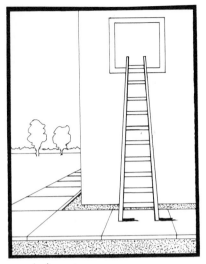

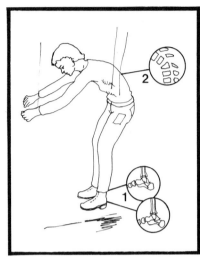

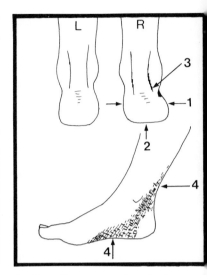

29. *Calcaneal fractures: mechanisms of injury* (1) The commonest cause of calcaneal fracture is a fall from a height on to the heels. Important factors include the height fallen, the nature of the ground, and the weight of the patient. The injury is common in slaters, window cleaners and construction workers. Rarely the injury may be produced by impact from below (e.g. a below-deck explosion on a ship).

30. *Mechanisms of injury* (2) Taking into account the commonest cause of injury, it is essential when examining a case of suspected calcaneal fracture that you do not overlook (1) a similar fracture on the other side (2) a wedge fracture of the spine. (Dorso-lumbar junction fractures are present in 5 per cent of calcaneal fractures.)

31. *Clinical appearance:* In major fractures, the heel when viewed from behind appears (1) wider, (2) shorter and flatter, and (3) tilted laterally into valgus. There is often tense swelling of the heel, marked local tenderness, and later bruising (4) which may spread into the medial side of the sole and proximally to the calf. Weight bearing is usually, but not always, impossible.

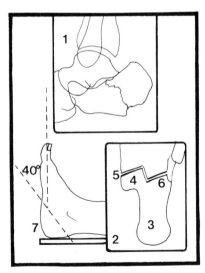

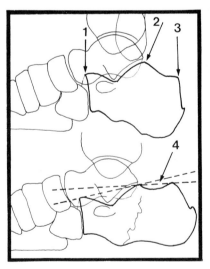

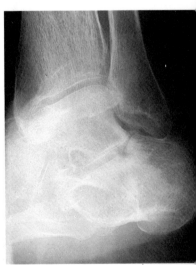

32. *Radiographs* (1) The most important view is a well centred and well exposed lateral projection (1) An axial projection (2) is helpful in visualising the pillar of the heel (3) the sustentaculum tali (4) the anterior talo-calcaneal joint (5) and the posterior talo-calcaneal joint (6). This film is taken with the tube tilted at 40° from the vertical (7).

33. *Radiographs* (2) A line may be drawn from the anterior articular process of the calcaneus (1) through the posterior articular surface (2) to intersect with a second line touching the superior angle of the tuberosity (3). This *Bohler's salient angle* is normally about 40°. It is decreased (4) in fractures which flatten the heel profile.

34. *Radiographs* (3) An oblique projection may be helpful if doubt remains: note in this radiograph the split in the posterior articular surface of the calcaneus.

Note that the key factor in assessing calcaneal fractures is whether or not there i involvement of the sub-talar joint.

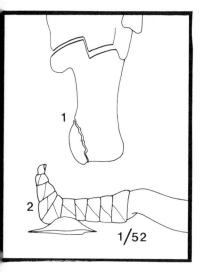

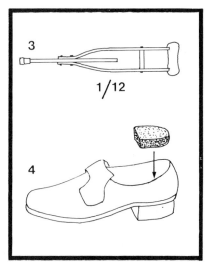

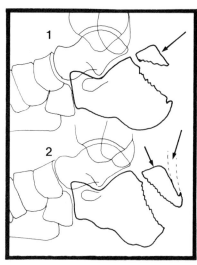

35. *Types of calcaneal fracture:* 7 common patterns of fracture have been described, and are arranged here roughly in order of increasing complexity. I. *Vertical fracture of the tuberosity:* The sub-talar joint is not involved and the prognosis is excellent (1). Nevertheless, swelling may be severe, and should be controlled by firm bandaging over wool and elevation of the limb (2).

36. *Vertical fractures* (2) Weight bearing, whilst not harmful, will be painful or impossible, and crutches will be required for some weeks; they may be discarded when pain settles (3). A crepe bandage or similar support may be worn till swelling subsides. Any long term heel pain may be controlled with a sorbo rubber heel cushion.

37. II. *Horizontal fractures* (1) These are of two types which must be distinguished. (1) The commoner injury involves the posterior superior angle of the calcaneus without disturbance of the Achilles tendon insertion: it is usually caused by local trauma (e.g. a kick). (2) The second is an avulsion fracture, produced by sudden muscle contraction.

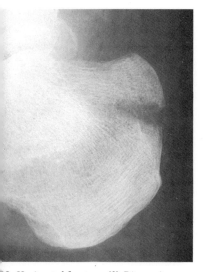

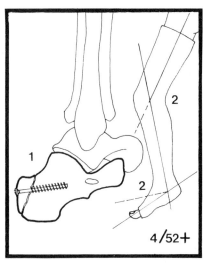

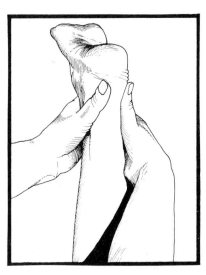

38. *Horizontal fractures* (2) *Diagnosis:* Differentiate between the two main types of horizontal fracture by (1) Noting the level of the fracture on the radiographs (Type 1 illustrated). (2) Studying the soft tissue shadows on the radiograph, looking for upward (proximal) retraction of the Achilles tendon. (3) Feeling for a gap between the tendon insertion and the point of the heel.

39. *Treatment* (1) (1) If the fracture is of the avulsion type (or if there is continued doubt) it should be openly reduced and fixed with a screw. (2) To remove stress from the screw, a long leg plaster should be applied with the knee and ankle in flexion. (3) After 4 weeks a below knee walking plaster may be substituted till union (about 8 weeks).

40. *Treatment* (2) (1) When the fracture is not of the avulsion type, it should be manipulated if severely displaced. Moderate residual displacement can usually be quite safely accepted. (2) Thereafter, a below knee padded plaster may be applied, and crutches used for the first week or so. (3) A further 5 weeks in a below knee walking plaster is then all that will be required.

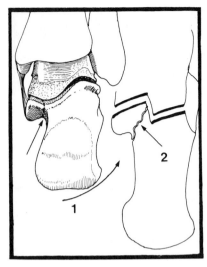

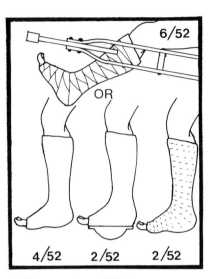

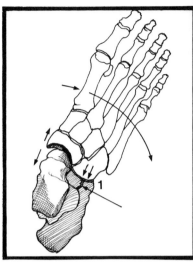

41. III. *Fractures of the sustentaculum tali* (1) These fractures result from eversion injuries (avulsion) (1). They are seen most clearly in axial projections, and indeed may be missed unless this view is taken and examined with care (2). Displacement is generally slight, and persisting disability is rare.

42. *Sustentaculum tali* (2) *Treatment:* Healing of the fracture is generally well advanced by 6 weeks. Prior to this the following treatments may be used. (a) A crepe bandage over wool pressure bandage and non-weight bearing with crutches for 6 weeks, or (b) a below knee padded plaster with crutches initially and then a walking heel; after 6 weeks a circular woven support for a further 2 weeks or so.

43. IV. *Anterior calcaneal fractures* (1) This fracture affects the anterior part of the calcaneus which articulates with the cuboid. It may result from (1) Forced abduction of the forefoot in which the cuboid strikes the calcaneus. (2) Forced inversion injuries which have the same effect. (3) As part of a mid-tarsal dislocation.

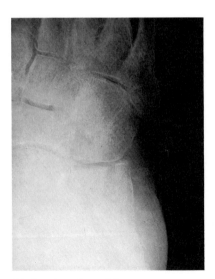

45. (3) If there is calcaneal shortening, the mechanisms of the mid-tarsal joint may be seriously disturbed, leading possibly to pain, restriction of movements in the foot, and osteo-arthritis. If the patient is elderly or has sustained multiple injuries, these risks may be accepted, and this injury also treated conservatively. In some other cases it may be possible by open operation and bone grafting to pack up the depressed articular fragments; this will improve function in the mid-tarsal joint and reduce the risks of secondary osteo-arthritis.

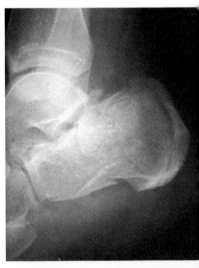

44. *Anterior calcaneal fractures: Treatment:* (1) If there is no significant compression or shortening of the calcaneus (as in the vertical split illustrated) the injury may be treated conservatively along the lines already indicated for fractures of the sustentaculum tali (42.). (2) If there is evidence of mid-tarsal instability, treat as for mid-tarsal dislocation.

46. V. *Fracture of the body of the calcaneus without involvement of the sub-talar joint* (1) The fracture line passes just posterior to the posterior talo-calcaneal joint. Frequently there is a decrease in the salient angle, and if this is the case (ill.) then flattening of the heel profile may lead to troublesome localised and persistent heel pain.

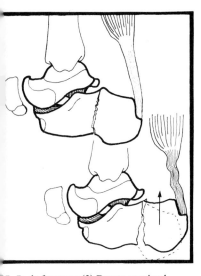

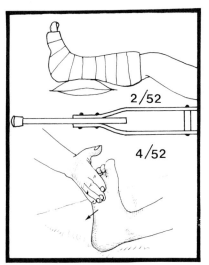

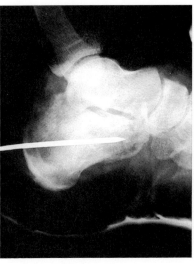

47. *Body fractures* (2) Due to proximal displacement of the portion of the calcaneus carrying the Achilles tendon insertion, there is slackening of the calf muscles, so that there is weakness of plantar flexion at the ankle, and loss of spring in the step. This slackness is eventually taken up, but recovery is facilitated by *prolonged, intensive physiotherapy* in the form of calf resisting exercises.

48. *Body fractures* (3) *Treatment* (1) If displacement is slight, good results may be obtained by conservative treatment along the following lines. (a) Pressure bandaging, bed rest, elevation and analgesics for two weeks. (b) Crutches until graduated weight bearing can be commenced at about 6 weeks. (c) Calf resisting exercises as soon as pain will permit, and continued physiotherapy till maximal recovery.

49. *Body fractures* (4) *Treatment* (2) More severely displaced fractures may be treated along similar lines or *alternatively* an attempt may be made to reduce the heel fragment. A Gissane spike may be driven into the heel which is then levered distally. The spike is incorporated in a plaster sabot which maintains the reduction while still permitting ankle movements.

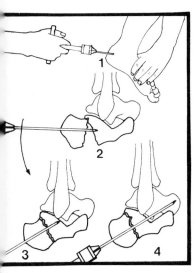

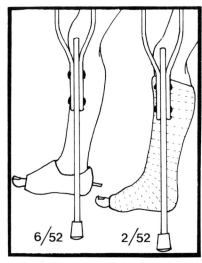

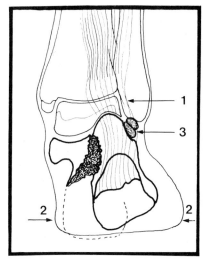

50. *Body fractures* (5) *Treatment* (3) If a suitable spike is not available, a large diameter Steinman pin may be used. Image intensifier control is helpful. The pin should be inserted a little to the lateral side of the heel (1). The heel fragment is engaged (2) and brought down (3). The pin may if required be driven across the sinus tarsi into the head of the talus (following the axis of the sub-talar joint) (4).

51. *Body fractures* (6) Treatment (4) The sabot and spike may be removed after 6 weeks and non-weight bearing exercises continued for a further 2 weeks before full weight bearing. Pin track infection is not uncommon, and at the first sign the pin should be removed and antibiotic treatment commenced. Because of this risk, this treatment should not be employed where there is any doubt about the peripheral circulation.

52. VI. *Calcaneal fractures with lateral displacement and involvement of the sub-talar joint* (1) Lateral displacement of the main fragment may cause (1) calf impairment and local heel pain as previously described; (2) broadening of the heel which may be unsightly and call for special footwear; (3) impingement symptoms from the lateral malleolus or squashed peroneal tendons.

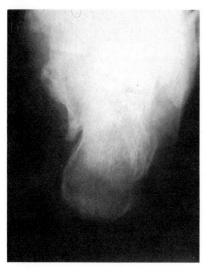

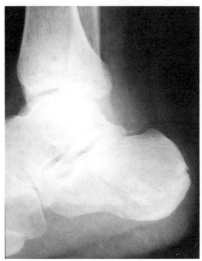

55. Nevertheless, the following alternative treatment may be considered. (1) Spike reduction of the major fragment (as in 49, 50). (2) *In addition* an attempt may be made to elevate any depressed lateral segment through a postero-lateral incision. If necessary, the depressed articular surfaces may have to be packed up with bone grafts to maintain their position.

53. *Sub-talar joint involvement* (2)
(4) Disruption of the sub-talar joint is often most obvious in the tangential projection; there may be depression of the posterior joint on the lateral side, leading to fibrous adhesions and loss of inversion/eversion movements. (5) Secondary osteo-arthritis is extremely common, giving persistent pain and lack of confidence in walking. This plus an acquired fear of heights may lead to loss of work and alcoholism.

54. *Sub-talar joint involvement* (3)
Treatment (1) (a) Where deformity is not marked (ill.) *or* where the peripheral circulation is poor *or* the patient elderly, the fracture should be treated along conservative lines as described at 48. (b) In other cases, conservative treatment may also be employed. Although morbidity is high, the results of more active treatment are somewhat uncertain.

Treatment after union: (a) Physiotherapy and occupational therapy should be continued until nothing more can be gained.
(b) Pain under the heel should be treated by a sorbo pad.
(c) Broadening of the heel may require surgical footwear.
(d) Impingement symptoms with sharply localised pain and tenderness beneath the lateral malleolus may respond to local surgery (excision of any exostosis and freeing the peroneal tendons).
(e) Persistent pain and limp, due possibly to secondary sub-talar osteo-arthritis, require careful assessment. Symptoms should be unremitting, persistent for 6–9 months *at least* after injury, and unresponsive to physiotherapy, before surgery is contemplated. Fresh radiographs should be compared with the original films to confirm sub-talar joint involvement, and assess the calcaneo-cuboid joint.
  If the sub-talar joint only is involved, a sub-talar fusion is advised. If there is any involvement of the calcaneo-cuboid joint, a full triple fusion will be necessary (fusion of the sub-talar, calcaneo-cuboid and talo-navicular joints).

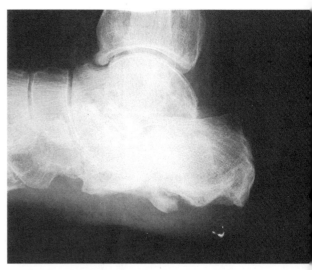

56. VII. *Central crushing fractures:* In the most severe of calcaneal fractures, the talus drives like a wedge through the central part of the calcaneus, leading to comminution of a severe degree and disruption of the sub-talar and calcaneo-cuboid joints. (In the united fracture illustrated, note the changes in the calcaneo-cuboid and mid-tarsal joints.) Surgical reconstruction is generally impossible and complications are common. Nevertheless a number do well without requiring late fusion if treated wholly conservatively or by spike reduction.)

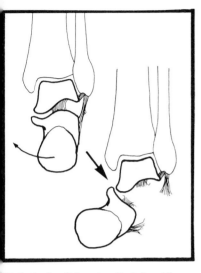

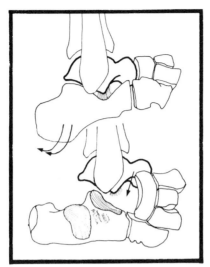

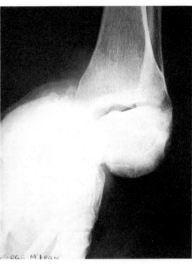

57. *Peri-talar dislocation: Pathology* (1) Forcible inversion of the plantar flexed foot throws stress on the lateral ligament of the ankle and the talo-calcaneal ligament. If the strong talo-calcaneal ligament ruptures, the talus remains in the ankle mortise and a sub-talar dislocation results.

58. *Pathology* (2) The forefoot remains with the calcaneus and the talo-navicular joint dislocates: as the talus remains in position this injury is often described as a peri-talar dislocation. It may be accompanied by fractures of the malleoli. The talus, freed from its attachments, goes into plantar flexion (and this is the position in which the foot must be placed during the initial stages of reduction).

59. *Diagnosis:* The diagnosis may be suspected clinically, but is always confirmed by radiographs. Note in the example how the talus has maintained its normal relationship with the tibia and fibula (somewhat concealed by the slight obliquity of the radiographic projection). Note that avascular necrosis of the talus does not occur, but late sub-talar osteo-arthritis is common.

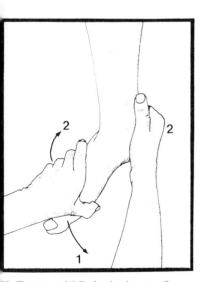

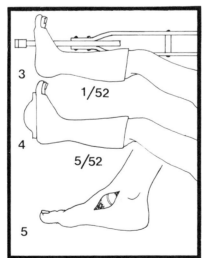

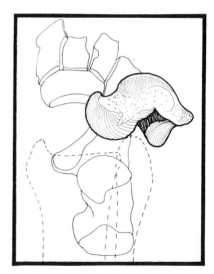

60. *Treatment* (1) Reduction is generally easy: under general anaesthesia (1) Plantar flex the foot. (2) Grasp the heel and the forefoot, apply a little traction, and swing the foot into eversion. Thereafter (3) Apply a padded below knee plaster with the ankle at right angles and the foot in slight eversion.

61. *Treatment* (2) (4) A walking plaster may be applied after a week and retained for a further 5 weeks.

Open reduction is necessary if manipulation fails, and the talo-navicular joint should be exposed first (5) as difficulty is usually due to button-holing of that joint. Instability may be controlled with Kirschner wires.

62. *Total dislocation of talus: Pathology:* With greater violence than shown in 57, there is complete rupture of all the other ligamentous attachments of the talus. The talus dislocates out of the ankle mortise and comes to lie subcutaneously in front of the ankle and on the lateral side of the foot. The head of the talus points medially and its calcaneal surface is directed posteriorly. (Very rarely eversion injuries may lead to medial dislocation of the talus.)

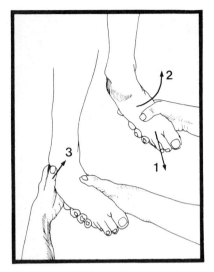

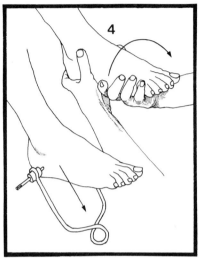

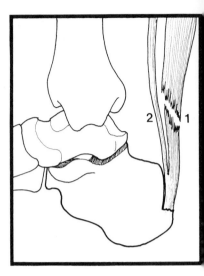

63. *Treatment* (1) Manipulative reduction should be attempted under general anaesthesia. It is imperative that delay is avoided, as there is always risk of skin sloughing where it is tightly stretched over the talus. The following technique may be employed. (1) Plantar flex the foot. (2) Invert the foot strongly. (3) The posterior part of the talus, lying laterally, should be pushed in a postero-medial direction.

64. *Treatment* (2) (4) When the talus starts to move into place, evert the foot.

If these measures fail, use a Steinman pin through the calcaneus to apply preliminary traction and control inversion. Occasionally open reduction may be required.
(5) Thereafter apply a padded plaster. Avascular necrosis is almost inevitable. (Further care as 19.)

65. *Acute rupture of tendo-calcaneus:* Rupture may follow sudden muscle activity (e.g. jumping or sprinting). It is especially common in the middle aged when degenerative changes are appearing in the tendon. It may be precipitated by local steroid injections. Usually the site is 4–8 cm above the insertion: rupture is complete (1) and the plantaris is spared (2). There is sudden pain with difficulty in walking and standing on the toes.

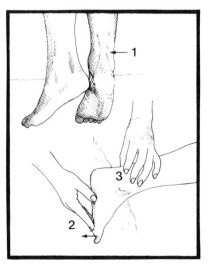

66. *Diagnosis:* The history and age of the patient may be suggestive. Clinically there may be (1) a visible gap in the tendon (2) weakness of plantar flexion against resistance (3) lack of 'firmness' on side-to-side pressure at the site of the rupture, again when the foot is being plantar flexed against resistance. Soft tissue radiographs may show a defect in the continuity of the tendon in the lateral projection.

67. *Treatment:* Both surgical and conservative measures have their advocates, but neither guarantee freedom from complications. *Surgery:* Operative treatment is most appropriate for the comparatively young and fit patient. The tendon is approached through a vertical incision, a little to the side of the mid-line. A general anaesthetic, a tourniquet, and the prone position are advisable. The ends of the ruptured tendon will be found to come together when the foot is plantar flexed. It is held in that position during suturing. Absorbable, non-absorbable or Bunnell pull-out sutures may be inserted: all have their advocates and all are effective. Fascia lata may be used if there is much fraying of the tendon. After wound closure a long leg padded plaster is applied with the knee and ankle in flexion. At 3 weeks skin sutures may be removed and a below knee plaster applied for a further 3 weeks with the ankle in a more neutral position. Complications are common and include wound break-down (sometimes severe enough to require grafting, and an argument in favour of absorbable sutures), deep venous thrombosis and secondary tendon rupture.

Conservative treatment: This is particularly suited to the elderly or frail patient. The aim of treatment is to hold the foot in plantar flexion in order to approximate the tendon ends and to hold them there until healing is advanced. A long leg plaster is applied, again with the knee and ankle flexed. This is retained for 4 weeks; a below knee plaster is then substituted, with the ankle still in a little plantar flexion. After a further 4 weeks the plaster can be discarded, weight bearing permitted, and physiotherapy to improve the gait and calf strength commenced.

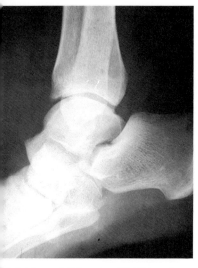

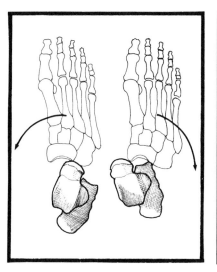

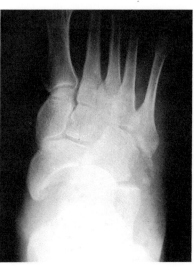

68. *Mid-tarsal dislocations* (1) Dislocation of the talo-navicular portion of the mid-tarsal joint may accompany sub-talar dislocations. The inversion mechanism has been described. (See 58.) As illustrated here, the sub-talar joint may reduce (incompletely) spontaneously, so that the talo-navicular dislocation is the main feature.

69. *Mid-tarsal dislocations* (2) The mid-tarsal joint lies between the talus and calcaneus posteriorly, and the navicular and cuboid anteriorly. *Both* elements of the joint may be disrupted as a result of (1) adduction (2) abduction forces applied to the forefoot.

70. *Mid-tarsal dislocations* (3) As in any other dislocation, abduction or adduction mid-tarsal dislocations are associated with ligament rupture or small avulsion fractures, but the talus, calcaneus, navicular and cuboid may escape significant fracture (illustrated: adduction mid-tarsal dislocation with small avulsion fracture of cuboid).

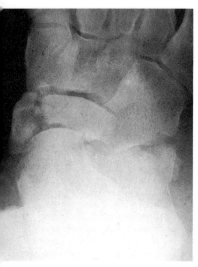

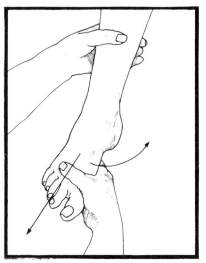

73. (4) A padded plaster is applied and split, and the limb elevated. (5) Non-weight bearing with crutches may commence after 1–2 weeks; any wires may be removed at 3–4 weeks. *Weekly* radiographs should be taken to detect late subluxation. (6) Plaster fixation may be discarded after 6–8 weeks and mobilisation commenced.

Complications: (1) Stiffness of the foot and ill-localised pain are common. This may be followed by (2) Secondary osteo-arthritis. If this is confined to the calcaneo-cuboid joint, it may be treated by a local fusion: otherwise a full triple arthrodesis (arthrodesis of sub-talar and mid-tarsal joints) may be required because of the functional interdependence of these joints. (3) Rarely medial plantar nerve palsy may be seen with intrinsic muscle wasting.

71. *Mid-tarsal dislocations* (4) On the other hand, a mid-tarsal dislocation may be associated with fracture of any of the components of the joint. The navicular is most frequently involved. (The radiograph shows an abduction type mid-tarsal dislocation with fractures of the navicular and cuboid.) When this is the case, reduction is more likely to be unstable, and secondary arthritic changes commoner.

72. *Treatment:* (1) Under general anaesthesia, traction is applied to the forefoot. (2) Maintaining traction, the forefoot is aligned with the hindfoot (abduction injury illustrated). (3) If there is evidence of instability, the forefoot should be stabilised with percutaneous Kirschner wires. If manipulation fails, open reduction may be required; a large navicular fracture may sometimes merit screw fixation.

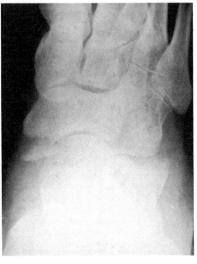

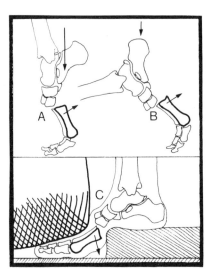

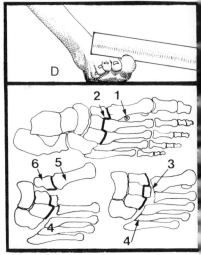

74. *Isolated fractures of the navicular:* (Do not mistake the common accessory centre of ossification for a fracture.) (1) The tuberosity may be fractured (ill.) by avulsion of the tibialis posterior; this and other undisplaced fractures may be treated conservatively (e.g. by 6 weeks in plaster). (2) Body fractures may be accompanied by dorsal extrusion of a large fragment which should be accurately reduced and fixed surgically.

75. *Tarso-metatarsal dislocations:* Injuries to the tarso-metatarsal region are infrequent and the mechanism of injury is not always clear. Dislocation of one or more metatarsals may follow (A) A fall on the plantar flexed foot or a blow to the forefoot as in road traffic accidents. (B) A blow on the heel when in the kneeling position, e.g. when a horse falls on top of a thrown rider. (C) Run-over kerb-side accidents.

76. *Tarso-metatarsal dislocations:* (D) Forced inversion, eversion or abduction of the forefoot as, for example, in a fall with the foot trapped. Note: (1) The dorsalis pedis/medial plantar anastomosis may be in jeopardy; (2) the metatarsal bases are keyed into the cuneiforms, and fracture of the second metatarsal base: (3) will allow lateral drift (4). In eversion injuries, the first metatarsal may drift medially (5) and may be accompanied by the cuneiform (6).

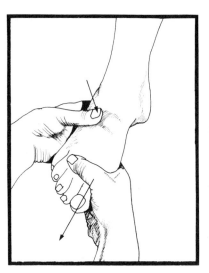

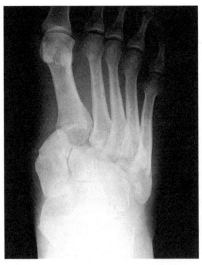

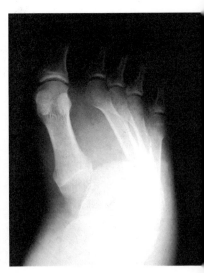

77. *Treatment:* Reduction should be attempted promptly because of the risks of oedema and circulatory impairment. (1) If the deformity is a single, multiple, dorsal or plantar dislocation without fracture, reduction can often be achieved by applying traction in the line of the metatarsals and pressure over their bases. If stable, a padded plaster is used for 8 weeks before weight bearing and mobilisation.

78. *Treatment* (2) Where there is lateral drift of all the metatarsals, fracture of the second metatarsal base (not always obvious on a single projection as here) may make reduction difficult and unstable. Open reduction and Kirschner wire fixation is advisable, (carried out through a longitudinal incision lateral to the dorsalis pedis artery). Thereafter plaster fixation for 6 weeks.

79. *Treatment* (3) Where the first ray is displaced medially, this should be reduced first (by traction and inversion, or through a small medial incision. If unstable, Kirschner wire fixation is advised.) Thereafter, proceed as 77 and 78. Anatomical reduction of all tarso-metatarsal dislocations should be the aim for reasonable results in terms of pain, stiffness and freedom from limp.

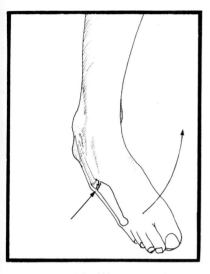

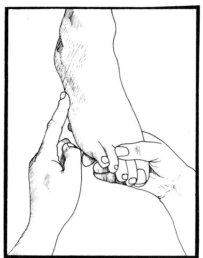

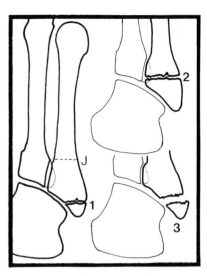

80. *Fractures of the fifth metatarsal base:* The commonest fracture of the lower limb is an avulsion fracture of the fifth metatarsal base: and it is often overlooked. It follows a sudden inversion strain (as, for example, from walking over uneven ground). In an effort to correct the progressive inversion of the foot, the peronei contract violently, and the peroneus brevis avulses its bony attachment.

81. *Diagnosis* (A) Tenderness is marked and well localised over the fracture, so that diagnosis should be easy. As the fracture results from an inversion injury, the patient often complains of having sprained his ankle. If an adequate clinical examination is not carried out and radiographs taken of the ankle only, *the fracture line will not be visualised.* The diagnosis is confirmed by the correct radiographic projections.

82. *Diagnosis* (B) Note in the radiographs that the fracture line runs at right angles to the axis of the metatarsal shaft. The fracture involves the joint (1) with the cuboid, if the fragment is small, and (2) with the fourth metatarsal, if the fragment is large. In the former case (3) separation of the fragments may occur. (Note that the classical (unrelated) Jones fracture (J) is situated distal to the intermetatarsal joint.)

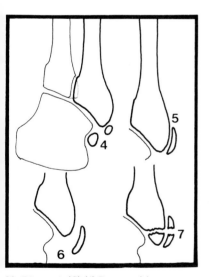

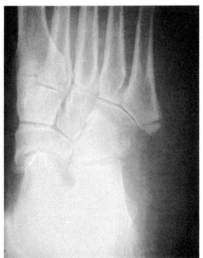

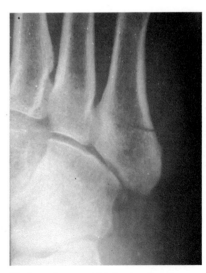

83. *Diagnosis* (C) (4) Do not misinterpret the rounded shadows of accessory bones (e.g. the os peroneum in peroneus longus, the os Vesalianum in peroneus brevis). In children (5) the epiphysis lying *parallel* to the shaft may also be wrongly taken for fracture. Nevertheless (6) separation or (7) fracture of the epiphysis may occur.

84. *Treatment:* Most fractures are undisplaced (ill.) but even marked displacement does not merit reduction. If symptoms are slight, give a crepe or similar support for 2–3 weeks, and if marked a walking plaster for 5–7 weeks. Pain from the occasional non-union may be expected to resolve spontaneously; but Sudeck's atrophy is common and may require prolonged treatment.

85. *Jones fracture:* This fracture is not associated with inversion injuries, but tends to occur in athletes during intensive training. Some of the radiological features resemble stress fractures. Healing may follow conservative management (as 84) but non-union is common and may require treatment. In the professional athlete, intramedullary A.O. cancellous bone screw fixation has been recommended.

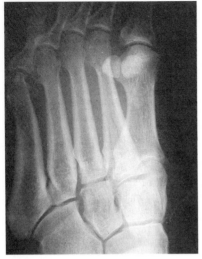

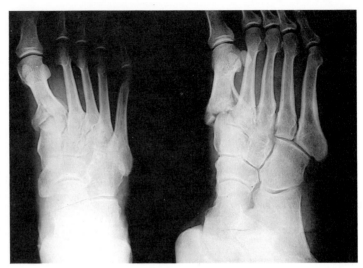

86. (1) *Metatarsal shaft and neck fractures:* These frequently result from crushing accidents, and any associated soft tissue injury will require careful surveillance (see 96). Spiral fractures generally result from forced inversion or eversion of the forefoot. If the fracture is undisplaced (ill: 2nd metatarsal fracture) without soft tissue damage, treat symptomatically—viz. a crepe bandage support, or a walking plaster if pain is severe.

87. (2) *First metatarsal:* (1) A.P. and oblique projections illustrate a slightly displaced first metatarsal fracture. In this type of injury, damage to the peripheral circulation and post traumatic oedema may present problems. Admission for a short period of elevation and observation, with the limb supported in a well padded split plaster is indicated. (Thereafter a below knee walking plaster for 5–6 weeks.) (2) If there is marked displacement with off-ending, reduction should be carried out to avoid disturbance of the mechanics of the forefoot. Traction to the toe, with local pressure over the displaced metatarsal may suffice, but open reduction (and sometimes wire fixation) may be necessary. (After care as above.) (3) Hair-line fractures without soft tissue crushing may be treated without preliminary elevation, while (4) compound injuries will require the appropriate wound treatment.

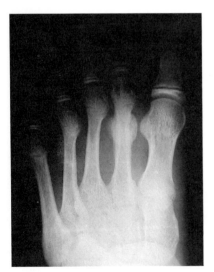

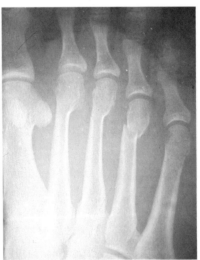

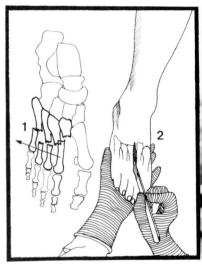

88. (3) *March fracture:* Fatigue fractures, usually of the second metatarsal neck or shaft, are not often seen until callus formation has occurred; reassurance, with at most a light support for 2–3 weeks, is all that is indicated. If seen at an early stage, severe pain will occasionally merit treatment in a below-knee walking plaster till union has taken place.

89. (4) *Multiple undisplaced fractures:* The radiograph shows fractures of the necks of the 2nd, 3rd and 4th metatarsals (the clue to the second metatarsal fracture is the kinking of the cortical shadow). Multiple fractures of this type without much displacement may be treated conservatively by plaster support (as 87, 1 or 3).

90. (5) *Multiple displaced fractures:* Fracture of the 4 lesser metatarsals is frequently accompanied by lateral drift, an unstable situation (1). Open reduction and internal fixation is advisable; frequently reduction and stabilisation of the second metatarsal will suffice as the intermetatarsal alignment is preserved. An approach (2) between the second and third metatarsals gives access to both and avoids the arterial anastomosis.

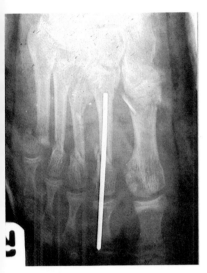

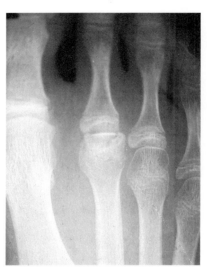

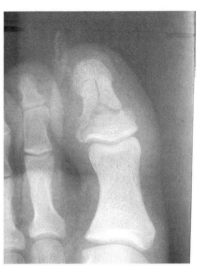

91. *Multiple displaced fractures* (2) Stability may be preserved with an intramedullary wire and plaster fixation. (After care as 87, 1.) *Displaced neck fractures* may be manipulated, but open reduction and Kirschner wire fixation is often required. A second incision may be needed to gain access to the 4th and 5th metatarsals. Mal-union may be treated by local trimming of any metatarsal head prominences in the sole.

92. *Freiberg's disease:* Osteochondritis of a metatarsal head (usually the second) may cause confusion in diagnosis. Although this condition may result from local trauma, symptoms are usually of gradual onset. An osteochondritic segment may be present, or more commonly there is narrowing of the M.P. joint and widening and flattening of the head. Persistent symptoms may require excision of the head.

93. *Phalangeal fractures:* Fractures of the terminal phalanx of the great toe are common in men and usually result from a heavy weight falling on the foot unprotected by industrial footwear. The fracture may involve the distal tuft only, but often runs into the I.P. joint. The fracture is often compound.

94. *Treatment:* (1) All wounds should be cleaned and the edges loosely approximated. (2) The nail should be retained unless virtually separated. Some advocate evacuation of the subungual haematoma. (3) Thereafter the fracture may be supported by (a) adhesive strapping to the adjacent toe or (b) a light dressing and the wearing of a stout shoe with, if necessary, a cut-out for the toe or (c) a walking plaster with toe platform—all for 2–4 weeks. *Fractures of the terminal phalanges of the lesser toes* may be treated in a similar manner. *Fractures of the middle and proximal phalanges* should be treated by strapping to the adjacent toe for 3–4 weeks; but if there is marked displacement with obvious deformity of the toes, they should first be reduced by traction. *In the case of the great toe,* a walking plaster with toe platform for 4 weeks may give greater relief of symptoms. *Note in all cases the circulation must be carefully assessed and additional precautions taken where necessary* (e.g. admission for elevation, etc.).

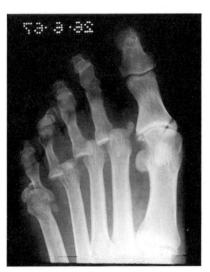

95. *Toe dislocations:* These should be reduced by traction. (ill. shows dislocations of the 4 lateral M.P. joints, with fractures of all proximal phalanges except the third.) If there is instability Kirschner wire fixation may be needed. Single dislocations may be reduced under local anaesthesia and supported by strapping to the adjacent toe: multiple dislocations will require general anaesthesia and a walking plaster with a toe platform for 4 weeks.

96. *Crushing injuries of the foot without fracture:* The foot is a resilient structure; it may be run over by a heavy vehicle or be severely crushed without sustaining any obvious fracture. If a history of this type of injury is obtained, admission is nevertheless advisable for (1) light pressure bandaging by crepe bandage over several layers of wool (2) elevation (3) observation of circulation. Sloughing of the skin over a heart-shaped area on the dorsum is not uncommon, but the area requiring de-sloughing and skin grafting will be minimised by prompt early care.

De-gloving injuries of the foot are potentially serious, especially when sole skin is involved, and require prompt plastic surgical attention.

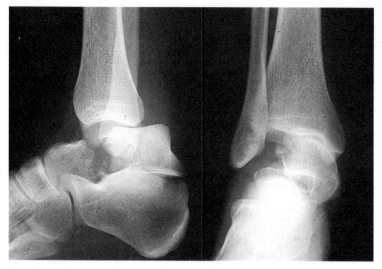 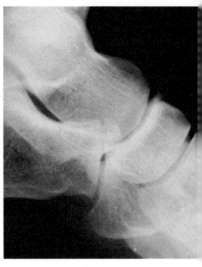

97. What is this injury? What complication is likely to develop?

98. What abnormalities are shown on this radiograph?

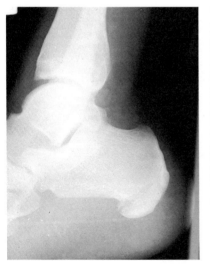 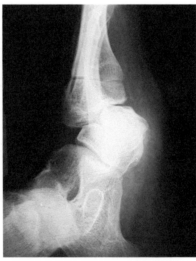 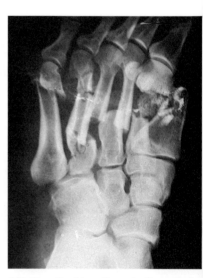

99. What injury is present? What is the most likely late complaint? Why is the ultimate prognosis good?

100. Manipulation has failed to reduce this deformity: what is the injury and what treatment would be advised?

101. Describe this radiograph of a crushed foot. What would be the main principles of treatment?

97. Type III fracture of the neck of the talus. The incidence of avascular necrosis in this type of injury approximates to 85 per cent.

98. There is an undisplaced fracture of the anterior process of the calcaneus as a result of recent trauma. In addition there is a small avulsion fracture of the dorsal aspect of the navicular, probably of long standing.

99. Fracture of the tuberosity of the calcaneus. Local heel tenderness may persist for some time, but the ultimate prognosis is good because the sub-talar joint is not involved in this class of fracture.

100. Tarso-metatarsal dislocation: if a recent injury, open reduction would be advised; if an old injury, surgical wedge correction with a tarso-metatarsal fusion might be indicated.

101. Comminuted fracture of the first metatarsal. Fractures of the shafts of the second and third metatarsals. Double fracture of the fourth metatarsal. Fracture of the neck of the fifth metatarsal. Lateral displacement. The injury is compound (horizontal streaks of ingrained dirt can be seen). Treatment: if viable, (1) Debridement. (2) Reduction and Kirschner wire fixation of the first and then the second metatarsals. (3) Plaster back shell or split padded plaster, elevation, observation, infection prophylaxis (including anti-tetanus), etc.

Index